Taking Control Of Your Diabetes

4th Edition

Steven V. Edelman, MD

Founder and Director of
Taking Control Of Your Diabetes

Professor of Medicine
Division of Endocrinology and Metabolism
University of California, San Diego

Director, Diabetes Care Clinic
Veterans Affairs Medical Center
San Diego, California

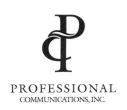

PROFESSIONAL
COMMUNICATIONS, INC.

Published by
Professional Communications, Inc.

400 Center Bay Drive
West Islip, NY 11795
(t) 631-661-2852
(f) 631-661-2167

PO Box 10
Caddo, OK 74729-0010
(t) 580-367-9838
(f) 580-367-9989

For orders, please call
1-800-337-9838
Or visit our website at
www.pcibooks.com

ISBN: 978-1-932610-87-1

Printed in the United States of America

DISCLAIMER: THE OPINIONS EXPRESSED IN THIS PUBLICATION REFLECT THOSE OF THE AUTHOR. HOWEVER, THE AUTHOR MAKES NO WARRANTY REGARDING THE CONTENTS OF THE PUBLICATION. THE PROTOCOLS DESCRIBED HEREIN ARE GENERAL AND MAY NOT APPLY TO A SPECIFIC PATIENT. ANY PRODUCT MENTIONED IN THIS PUBLICATION SHOULD BE TAKEN IN ACCORDANCE WITH THE PRESCRIBING INFORMATION PROVIDED BY THE MANUFACTURER.

This text is printed on recycled paper.

This book is written for and dedicated to people living with diabetes and their loved ones, as well as to diabetes health care professionals who have dedicated their careers to diabetes.

To my supportive family and friends for their never-ending support of my health, happiness, and professional work and living with my diabetes.

To my incredible daughters, Talia and Carina, of whom I am so proud, and to my lifelong friend, Ken Facter, MD, MBA, JD. May he rest in peace.

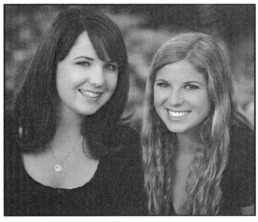

Talia and Carina Edelman

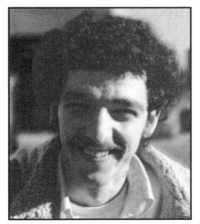

Ken Facter

Acknowledgments

The basis for this book embodies the philosophy of the large patient-oriented conferences and health fairs that all of us at Taking Control Of Your Diabetes have been presenting across America since 1995.

I would like to express my appreciation to Sandy Bourdette, Jill Yapo, Michelle Day, Antonio Huerta, Jennifer Braidwood, Roz Hodgins, Jimm Greer, Robyn Sembera, Michelle Feinstein, David Snyder, and Scott Allen for their hard work and dedicated service to Taking Control Of Your Diabetes. My thanks also go to Malcolm Beasley, Phyllis Jones Freeny, and Nikki D Merrill of Professional Communications, Inc. for their friendly and expert advice and help in putting together this book.

Thanks to Janice Baker, Jamie Blose, Mandy Bentley, Heidi Rataj, Ian Blumer, Juan Frias, and the folks at TCOYD for helping me review the various chapters in the 4th edition.

Special Acknowledgement

A very special acknowledgement goes to Sandy Bourdette for her never-ending devotion to Taking Control Of Your Diabetes and the people we serve. I came to Sandy in 1995 and asked her to help me make my vision of holding a patient-oriented educational conference a reality. That first conference is what ultimately led to TCOYD becoming the organization it is today. Not only did Sandy give up her successful meeting planning business to work solely for a grassroots, not-for-profit organization, she also sacrificed her home, which served as our office in the early years of the organization's history. Since those early days over 17 years ago, Sandy has maintained the infrastructure of TCOYD and has consistently produced the unprecedented high-quality programs that have truly made TCOYD the premier, nationwide, patient-education organization.

Contents

Contents

Contributors

Timothy S. Bailey, MD, FACP, FACE, CPI
San Diego, California
Associate Clinical Professor of Medicine
University of California, San Diego
Dr. Bailey is a practicing clinical
endocrinologist in San Diego.

Ian Blumer, MD
Ajax, Ontario, Canada
Lecturer, University of Toronto; Medical
Advisor, Charles H. Best Diabetes Centre.
Dr. Blumer's website (www.ourdiabetes
.com) is devoted to empowering people
living with diabetes.

Patrick J. Boyle, MD
Depoe Bay, Oregon
Emeritus Professor of Medicine
University of New Mexico Health Sciences

Deborah Cohen, PT, MS, CSCS, COMT,
WCS
San Diego, California
Physical Therapist, San Diego Pelvic
Rehab
Debbie Cohen is a pelvic floor physical
therapist, a certified strength and
conditioning specialist, a certified
orthopedic manual therapist, and women's
health clinical specialist.

Sheri R. Colberg, PhD, FACSM
Norfolk, Virginia
Professor of Exercise Science,
Old Dominion University
Dr. Colberg is an exercise physiologist
with a doctorate from UC Berkeley.

Lorena Drago, MS, RD, CDN, CDE
Forest Hills, New York
Lorena Drago is a registered dietitian, a
certified diabetes educator, and author
of the bilingual book Beyond Rice and
Beans: The Caribbean Latino Guide to
Eating Healthy With Diabetes, Cultural
Food Practices, *and* The 15-Minute
Consultation: How to Enhance Learning
and Get Your Message Across Every
Time.

Cyndee R. Fena, RDH, MT
Carlsbad, California
Cyndee Fena was a certified dental
hygienist who had type 1 diabetes. She
was also a professional belly dancer and
was featured on the cover of Diabetes
Forecast *magazine. Sadly, Cyndee*
passed away before the publication of the
3rd edition.

Juan Pablo Frias, MD
Clinical Faculty, University of California
San Diego; Chief Medical Officer Tethys
BioScience, Division of Endocrinology and
Metabolism.

Catherine Gagnon, CNP
San Diego, California
Sex Therapist, San Diego Sexual
Medicine
Catherine Gagnon is a certified nurse
practitioner who has worked in private
practice and Planned Parenthood, as
well as having prior experience as an ICU
nurse.

Irwin Goldstein, MD
San Diego, California
Director of Sexual Medicine at Alvarado
Hospital; Clinical Professor of Surgery
at University of California, San Diego;
Director of San Diego Sexual Medicine;
Editor-in-Chief of *The Journal of Sexual*
Medicine; author of *The Potent Male* and
co-author of *When Sex Hurts*.

Sue Goldstein, BA, CCRC, IF
San Diego, California
Sue Goldstein is an AASECT Certified
Sexuality Educator; Program Coordinator
at San Diego Sexual Medicine where she
manages the clinical research department
and directs educational programming; and
co-author of When Sex Isn't Good.

Contributors

Susan Jung Guzman, PhD
San Diego, California
Director of Clinical Services, Cofounder,
Behavioral Diabetes Institute
*Dr. Guzman is a licensed clinical
psychologist specializing in emotion and
behavioral aspects of diabetes.*

Kriss S. Halpern, JD
Santa Monica, California
*Kriss Halpern is a trial attorney in Santa
Monica, California, specializing in the
rights of consumers. He has type 1
diabetes, often contributes to Diabetes
Interview on legal issues, received the
Charles H. Best award from the American
Diabetes Association as a volunteer with
the Diabetes Control and Complications
Trial, and is a member of the Diabetes
Coalition of California.*

Rose Hartzell, PhD, EdS
San Diego, California
Sex Therapist, San Diego Sexual
Medicine
*Rose performs psychotherapy and is a
sexuality researcher at San Diego Sexual
Medicine.*

Francine R. Kaufman, MD
Los Angeles, California
Chief Medical Officer and Vice President
of Global Medical, Clinical, and Health
Affairs at Medtronic Diabetes
Distinguished Professor Emerita of
Pediatrics at USC and Children's Hospital
Los Angeles

Mayssoun S. Khoury, DDS
Newport Beach, California
*Dr. Khoury is a dentist, educator, bureau
speaker for the American Diabetes
Association, and author.*

Rachel Peterson Kim, MD
San Diego, California
*Dr. Kim is a rheumatologist and Medical
Director of Medikinetics.*

Ingrid Kruse, DPM
San Diego, California
Staff Podiatrist, VA San Diego Healthcare
System; Clinical Instructor, Department of
Family and Preventive Medicine, UCSD
*Dr. Kruse has specialized in high-risk
diabetic foot care for the past 25 years
and has set up multiple diabetic foot
clinics during that time. She currently
practices at the San Diego Veteran's
Hospital.*

Urban Miyares
San Diego, California
President, Disabled Businesspersons
Association
*Urban Miyares is a nationally recognized
disabled Vietnam veteran, entrepreneur,
lecturer, writer, inventor and patent holder,
television personality, and world-class
athlete. He was diagnosed with diabetes
during the Vietnam War.*

Aaron B. Morse, MD, FCCP
Santa Cruz, California
Diplomate of the American Board of Sleep
Medicine and Medical Director of the
Central Coast Sleep Disorders Center

Adrienne Nassar, MD
San Diego, California
Department of Endocrinology, University
of California, San Diego

Jeremy H. Pettus, MD
San Diego, California
Department of Endocrinology, University
of California, San Diego

Contributors

William H. Polonsky, PhD, CDE
San Diego, California
Assistant Clinical Professor in Psychiatry,
University of California, San Diego;
Founder, Behavioral Diabetes Institute;
and author of *Diabetes Burnout: What to
Do When You Can't Take It Anymore.*

Ruth Roberts, MA
San Diego, California
Director of Diabetes Services, Inc.
*Ruth Roberts is a medical writer,
publisher, and internet entrepreneur.*

Janice Roszler, MSFT, RD, CDE, LDN
Miami Beach, Florida
*Janice Roszler is a registered dietitian,
certified diabetes educator, marriage and
family therapist, and was the AADE 2008-
2009 Diabetes Educator of the Year.*

Amy Tenderich, MA
San Francisco, California
Founder and Editor of *www.diabetesmine
.com*, Vice President of Patient Advocacy
at Alliance Health Networks.
*Amy Tenderich is a journalist/blogger and
well-known public speaker and patient
advocate; co-author of the book* Know
Your Numbers, Outlive Your Diabetes.

Paul E. Tornambe, MD
San Diego, California
Director, San Diego Retina Research
Foundation; President, Retina Consultants
in San Diego; and past President of the
American Society of Retina Specialists
*Dr. Tornambe is in active practice, limited
to medical and surgical diseases of the
retina and vitreous.*

Janet M. Trowbridge, MD, PhD
Edmonds, Washington
Staff Physician, Puget Sound Dermatology

John Walsh, PA, CDE
San Diego, California
Clinical Diabetes Specialist, Advanced
Metabolic Care + Research, Escondida,
California, President, Diabetes Services,
Inc.
*John Walsh has been a pump wearer
since 1983 when he started to develop
protocols to make pumping easier and
more effective for his patients.*

James D. Wolosin, MD
San Diego, California
Chief, Division of Gastroenterology;
Chairman, Department of Medical
Specialities at Sharp Rees Stealy Medical
Group

Taking Control Of Your Diabetes, or TCOYD, our nonprofit organization, has been in existence now for over 17 years. Through our nationwide series of educational and motivational conferences, we have directly touched the lives of well over 200,000 people with diabetes and their loved ones. I have always known that when it comes to effective self-management of diabetes, there is nothing better than personal interactions with diabetes experts in order to become educated and motivated to do well with diabetes. With over 137 conferences completed to date, more and more people with diabetes continue to attend our programs and tell us what a difference TCOYD is making in their lives and in their ability to take control of their diabetes. With the education and support provided by TCOYD, people with diabetes learn to look at life differently and to appreciate what people who don't have diabetes tend to take for granted. "I can live a normal life and do anything I want to do without letting diabetes get in my way," is the mindset that is encouraged through every TCOYD conference.

This book is written with the same spirit and delivers the same messages as our live events. I was inspired to write this 4th edition of the TCOYD book because of the many new advances that have become available since the previous edition was published and also because of the many joyful and moving experiences I've had during the past 18 years directing TCOYD. It is my privilege to

Team TCOYD

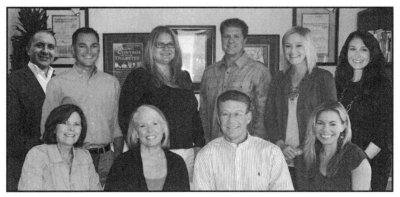

Left to right: *(top)* Antonio Huerto, David Snyder, Jill Yapo, Jimm Greer, Jennifer Braidwood, and Michelle Feinstein; *(bottom)* Roz Hodgins, Sandy Bourdette, Steve Edelman, and Michelle Day.

work side by side with so many diabetes professionals who volunteer their time and expertise in order to help TCOYD achieve and maintain our status as the premier patient-education organization worldwide. Our super dedicated, talented, and hard-working TCOYD team supports me by continuously transforming the mission and vision of TCOYD into reality. And, of course, without the support of my family, none of this would be possible.

This edition consists of new and updated chapters written by professionals, many of whom have diabetes and are dedicated to helping people with diabetes live healthier, happier, and more productive lives. I am confident that the material in this book will help you become more educated and motivated to be the most active member of your own health care team.

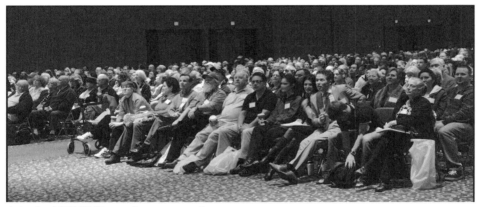

A typical TCOYD conference audience.

1

Taking Control of Your Diabetes

My Story

Let me start from the very beginning... I was born on Labor Day, September 6th, 1955. I was a typical kid until I was 15 years old, when I started to develop the classic symptoms of weight loss, excessive thirst, tiredness, and poor wound healing. I clearly remember at that time having a scab on my knee that just would not heal. In between my middle school classes at Patrick Henry Junior High in Los Angeles, I would run to the restroom to urinate and relieve my distended bladder, then slurp up as much water as possible at the drinking fountain. I could not quench my thirst and I remember all of the kids in line behind me yelling at me because I took so long. Then halfway through my next class, I would have to urinate again and almost desperately seek out the nearest drinking fountain. My teachers were annoyed with me because I was the only kid to ask for the bathroom pass every single day. I was also reprimanded several times for falling asleep in class. I just could not keep my eyes open, and I had hardly any energy at all. By the time that class was over, my bladder was bursting again, and I would be dying of thirst. I would come home from school and go to bed at 3 o'clock in the afternoon and sleep until the next morning. I lost 20 pounds in a few weeks, which I loved because I was always a little chunky. My nickname at school was "the stump." I also remember a family vacation in Mexico when I drank nothing but bottle after bottle of soft drinks, which are packed with sugar and, of course, made matters worse. Even if diet drinks had been available, I would not have ordered one, because I did not know I was developing diabetes.

Finally, I realized something was wrong and I asked my mother to take me to the doctor. We went to the urgent-care unit of my health maintenance organization (HMO) and had my blood and urine collected for tests. The doctor spent a few minutes with me asking medical questions. After looking at the results of my tests, he called in an army of nurses who urgently wheel-chaired me off to the intensive care unit (ICU) to give me intravenous (IV) fluids and insulin. I was in the hospital for 1 week and during my stay, all kinds of people came to my bedside to tell me about diabetes. Several nurses kept telling me, "You can live a normal life"; I had no clue what they were talking about. When you are first diagnosed and in emotional shock, retaining information is pretty difficult. I do remember attending a diabetes class during the first week in the hospital. There I was, a newly diagnosed, young, naïve teenage boy with type 1 diabetes, sitting in a room with about 25 very obese, older people, all with type 2 diabetes (adult onset). The single fact I remember from that class in 1970 was that ketchup has a lot of sugar in it. I kept thinking, "What am I going to dip my French fries in now?" I had lots of fun practicing how to give insulin injections into an orange, but the fun ended when it got to be my leg.

The other big fiasco that I remember at that time was the first injection I received from a new nurse after I was moved to a regular hospital room from the ICU. She came in with what looked like a horse syringe. It was huge and reminded me of a large pump squirter that I used for water fights with the kids on my block. The nurse proceeded to inject me with this large syringe, which really hurt because of the large volume of insulin that was forced into my thigh. A short time later, the doctor who was assigned to take care of me, who was not a diabetes specialist, came in to see me. I asked him why the shot was so large and he was also puzzled. To make a long story short, the nurse had misread the doctor's order. Instead of giving me 15 units of insulin (handwritten very sloppily as 15U), she gave me 150 units of insulin. Then all hell broke loose. They put me back in the ICU, stuck some more IV lines in me, made me drink very sweet fluids, and tested my blood glucose every 5 or 10 minutes for several hours. All hospitals now have a rule that the word Units must be written out completely and not indicated by just a capital U.

Even while attending the diabetes class that first week while in the hospital, my instincts told me that this was not the best learning environment for someone like me, and there had to be a better way. Eventually I was discharged to go home on only one shot a day in the morning of NPH and Regular, and I was given a strict diet using the old exchange system, by which I would weigh all of my portions of protein, carbohydrate, and fat on a little scale. What a pain! I was also supposed to test my urine for glucose 4 times a day and keep records of everything. At first, with the help of my mother, I did everything by the book, but eventually I lost interest. I did not realize why it was so important and I certainly was not informed or motivated to take control of my diabetes. My father, who was not around very much, did not believe I had diabetes. That part of my family life deserves a separate book.

I would see my doctor every 3 months, have my blood and urine collected in the morning, and then wait the usual 2 to 3 hours for the results to come back from the lab. My doctor would come into the room, look at the results, and say the same thing every time: "Steve, you are doing fine. I will see you next time." In addition, I never went to a camp for diabetic kids or spent any time in support groups or classes for young people with diabetes. I was never educated about how to take an active role in my own diabetes care, and as a result, my control started to slip.

I worked at a boys' camp in Los Angeles every summer and almost every weekend during the rest of the school year as a camp aid, cook, and counselor. Every week we had a contest called, for lack of a better term, "The Pissing Contest." The contest was to see who could urinate for the longest period of time. We took this event seriously. We used a stopwatch that measured to 1/100th of a second. During competition, you had to have one continuous stream and you had to keep your hands behind your back so you could not do any type of weird manipulation to artificially increase your time. Well, I remember winning week after week after week, and I still hold the camp record to this day. Just try urinating continuously for 1 minute and 15 seconds straight, without stopping! Time yourself the next time you go. The not-so-funny thing about this story is that my diabetes was horribly out of control, resulting in excessive thirst and urination. I am sure I also stretched my bladder terribly back then, and I am paying for it now. Home glucose monitors and the hemoglobin A1C test had not been invented at that time.

It took me several years before I realized that I should do something about the fact that I was probably not doing well, despite the repeated comments at every visit from my doctor that I was "doing fine". I truly did not know that I was doing harm to my body. I was not a rebellious teen-

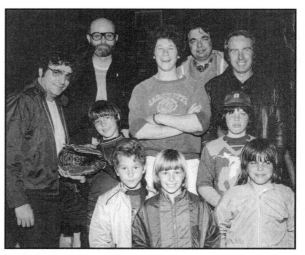

Griffith Park Boys Camp: Father-son weekend. Can't remember what I was laughing at.

ager who purposely went out of control to gain attention. I simply was never told in a way that I understood what my goals of control should be and why it was so important.

On one occasion, I decided to test my doctor, because what he was saying to me at every visit did not make sense. On the morning of my next appointment, I went to Winchell's Donut Shop and ate five donuts, including two glazed, two chocolate cake, and one maple bar (my favorite)! I then proceeded to give my urine and blood samples at the office as usual. I remember using my own urine test strips in the hospital bathroom to test the sample I turned in for analysis. The strip turned black in about 3 seconds, indicating that my urine was packed with sugar. I waited the usual 2 or 3 hours, and finally my doctor walked into the examination room holding his clipboard and studying the results of the blood and urine tests. He looked me straight in the eye and said, "Steve, you are doing fine. I will see you next time." From that point onward, I knew I could not trust him to take care of me, and I made a decision never to see that doctor again.

The bad news is that those early years of poor control contributed greatly to my development of several diabetic complications. I have proliferative diabetic retinopathy, an advanced form of diabetic eye disease, and I have received extensive laser surgery to both eyes in order to stabilize the problem. I have diabetic kidney disease, causing protein to spill into my urine and give me high blood pressure, for which I take three different medications to control the situation. I also have some manifestations of diabetic neuropathy (hypoglycemia unawareness and gastroparesis). The good news is that I sought out incredible diabetes specialists, such as Doctors Mayer Davidson and Richard Berkson, and started to receive the appropriate treatment to minimize and slow down the progression of these complications. I feel fortunate that I was able to improve my control at a time when my complications were not extremely advanced.

I was always interested in science and decided to go to medical school. At the University of California at Los Angeles (UCLA), where I did my undergraduate premedical studies, I became more interested in medicine and, specifically, diabetes. I worked in a diabetes research laboratory and observed patients in diabetes clinic. During that time, I also realized that one shot a day was totally inadequate, and I improved my regimen to allow for better control. Later, during my last year in medical school, I went on an insulin pump and became "fuel injected." Over the past several years, I have experimented with the new rapid-acting and long-acting designer insulin analogues, Symlin (another important hormone that I will discuss in *Chapter 8*), and continuous glucose monitoring in trying to find a regimen that fits my lifestyle the best.

I remember quite vividly when I studied physiology during my first year of medical school in 1978 at the University of California, Davis campus. The professor was citing statistics from old textbooks about the high death rate in people with diabetes. He stated that 50% of people with diabetes die from diabetic kidney disease within 20 years after the initial diagnosis. During the lecture, my classmates were trying to avoid eye contact with me or attempted to give me some type of visual sympathy from across the lecture hall (both situations made me feel uncomfortable). That afternoon we had a physiology laboratory and had to dissect the cadaver of a 25-year-old male who had died of diabetic kidney disease. At the time, I was 23 years old with 8 years of diabetes behind me. My best friend, Ken Facter, always tried to comfort me by saying that at least I knew what I was going to die of! These early experiences motivated me to take better care of myself and to devote my career to helping people with diabetes. Ironically and tragically, Ken died suddenly of

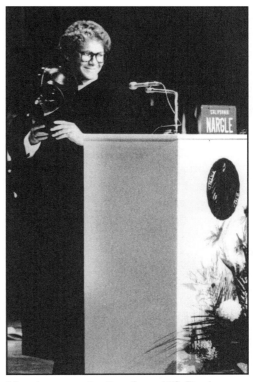

Me at my graduation from UC Davis Medical School as I gave the Valedictorian address.

a heart attack at the age of 40. His death was a painful wake up call to me that we must live every day to the fullest and not take one second of life for granted.

After my medical residency at UCLA, I did the first part of my diabetes specialty training (fellowship) at the famous Joslin Diabetes Clinic in Boston. I learned a great deal about all aspects of diabetes care as I worked and gained experience in the various departments that dealt with pregnancy, the kidneys, the eyes, young children with diabetes, the feet, the heart, and general care. I also gave lectures to the patients admitted to the Joslin Clinic and spent a lot of time answering questions about diabetes. I was always impressed by how thirsty the patients were for information about their condition. Those early interactions with patients had a profound impact on my career as an educator.

I eventually ended up in San Diego, where I am a professor at the University of California San Diego School of Medicine and a staff member of the Veterans Affairs Medical Center. Here, I met two of my mentors and very close friends, Alain Baron and Bob Henry. They were two incredible role models who have selflessly supported the development of so many young people needing guidance in their career. I also have had the honor and privilege of serving our country's veterans living with diabetes. This is such a special population of real heroes.

Ingrid Kruse, a podiatrist specializing in diabetic foot conditions and I have two incredible daughters, Talia and Carina. When I think about it, our kids have lived their entire lives in an environment surrounded by diabetes professionals and diabetes-related products, information, and social events. I can't tell you how many times I have dragged them to a diabetes function or conference.

Taking Control Of Your Diabetes: the Beginning

As a young faculty member, I spent a lot of time and energy, after the results of the Diabetes Control and Complications Trial were released in 1993, trying to educate health care providers on how to take better care of their patients with diabetes. However, it was slow going and diabetes care was not improving fast enough at the community level. I realized there were many barriers at that time that limited successful diabetes management. Here are a few:

- Managed care was beginning to hamper proper medical care in a major way.
- As a caregiver, I was fairly helpless in trying to fight the system.
- There was very little education directed toward people with diabetes.

Lastly, it took too long for information to filter down from the major research institutions to the specialists and then to the health care provider who, in turn, had to change their practice habits before their patients could be the recipients of a proven treatment strategy, new device, or medication. For these reasons, I decided to take the most important messages directly to those who were most affected by this condition.

In 1995, I had the idea of putting on a large conference for 1000 people with diabetes called "Taking Control Of Your Diabetes"

(TCOYD). I joined forces with my long-time colleague and friend, Sandy Bourdette, and we produced our first conference at the San Diego Convention Center, focusing on education, motivation, and self-advocacy. I realized early on that this approach could make a significant impact on diabetes care in this country, and it was a large piece of the diabetes-care puzzle that was missing.

Since the beginning of TCOYD in 1995, we have been pushing these three important themes and they have never lost their importance or magnitude:

1. *You have the main responsibility for taking control of your diabetes.* This is your life, and no one should be more interested in getting the best health care than you. The responsibility does not lie with your wife, husband, mother, father, sister, brother, or doctor. Your doctor does not bear the main responsibility for your health; that is your responsibility. It is you who will personally suffer if you develop blindness or kidney failure, not your physician.

2. *You are your own best advocate.* In these days of managed care and the shrinking health care dollar, it is becoming more and more difficult to obtain the proper care you deserve and need to stay healthy. You must become knowledgeable about and get involved with the administrative aspects of your health care system so that you have timely access to the proper tests, most effective medications, and latest medical devices. This can be a frustrating and time-consuming process that can wear you down, but in the end, you will win if you are persistent.

3. *Be smart and be persistent.* Educate yourself about preventive measures to avoid eye, kidney, nerve, and heart disease. Be knowledgeable about the screening tests used to diagnose diabetes-related problems early so that you can obtain proper treatment in time. Be up-to-date on all of the various treatment options available to aggressively treat any complication that you have so that its progression will be slowed or halted.

Simply stating these themes is one thing, but getting folks to take ownership of their health is another. That was the challenge. At that very first conference in 1995, I realized how thirsty people with diabetes were for information about their condition and how much more needed to be accomplished. Getting people to put diabetes high on their priority list is such a key component for long-term success and depends so much on individualizing communication and education styles, as well as therapeutic strategies.

TCOYD became a not-for-profit organization and has steadily grown, while maintaining a high level of quality and impactful programs across the United States, including our flagship face-to-face conferences. We also developed a television show, award-winning newsletter, website, and other innovative programs such as *Extreme Diabetes Makeover* and *The Edelman Report* (please, do not pronounce the T), all found on our website (*www.tcoyd.org*).

Several years ago, I realized there was another piece of the diabetes-care puzzle that was still missing. It was related to the communication and understanding between the caregiver and the person with diabetes.

A huge challenge is to improve the attitudes of caregivers toward their patients struggling with diabetes and create an empathetic atmosphere with more open communication, avoiding the inappropriate labeling of patients as "noncompliant." I have never met a patient who did not want to live a long and healthy life. Our unique *Making The Connection* initiative puts the doctor's learning environment smack in the middle of a TCOYD patient conference. For part of the day, they are in their own room receiving several cutting-edge lectures from experts in the field. They also join the people with diabetes attending the patient conference during several parts of the day.

During the afternoon, the professionals attend a workshop together with a large group of patients that is led by one of our "touchy, feely" faculty, typically Bill Polonsky, who is an incredible person, dedicating his career to helping people overcome the emotional and behavioral barriers of living with diabetes. This is always interactive and enlightening for both the people with diabetes and the caregivers, because they have the opportunity to express both sides of the doctor-patient relationship and come to an understanding of the frustrations faced by both groups.

At the end of the day, the professionals have a better understanding of what it is like to live with diabetes on a day-to-day basis. In turn, the people with diabetes realize that our health care system is in need of repair and that the providers are under lots of different pressures. Most of all, the people with diabetes learn that their health care providers are on their side.

I believe that teaching institutions should educate both the professionals and patients together on a parallel track and encourage a bidirectional exchange of information between the caregivers and the people with diabetes. The key message here for people with diabetes is to help your caregiver take better care of you.

Our mission statement says it all...

Guided by the belief that every person with diabetes has the right to live a healthy, happy, and productive life, TCOYD educates and motivates people with diabetes to take a more active role in their condition and provides innovative and integrative continuing diabetes education to medical professionals caring for people with diabetes.

The main message I want to convey to you is that you can take control of your diabetes, even if you already have complications. It is never too late to get in control, both mentally and physically. The concept of TCOYD embodies the philosophy of self-help and self-advocacy.

Summary

Who should take care of the people with diabetes in this country? I say anyone who is interested, and the most interested person should be you! Taking control of your diabetes is simply being an informed health care consumer. The first step is to become motivated to take care of yourself so that you can live a happier, healthier, and more productive life. You have a responsibility to yourself and to your loved ones to take the best possible care of yourself. The second step is to become informed about what you need to do to get in control of your diabetes and stay there. Education is the key to survival both mentally and physically, and you must not rely on anyone else to do this for you. If the proper therapy is not instituted in a timely manner, the person who will suffer is you. The third step is to be a self-advocate. In the current times of managed care and the shrinking health care dollar, you may need to fight for what you need and deserve.

Taking control of your diabetes requires a healthy mind-set that you can live a normal life and do anything that you want to do without letting diabetes get in your way. You must take the attitude that by having diabetes, you will look at life differently and appreciate the things that others take for granted. Don't be afraid to learn as much as you can about diabetes and, please, do not hesitate to be aggressive in order to obtain the medications, tests, devices, and examinations that you will need to stay healthy. Teach others, spread the word about diabetes, and motivate your friends and family members who have any chronic condition to take an active role in their health care. Please learn about all the new programs that TCOYD provides to help you take control of your diabetes. Remember that you have the main responsibility for taking control of your diabetes. You are your best self-advocate, and be smart and be persistent. Take control of your diabetes—you owe it to yourself and to your loved ones.

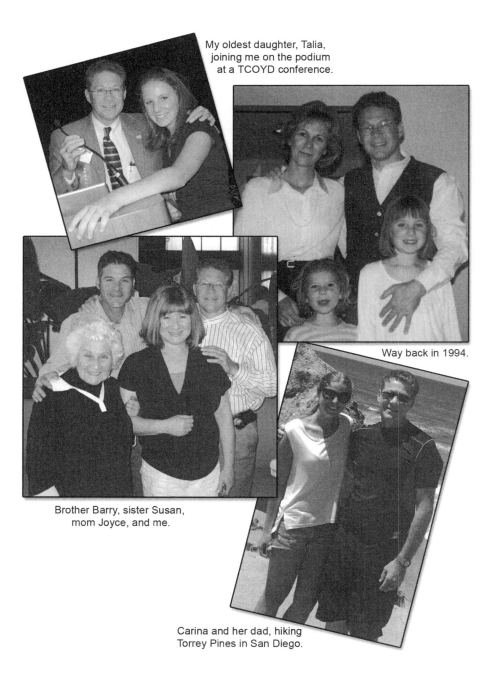

My oldest daughter, Talia, joining me on the podium at a TCOYD conference.

Way back in 1994.

Brother Barry, sister Susan, mom Joyce, and me.

Carina and her dad, hiking Torrey Pines in San Diego.

2

You Need to Know More Than Your Caregiver About Diabetes

The Hard Core Facts

As I mentioned in *Chapter 1*, I have never met a person with diabetes that did not want to live a long and healthy life, and by the same token, I have never met a health care professional who did not want to help his/her patients get and stay healthy. So why do you need to know more than your caregiver? Many health care providers, bless their souls, do not know much about diabetes. In most current medical school curriculums, only a fraction of the education time (less than 4%) is reserved for teaching diabetes, yet 25% to 30% of their patients will have this very common and complicated condition, no matter what type of adult medicine they go into. Remember that doctors are on your side, so help them take better care of you.

The Different Types of Diabetes

I always like to clarify up front about the different types of diabetes. Many folks become confused about what type of diabetes they have. Knowing and understanding what type of diabetes you have really sets the foundation of what you need to know throughout the rest of the book, because there are important differences in screening, prevention strategies, and treatment regimens for type 1 and type 2 diabetes. The classification of the different types of diabetes has changed many times in the past several years, leading to lots of confusion. There are many different types of diabetes, but the most common are type 1 diabetes, latent autoimmune diabetes in adults (LADA), type 2 diabetes, and gestational diabetes (**Table 2-1**).

Type 1 Diabetes

Type 1 diabetes was formerly called insulin-dependent diabetes mellitus (IDDM), juvenile-onset diabetes, brittle diabetes, or unstable diabetes. While type 1 diabetes usually develops before the age of 20, one can develop type 1 diabetes at any age, hence the term juvenile-onset is misleading. I do not like the words "brittle" and "unstable." These terms refer to the fluctuation in blood glucose values throughout the day that are commonly experienced by people with type 1 diabetes. At the time of diagnosis, people with type 1 diabetes are usually thin or of normal weight and there are usually no other associated conditions, such as high blood pressure or abnormal cholesterol levels, that are commonly seen in type 2 diabetes (**Table 2-2**). Only about 10% of all people with diabetes in the United States have the type 1 variety. Type 1 diabetes does run in families, although not nearly as strongly as is observed with type 2 diabetes. There have been case reports of several children in the same elementary school class coming down with type 1 diabetes within a short period of time. One of my female patients has type 1

Table 2-1

The Different Types of Diabetes[a]

Type 1 Diabetes
Previously called insulin-dependent diabetes mellitus (IDDM), juvenile-onset diabetes, brittle diabetes, unstable diabetes, and ketosis-prone diabetes

Type 2 Diabetes
Previously called non–insulin-dependent diabetes mellitus (NIDDM), adult-onset diabetes, old-age diabetes, stable diabetes, and non–ketosis-prone diabetes

Gestational Diabetes
Also called diabetes of pregnancy

LADA
Latent autoimmune diabetes in adults or late-onset type 1 diabetes

[a] Although there are many other types of diabetes, they are not as common.

diabetes and all three of her children developed type 1 diabetes before the age of 7. These later scenarios are less common than the sporadic cases. I am the only person in my family who developed type 1 diabetes, which is the more typical situation. People with type 1 diabetes have "first-degree" relatives (parents, siblings, or children) with type 1 diabetes approximately 4% to 8% of the time.

The cause of type 1 diabetes is not entirely known, but it is believed that for some reason (genetic, viral, or environmental), antibodies are produced that specifically destroy the pancreas. Any condition in which antibodies are produced that attack the body is called an autoimmune condition. Antibodies are the cells in the body that normally attack and destroy anything foreign, and the pancreas is the organ that produces and secretes insulin. Insulin is needed to help the glucose molecules that appear in the blood after eating to get into the cells of the body to be used and stored for energy. If there is not enough insulin, the glucose stays at high levels in the bloodstream and circulates to all of the organs of the body, including the eyes, kidneys, heart, blood vessels, and nerves. It is the chronic elevation of blood glucose levels over many years that leads to damage of these organs and the classic complications of diabetes.

Table 2-2

Main Differences Between Type 1 and Type 2 Diabetes

Characteristics	Type 1 Diabetes	Type 2 Diabetes
Age at onset	Usually less than 20 years	Usually over 35 years
Body habitus	Typically thin or not obese	Typically obese
Other family members also with diabetes	Approximately 4% to 8%	Approximately 70% to 90%
Ethnic groups	Typically white	African American, Asian American, Hispanic, Pacific Islander, Native American
Cause of diabetes	The insulin-producing cells of the pancreas are destroyed by antibodies	The body is resistant to the glucose-lowering effect of insulin—insulin resistance
Type of therapy required	Insulin	Diet alone and/or pills and/or insulin
Associated conditions at the time of diagnosis	Usually none	High blood pressure, high cholesterol levels, heart disease
Total diabetes in the United States	Approximately 10%	Approximately 90%

The main problem in type 1 diabetes is a lack of insulin, not insulin resistance, which is the main cause of type 2 diabetes. This is why people with type 1 diabetes always need insulin, and the diabetes medications that we use for type 2 diabetes typically do not work and certainly are not a replacement for insulin. Insulin must be injected because if it is swallowed, the enzymes in the stomach will digest and inactivate it before the insulin enters the bloodstream.

An important subcategory of type 1 diabetes is called LADA (latent autoimmune diabetes in adults). This is the most missed diagnosis in diabetes! This is basically when someone is diagnosed with type 1 or autoimmune diabetes later in life as an adult. Barbara is one of my good friends and a patient diagnosed with type 1 diabetes at the age of 64. The destruction of the insulin-producing cells of the pancreas (beta cells) is slower in LADA patients, so the symptoms are not as severe as they would be in a newly diagnosed teenager with extreme thirst, urination, and weight loss. This type of presentation of elevated blood glucose levels in an adult with not-so-severe symptoms can fool the caregiver into thinking the patient has type 2 diabetes. The person may be prescribed oral medication commonly used for type 2 diabetes, which does not work well. Eventually the need to start insulin will arise fairly quickly. I tell practitioners at the medical education lectures that I give around the country to look out for LADA patients and to order a test called the GAD antibodies test. GAD stands for glutamic acid decarboxylase (see why I use GAD instead) and can be easily measured by most laboratories. If positive, the patient most likely has type 1 diabetes. Knowing what type of diabetes you have is important, because it has important genetic and treatment implications.

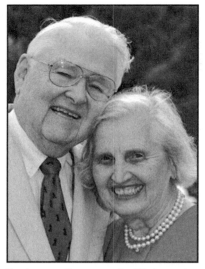

Barbara, diagnosed with type 1 diabetes at the age of 64, with her husband, Dave.

The ultimate cure for type 1 diabetes will most likely come from stem cell research. Developing a vaccine that allows for immune protection against the autoantibodies that attack the pancreas is another approach being studied. At the time of this edition, there have been no major advances in preventing type 1 diabetes that will affect a large number of people. A more detailed description is found in *Chapter 32* on the prevention of diabetes. In the meantime, it is important to stay as healthy as possible so that when a cure comes along, you will be a good candidate.

Type 2 Diabetes

Type 2 diabetes was formerly called non–insulin-dependent diabetes mellitus (NIDDM), adult-onset diabetes, and stable diabetes. This terminology of "non–insulin-dependent" led to confusion because many people with type 2 diabetes are treated with insulin, usually after the oral diabetic mediations have lost their effectiveness. In addition, blood glucose levels of people with type 2 diabetes can be just as unstable or brittle as those of type 1 diabetics. People who develop type 2 diabetes are usually over the age of 35, but one can develop type 2 diabetes at any age, as is the case with type 1 diabetes. People with type 2 diabetes are usually overweight and commonly have high blood pressure and abnormal cholesterol levels at the time of diagnosis. Type 2 diabetes is also commonly found in certain ethnic groups, such as African Americans, Native Americans, Asian Americans, Pacific Islanders, and in people of Hispanic descent. In contrast, type 1 diabetes is predominantly a white man's disease. Approximately 90% of all people with diabetes are of the type 2 variety. In addition, type 2 diabetes runs strongly from generation to generation. Approximately 70% to 90% of people with type 2 diabetes have a family history of diabetes, whereas only about 4% to 8% of type 1 diabetics have someone else in their family with the same type of diabetes (**Table 2-2**).

The cause of type 2 diabetes could not be more different than that of type 1 diabetes. However, many of the complications are similar because both types of diabetes lead to high blood glucose levels. At the time of diagnosis in people with type 2 diabetes, there is usually an excess amount of insulin, which is in striking contrast to what is observed in type 1 diabetics. The problem is that the tissues of the body are resistant to the normal glucose-lowering effects of insulin; thus the medical phrase "insulin resistance."

In the early prediagnosis stage, insulin resistance can be found in high-risk individuals who will eventually develop type 2 diabetes. When insulin resistance is present, the blood glucose values start to climb because the insulin is not totally effective at getting the glucose molecules into the cells of the body for energy. As a compensatory mechanism, the pancreas secretes more and more insulin in an effort to overcome this insulin resistance. For many years, this physiologic adaptation works well and the individual's glucose values are near normal. This is why it commonly takes many years to diagnose type 2 diabetes. It is often said that of the estimated 26 million people with diabetes in this country, only two thirds of them know they have the condition. It is important to note that in the early stages of type 2 diabetes there are no symptoms, such as excessive thirst and urination, and this is why screening is so important.

As time goes on, the pancreas gets tired of overproducing excess amounts of insulin to overcome the insulin resistance and eventually burns out or becomes exhausted. When this occurs, the blood glucose levels really go through the roof, and this is normally when the oral medications start to lose their effectiveness, and the patient needs insulin and/or an incretin, such as Byetta, Bydureon or Victoza, in order to control the glucose levels (discussed in *Chapter 7* and *Chapter 8*). How long does it take for the pancreas to become exhausted? It is different for everybody, depending on how early they were diagnosed and what they were treated with, but it is usually 5 to 15 years from the time of diagnosis. This scenario of events that occurs in type 2 diabetes is commonly referred to as "the natural history of type 2 diabetes" (**Figure 2-1**). It is my belief that the earlier the diagnosis is made and the better the glucose control from the time of diagnosis, the longer someone

Figure 2-1

The Natural History of Type 2 Diabetes

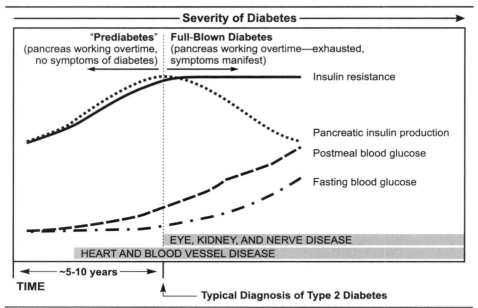

Insulin resistance can be present for many years before the diagnosis of diabetes. Blood glucose levels are not markedly elevated in the early stages of diabetes. Once the pancreas becomes exhausted, the blood glucose values go through the roof. As the pancreas becomes exhausted, the chance of achieving good glucose control with diet and exercise alone or with one oral agent goes down. The need for insulin therapy normally goes up over time as well.

with type 2 diabetes can control their diabetes with an exercise program and realistic meal plan with or without medication(s). The various types of therapy available for type 2 diabetes may also influence this "natural history" and will be discussed later in the book. An important point is that glucose control is the most important issue, even if you need "tons" of medication to achieve your goals. You will be much better off and have less complications than someone with diabetes who brags that they take no medications and has horrible glucose control.

Gestational Diabetes

Gestational diabetes is another common type of diabetes. It usually occurs in women… (get it?). It refers to the development of diabetes while a woman is pregnant. The cause of gestational diabetes is more closely related to type 2 diabetes in that insulin resistance is present with the added influence of female hormones that rise during pregnancy. Most women revert to normal glucose levels after delivery. However, women with a history of gestational diabetes also have a higher chance of developing type 2 diabetes with subsequent pregnancies and later in life. It is also extremely important to keep blood glucose levels under control during pregnancy to prevent fetal abnormalities and problems with the delivery. One of the problems at delivery is that the baby is too large physically but internally underdeveloped so the rate of C-sections goes up and the length of time that the baby needs to stay in the hospital is longer. If you have type 1 diabetes and you become pregnant, in reality you do not have classic gestational diabetes. You are simply diabetic and pregnant. Treatment for gestational diabetes is somewhat different than it is for type 2 diabetes. In general, insulin is used most of the time; however, use of oral medications, such as the sulfonylureas (SFUs) and metformin, are being used more and more as their safety in offspring is being monitored closely. As in all types of diabetes, diet and exercise regimens are extremely important. Dr. Lois Jovanovic is an international expert on gestational diabetes. Lois runs the Samsun Diabetes Research Institute in Santa Barbara, California and has been a speaker for TCOYD. (Please see *Diabetes & Pregnancy: What to Expect* and *Gestational Diabetes: What to Expect* by the American Diabetes Association and *Medical Management of Pregnancy Complicated by Diabetes*, 3rd edition.)

Diagnosis of Diabetes

If you are reading this book, you probably already have diabetes, but I think it is important to discuss how diabetes is officially diagnosed. This may be important for your friends or family members who are at risk for developing diabetes. The criteria for diagnosis by the American Diabetes Association are shown in **Table 2-3**. It is important to note that these criteria are only for the diagnosis of diabetes in people who previously did not know they were diabetic and are not the treatment goals for people already living with diabetes.

The most common and easiest way to make the diagnosis is by measuring the fasting blood glucose (FBG), which refers to the glucose value in the morning after an overnight fast and before breakfast. If the blood glucose value is 126 mg/dL or higher, the diagnosis of diabetes can be made. FBG levels less than 100 mg/dL are considered normal. It is important to point out that any FBG over 100 mg/dL but less than 126 mg/dL is abnormal and should warrant close follow-up. The official phrase for FBG in this gray zone is "impaired fasting glucose" or "prediabetes" (**Figure 2-2**).

The newest test to be officially used to diagnose diabetes is the hemoglobin A1C or A1C (a blood test that gives an estimate of what the average blood glucose value has been over the preceding 2 to 3 months) discussed in detail later in this chapter. Values for normal individuals are defined as less than 5.7%, prediabetes between 5.7% and 6.4%, and anything above 6.4% is classified as diabetes (**Figure 2-2**). The A1C is a simple blood test that can be drawn anytime of the day with no need for fasting.

The postmeal (or postprandial) glucose value, taken 2 hours after the start of a meal, is

Table 2-3

Official Criteria for Diagnosing Diabetes[a]

- Any individual with the symptoms of high blood glucose (hyperglycemia) and a blood glucose value at any time of the day over 200 mg/dL

  OR

- A fasting blood glucose (FBG) test, which is done in the morning before anything to eat or drink other than water, that is 126 mg/dL or higher

  OR

- An abnormal oral glucose tolerance test (OGTT), defined as a 2-hour glucose value that is 200 mg/dL or higher (*see text*)

  OR

- Glycosylated hemoglobin (A1C) value above 6.5% (*see text*)

---

[a] These official criteria are from the American Diabetes Association. Available at *www.diabetes.org*.

Figure 2-2

Tests for Diagnosis of Diabetes

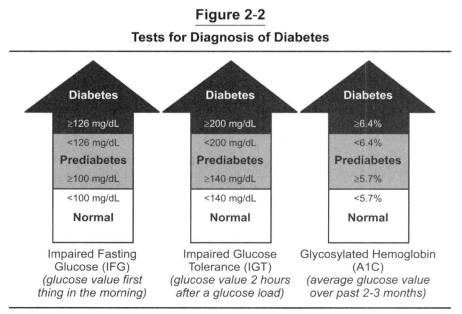

| Impaired Fasting Glucose (IFG) *(glucose value first thing in the morning)* | Impaired Glucose Tolerance (IGT) *(glucose value 2 hours after a glucose load)* | Glycosylated Hemoglobin (A1C) *(average glucose value over past 2-3 months)* |

normal below 140 mg/dL in individuals without diabetes. If the post-meal glucose value is consistently above 200 mg/dL, diabetes can be diagnosed. In addition, if one has symptoms of elevated blood glucose values, such as excessive thirst and urination, lethargy, poor wound healing, blurry vision, frequent urinary tract infections, and random glucose values over 200 mg/dL at any time of the day, diabetes is present and no further tests are needed for a diagnosis. If the postmeal glucose value is above 140 but less than 200 mg/dL, we classify these folks as having impaired glucose tolerance (IGT) or once again prediabetes (**Figure 2-2**). *Chapter 32* is devoted to the prevention of diabetes in people who have prediabetes.

The oral glucose tolerance test (OGTT) is an official diabetes diagnostic test, although not commonly needed. After an overnight fast, one swallows 75 grams of glucose (a large glass of very sweet syrup) in the morning, and the blood glucose levels are followed over the next 2 hours. The OGTT is mainly used for clinical research purposes. There is a modified OGTT that is now used for screening women who are at risk for developing gestational diabetes; it is performed at 26 weeks into the pregnancy. An individual is defined as being at risk for diabetes if she has had a prior episode of gestational diabetes, has given birth to an infant weighing over 9 pounds, has a family history of diabetes, is overweight, has high blood pressure or cholesterol levels, or is of an ethnic group with a high incidence of diabetes (**Table 2-4**).

Table 2-4

Risk Factors for Developing Type 2 Diabetes

- Having someone in your family with diabetes, especially a first-degree relative
- Being overweight, especially with central obesity, commonly referred to as a "beer belly"
- Having some or all of the other associated conditions commonly seen in type 2 diabetes, such as high blood pressure or high cholesterol levels (these conditions may appear before the diagnosis of diabetes)
- Being a member of an ethnic group that has a high incidence of diabetes, such as African American, Hispanic, Native American, Asian American, and Pacific Islander
- Developing diabetes during pregnancy (gestational diabetes)
- Giving birth to an infant weighing over 9 pounds. (If a woman has high blood glucose during pregnancy, the infant may be large physically although it is usually developmentally abnormal internally.)
- Being told by a caregiver that you have "a touch of diabetes" or "borderline diabetes." (There is no such thing.)

Why Is Glucose Control Important?

Why is everyone stressing that your glucose values should be as close to normal as possible? It is simply because high glucose values over an extended period of time can cause damage to the organs of the body. Certain organs seem to be more susceptible to elevated blood glucose levels or hyperglycemia than others, with the eyes, kidneys, nerves, and blood vessels being the most seriously affected. Remember that the blood bathes every organ in our bodies at all times, and anything that is toxic in the bloodstream will have a major impact on the health of our organs. It is also important not to panic if your blood glucose level gets too high occasionally, even if it is high for a few weeks or months. It is the chronic elevation over years and years that causes the real damage, leading to blindness, kidney failure, nerve disease, amputation, heart disease, and stroke. I feel that every person with diabetes needs to work out an individual treatment plan to get their blood glucose level as close to normal as possible. It is also important that in the quest for normal or near-normal glucose levels, the treatment plan should not be so rigid that there are major disruptions of one's lifestyle, including frequent episodes of hypoglycemia (blood glucose levels that are too low). Treatment plans need to be individualized based on your age, risk of hypoglycemia, normal daily eating and sleeping habits, other medical problems, including heart disease, etc. One size does not fit all!

For many years, most physicians did not stress good or "tight" glucose control in their diabetic patients because definitive, long-term clinical studies demonstrating the benefits of tight glucose control had not been undertaken and there was concern that all of the trouble and expense of controlling their patients' glucose values were not warranted until the benefits were proven. I was among a minority of physicians in this country at that time who believed that tight glucose control not only made one feel better on a day-to-day basis, avoiding short-term or acute complications, but that it also reduced the long-term complications. Long-term microvascular complications refer to the eye (retinopathy), kidney (nephropathy), and nerve (neuropathy) diseases commonly seen in people with diabetes.

My beliefs were based on my own experience as a patient and physician and on a fairly large body of medical literature already published supporting the notion that glucose control matters. The government initiated a long-term clinical trial to address this important issue. This study is called the Diabetes Control and Complications Trial (DCCT) and was completed in 1993. Even at the time of this 4th edition, it remains one of the most important studies in the field of diabetes. The

DCCT was one of the longest, most extensive, and expensive government studies. The DCCT was not the first study to show the importance of glycemic control in preventing and delaying the progression of microvascular complications of diabetes. The DCCT was, however, the most powerful and well-done study and has set the standard of care for the United States and the world. The DCCT, sponsored by the National Institutes of Health, was a 9-year, $160 million, multimember trial that studied over 1400 patients with type 1 diabetes.

The DCCT was designed to answer two main questions:

1. Whether intensive glycemic control could prevent the classic long-term microvascular complications of diabetes
2. Whether intensive glycemic control could delay the progression of microvascular complications already present in people with diabetes.

The DCCT also looked at the incidence of hypoglycemia (low blood glucose) and weight gain.

In the DCCT, patients were put into either an intensive treatment group or a conventional treatment group. The people randomized to the intensive treatment group were put on multiple insulin injections or insulin pumps and were required to perform frequent home glucose monitoring. The goal was to lower the glucose values to normal or near-normal levels. The treatment goal for the people in the conventional treatment group (who were put on one or two injections per day) was to avoid symptoms of extreme low and high blood glucose levels. Home monitoring with glucose meters was not encouraged.

The patients were further subdivided into a primary prevention group (those who had no evidence of microvascular complications when the study began) and a secondary intervention group (those who already had some evidence of eye, kidney, or nerve disease at the beginning of the study).

Figure 2-3 shows the glycosylated hemoglobin (or A1C; a long-term glucose control factor that will be discussed later) and daily average blood glucose values during the 9-year study in the intensively and conventionally treated groups. It is important to note that despite an enormous amount of attention and effort given by the DCCT study personnel and the use of multiple injection regimens, insulin pumps, and home glucose monitoring devices, the patients randomized to the intensive treatment group did not achieve completely normal glucose values or a normal A1C value (a blood test that determined the extent of blood glucose control over the preceding 3 months). The important

Figure 2-3

Glycosylated Hemoglobin (A1C) and Daily Average Blood Glucose Values During the 9-Year Diabetes Control and Complications Trial

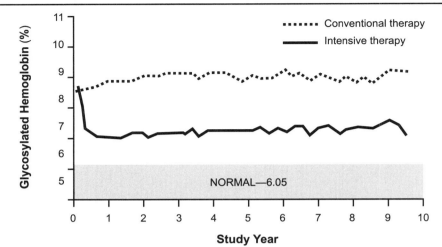

Diabetes Control and Complications Trial Research Group. *N Engl J Med*. 1993;329:977-986.

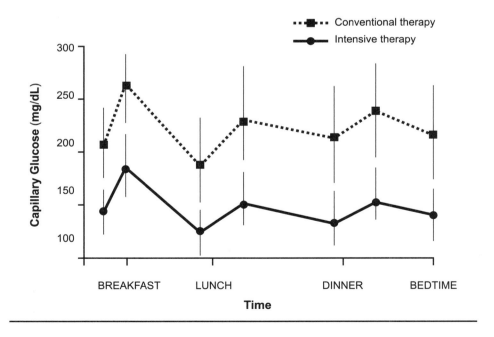

message here is that it is very difficult to achieve completely normal glucose values in the majority of people with diabetes compared with those who do not have diabetes. We now have designer insulin analogues and continuous glucose monitors (CGMs), which were not available at the time of the DCCT, that can help people more safely achieve even tighter control.

The average daily glucose value (before and after meals) for the intensively treated group was about 155 mg/dL. The average daily blood glucose value for the conventionally treated group was about 230 mg/dL. These are valuable numbers to keep in mind, especially if you have a glucose meter that keeps an average of your values. You can always compare your averages with the patients in the DCCT. Despite having poor glucose values in the conventionally treated group, on the average they still had better control than most people with diabetes in this country at that time. This, in my opinion, represented the sad state of diabetes care in the United States. Unfortunately, diabetes care did not change much during the ensuing years, which is one of the reasons I founded TCOYD. Finally after 2 decades, I feel that diabetes care is slowly improving in this country.

Intensive glycemic control reduced the risk of developing new retinopathy by an impressive 76% and delayed significant progression by 54% in people who already had eye disease. The benefits of intensive glucose control became apparent when the groups were compared after only 3 years of therapy. The reductions in kidney and nerve disease with intensive glucose control were also impressive, showing the same trends as seen with retinopathy.

It is clear that intensive glycemic control can prevent the onset and delay the progression of microvascular complications in type 1 diabetes. Further analysis also revealed that the risk for developing complications increased dramatically when the A1C was greater than two percentage points above the upper limit of normal (greater than 8% in the DCCT). It has been estimated that for every 1% rise in A1C above 8%, there is a 40% to 50% increase in the risk of developing retinopathy or eye disease.

The quality of life of the patients who achieved good glucose control was excellent, although as a group they experienced a small weight gain and a higher incidence of hypoglycemia (low blood sugar) compared with the patients with poor glycemic control. The patients who were intensively treated experienced a threefold incidence of severe hypoglycemic reactions requiring assistance from others, or they experienced unconsciousness. In addition, there were no differences between the two groups with respect to major accidents or deaths.

The gain in body weight (about 5 to 10 pounds) that occurred in patients in the intensive-therapy group is commonly observed when people with diabetes markedly improve their blood glucose control. Part of the reason for the weight gain in the well-controlled group is that less glucose was spilling over into the urine, and more was available for energy. Both hypoglycemia and weight gain can be minimized by diet control and exercise.

Both groups scored equally on the quality-of-life questionnaire despite the daily study demands imposed on the intensive treatment group. In other words, the group that achieved excellent control did not feel that their lifestyle was adversely affected. I believe that the patients who were performing home glucose testing and going through the rigors of an intensive diabetes regimen felt great and in control, both mentally and physically. A similar study was completed in the United Kingdom that demonstrated the same benefits in people with type 2 diabetes (the United Kingdom Prospective Diabetes Study, or UKPDS). The debate over the importance of good glucose control is over, and current studies are aimed at evaluating the various methods used to safely achieve glycemic goals in type 1 and type 2 diabetes.

In addition to the long-term microvascular complications of diabetes (eye, kidney, and nerve disease) that are minimized by improved glucose control, the acute short-term complications are also lessened. Acute complications, such as excessive thirst and urination, daytime tiredness, poor wound healing, blurry vision, urinary tract infections, and tooth and gum disease, affect how one feels on a day-to-day basis (**Table 2-5**). These acute complications of poorly controlled diabetes reduce the quality of life and adversely affect work performance in adults and school performance in children and young adults. The acute effects of hyperglycemia may manifest as frequent falls and mental impairment in the elderly. Many of the acute complications develop gradually, and it is only when good glucose control is achieved that one realizes how much worse

Table 2-5

Acute Complications of Poorly Controlled Blood Glucose Levels

- Excessive thirst, especially for cold drinks
- Frequent urination, including during the night
- Daytime tiredness and lack of energy
- Cuts, scrapes, and scratches take a long time to heal
- Frequent urinary tract and vaginal infections
- Tooth and gum disease
- Frequent falling and mental impairment may be seen in the elderly

they felt when in poor control of their diabetes. If hyperglycemia were painful, a lot more people with diabetes would be under better control and experience far fewer complications.

Achievable Goals of Glucose Control That Protect You From the Complications of Diabetes

The goals of glucose control for people with diabetes are quite different from the diagnostic criteria or the normal ranges that are seen in nondiabetic people. Glucose control goals, which have changed dramatically over the past few years, are shown in **Table 2-6**. The goals for glycemic control for people with diabetes keep getting lower and lower as the clinical researchers find out that we really should be shooting for totally normal blood glucose levels all of the time to avoid 100% of the complications. This is a tough goal to achieve but with all the new advances in diabetes care, a lot more people with diabetes are achieving better A1C values than ever before. Different organizations have different recommendations, but the bottom line is that we should all try to get our numbers as low as possible while avoiding frequent and severe hypoglycemia. An A1C of less than 7% is an excellent start, however, for some individuals who are older, prone to hypoglycemia, and/or have heart disease, the A1C goals needs to be individualized and may be higher than others.

Glycosylated Hemoglobin (A1C): The Long-Term Control Factor

The A1C is an important laboratory parameter that gives doctors and patients an idea of what the glucose control has been over the past

Table 2-6
Goals of Glucose Control for People With Diabetes

| Test | Typical Glucose Range (mg/dL) | |
	Normal (no diabetes)	People With Diabetes
Before-meal glucose level (preprandial)	<115	<120
After-meal glucose level (postprandial)	<140	<180
Bedtime glucose value	<120	100-140
A1C[a]	4% to 6%	<7%

[a] The normal range for glycosylated hemoglobin (A1C) is not standardized and may vary from lab to lab.

From the American Diabetes Association. Available at *www.diabetes.org*.

2 to 3 months. Remember that there are 1440 minutes in a day and a single glucose test only represents one moment in time and does not reflect the overall glucose control on the average for an extended period of time. I call the glycosylated hemoglobin (also known as A1C or HgbA1c) the "long-term glucose control factor." When the glucose level in one's blood is high for an extended period of time, the excessive glucose molecules stick or bind to many structures in the body, including the red blood cells, which contain an oxygen-carrying substance called hemoglobin and other proteins (**Figure 2-4**). The average life span of red blood cells, which are being produced and cleared from the body continuously, is about 2 to 3 months. When we measure the amount of glucose on the hemoglobin of the red blood cells, for example, it is called the glycosylated hemoglobin, and is indicative of the amount of glucose in the circulation over the past 2 to 3 months. We then compare this number with that of nondiabetic individuals. You can look at a chart to determine what your blood glucose average has been over a 2- to 3-month period by knowing your A1C values (**Figure 2-5**).

The Bayer A1C Now At Home Kit will allow the user to measure their A1C with a drop of blood in the privacy of your own home. The test kit will give you an accurate value in 5 minutes. You do not have

Figure 2-4

A1C Measures Glucose Levels Over a 2- to 3-Month Period

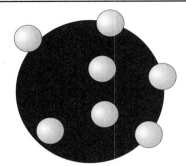

Normal Blood Glucose

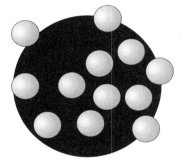

High Blood Glucose

● Red blood cell
◯ Glucose

Abbreviation: A1C, glycosylated hemoglobin (a test that measures how much glucose has been sticking to the red blood cells in the last 2 to 3 months).

Glucose irreversibly attaches to red blood cells in proportion to the average glucose concentration in the blood.

to wait a few days for the results, and best of all, you do not have to fight the usual medical office bureaucracy to get your own result. There is another long-term glucose control factor called fructosamine, which gives you an idea of the average blood glucose value of the past 2 to 3 weeks. It is normally used in women with diabetes during pregnancy because of the need to keep tight control during this important time period. Home glucose monitoring is probably the most important test to do when you are pregnant and have diabetes. GlycoMark (*www.glycomark.com*) is another very short-term glycemic control marker that gives you an idea of what your average blood glucose has been over a short period of time (2 days to 2

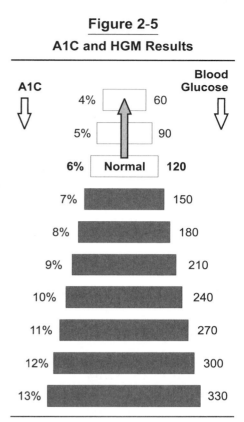

Figure 2-5
A1C and HGM Results

A1C		Blood Glucose
4%		60
5%		90
6%	Normal	120
7%		150
8%		180
9%		210
10%		240
11%		270
12%		300
13%		330

Abbreviations: A1C, glycosylated hemoglobin; HGM, home glucose monitoring.

This chart shows the relationship between A1C levels and average blood glucose readings; A1C measurement is presented as a percentage of glycosylation. A 6% A1C corresponds with a 120 mg/dL blood glucose level on average over the past 2 to 3 months.

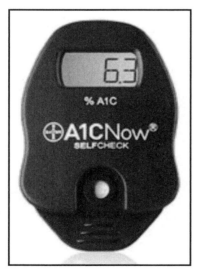

The A1C Now home glucose monitoring (HGM) device manufactured by Bayer.

weeks) and in addition, correlates well with your postprandial glucose excursions.

It is extremely important to realize that unlike the glucose value, the A1C value is not measured the same way everywhere in the United States. This is why there are different normal ranges depending on the laboratory technique used. Always compare your A1C value with the nondiabetic ranges. The normal ranges that are usually preprinted next to your value represent the ranges that nondiabetic people have. In general, your value should be less than 1 percentage point above the upper limit of normal. For example, if the normal range is 4% to 6%, your first goal would be to get below 7%.

Don't you love it when the front office clerk says, "You cannot have your results"? You can sign a release-of-information form that should allow them to release your lab results to you. Make sure you ask the office staff about this requirement at your next appointment. Many health care systems, including the Veterans Affairs Medical Centers, have online access for patients to see their laboratory values and other personal medical records. Do not trust others to interpret your laboratory values. You need to know your numbers and know what the numbers mean. Ask questions and do your own investigation and research. Remember that you are your own best advocate. Be smart and be persistent!

Home Glucose Monitoring: A Personal Laboratory in the Palm of Your Hand

Home glucose monitoring (HGM) has been one of the more important advances in the field of diabetes since the discovery of insulin in the 1920s. People with diabetes have been able to test their own blood sugar levels with these hand-held devices for almost the past 30 years. Before the availability of HGM devices, people with diabetes tested their urine for glucose, which is terribly inaccurate. When the glucose in the blood is too high, the kidneys try to filter it out in the urine, which can be measured either by test strips or chemistry pills that you put in a test tube with water. The results of these archaic urine tests do not give you an actual number but rather a very rough guide depending on the color change of the urine strip or test tube concoction. The problem is that when you measure glucose in your urine, it actually is a reflection of what your

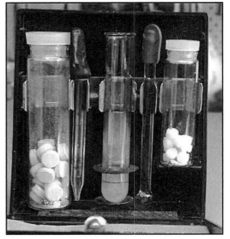

A urine test kit.

blood glucose was several hours prior to the test and does not reflect what is happening at the time of the test. Urine testing cannot be used effectively to make day-to-day decisions on insulin dosage and other self-management techniques. In addition, as one grows older, the ability of the kidneys to filter out the glucose in the blood declines so that the urine test may look good when the blood has excessive amounts of glucose.

Should all people with diabetes test their own blood levels at home? In my opinion, the answer is a strong, loud, and resounding YES! Some individuals who are elderly with consistent daily schedules and whose diabetes is quite stable on oral medications may only need to test once or twice a week at the most. On the other hand, others may be on a multiple-injection insulin regimen or an insulin pump, running around like a wild man or woman, working long hours, and exercising and eating at different times. These active people with diabetes, trying to lead normal lives, may need to test as often as 8 to 12 times a day in order to stay in good control. CGM now is available and can be a tremendous asset to folks on insulin. I have devoted an entire chapter to this topic (*Chapter 12*).

It is not enough to merely test your blood glucose at home or during daily activities. It is of utmost importance that you know what to do with the numbers and then act on those numbers. Don't test and just write the number down in your logbook for your caregiver to review. You should be thinking about what that number means, why you are at that glucose level, and what you should do to correct the number, if needed. You should also be thinking about how to avoid problems again in the future. If you are on insulin, you can always give yourself extra insulin (only if you have been educated to do so) to bring down a high blood glucose level. In addition, there is a whole list of nonpharmacologic maneuvers that do not involve pills or insulin adjustments that can help bring the glucose level into a more normal range. Techniques used to adjust for high premeal blood glucose levels are listed in **Table 2-7**. These techniques are important to minimize extreme hyperglycemia after eating and give you the power to act on the results of HGM, even if you are taking pills alone and not on insulin.

Even with HGM and the knowledge and ability to act on the results, it is difficult to mimic the metabolism of a nondiabetic individual. A normally functioning pancreas is a sophisticated organ with complicated and precise physiologic mechanisms to keep the blood glucose level in a tight range 24 hours a day, no matter what type of food is ingested. In a normal individual, the cells of the pancreas (beta cells) not only can detect changes in glucose on a second-to-second basis, but they can also identify and react to the rate of change of glucose during meals (how fast the blood glucose is rising or falling). There are other important glucose regulatory hormones such as amylin, glucagon, GLP-1, etc, that also play an important role and will be discussed in detail later in the book. This is one reason non-diabetic people can eat a hot fudge sundae and their blood glucose will never go above 140 mg/dL... those S.O.B.s!

If your physician does not offer you an HGM device, you need to be your own advocate and ask for one or get one on your own. Many patients do not like to prick their finger and test on a daily basis. I have heard many caregivers say, "I can't get my patients to test." I know why this is so; the patients may not have been given the knowledge to analyze and act on each individual number at the time of the test. I would give up test-

Table 2-7

Techniques Used to Adjust for High Premeal Glucose Levels

- Increase the time interval between consumption of the meal and the insulin shot (if you are on insulin)
- Eat less than your usual amount of food
- Eliminate or replace foods containing simple or refined sugars, such as fruits
- Delay your meal if possible
- Exchange the milk, or any beverage with calories in it, for a noncaloric drink
- Do not eat all of your meal at once if possible. Spread the calories over an extended period of time. For example, save the fruit or bread for later
- Do mild exercise, such as walking, after eating
- If you recognize a consistent trend of high glucose values at a particular time of day, you should notify your caregiver to make the appropriate change in your oral medication or insulin. You can also make the appropriate changes yourself if you have been properly educated to do so

ing myself if I didn't have the knowledge to act on it. Many patients become frustrated when their blood glucose levels are always high, and they are not given any instructions about how to bring them down. "So why test? It is always high!" is a common complaint. Throughout the rest of the book, and especially in the chapters on therapy, I will be explaining how I manage my diabetes and the diabetes of my patients using HGM and CGM results. In addition, there are definitely proper techniques to make the fingerstick less painful.

In people with diabetes, emotional issues also play a big role in not utilizing this valuable tool of HGM to control their diabetes. We all want to "do good" for our doctors and are ashamed that we did not test often enough or that our glucose values were too high. I have collected some of my favorite and most common excuses that my patients have used when they "forgot" to bring their HGM logbook to clinic… once again!

- "My meter was stolen." (The Rolex watch was next to the meter but the thief just took the meter… give me a break.)
- "Oh, gosh, I forgot it again!"
- "My dog ate it."
- "Darn… I left it in the car." At this point, I usually tell my patient to go out to the parking lot to get it. Then there is the usual reply, "I took the bus today."
- "Oh, I didn't think you wanted to see it!" This one really bugs me. My usual reply is, "I am the diabetes doctor, this is a diabetes clinic, I am the one who asked you to test your blood glucose at home, and I would really be interested in seeing the results. Now why wouldn't you think I wanted to see it?"
- "My wife was supposed to bring it." This excuse gets back to one of my three main themes of this book: *You* have the main responsibility of taking control of your diabetes.
- "I went on vacation and did not take my meter." She also left her diabetes at home, too? I would think that one of the more important times to test is while on vacation when you are not eating, exercising, and sleeping as you normally do.

To make life easier and more comfortable, many companies have developed meters that require a very small amount of blood. This means that the traditional and sometimes painful "fingerstick" can now be done on the forearm or thigh, which turns out to be a gentler, more preferred area from which to obtain blood. There are many glucose meters and you can find one that best fits your needs. There are very simple ones with large easy-to-read screens. There are meters with lots of bells and whistles that help you analyze and track your numbers, and identify trends and patterns at different times of the week. There are meters that do not require coding with each package of strips that you use and meters that communicate with other devices like insulin pumps. Please, see **Table A-1** on the various meters in the *Appendix*.

I have observed many children and adults "dry lab it." "Dry labbing" is when a person fills up his or her logbook with falsely normal or near-normal glucose values (smart patients will put an occasional high level in to throw off the caregiver). The numbers are written with the same colored pen, there is no food or blood on the sheets, and there is not much variation in the numbers, which is unusual in real life. In addition, certain numbers repeat themselves too often, which is statistically highly unlikely. Now that long-term glucose control factors such as the A1C are widely available to caregivers, it is difficult to avoid getting caught faking your results (darn it!). **Figure 2-6** is the logbook of someone who has been dry labbing it. The funny thing about this guy is that the clinic date was in the afternoon on the 8th and when he was making up the numbers he went past the 8th and when he realized it, he simply crossed off the number on the 9th and did not think I would notice it. Look how many times he logged a value of 144 or numbers ending in zero or 5.

Figure 2-6

Glucose Logbook Example of Dry Labbing by an Adult Patient With Type 2 Diabetes

Usual Target Before Meals: 70-130				**BLOOD GLUCOSE**					Usual Target 1-2 Hours After Meals: 70-180		
DATE	INSULIN			BREAKFAST		LUNCH		DINNER		BED TIME	OVER NIGHT	COMMENTS
				BEFORE	AFTER	BEFORE	AFTER	BEFORE	AFTER			
3	TYPE	AM	PM	160		135		121				
4	TYPE	AM	PM	157		144		135				
5	TYPE	AM	PM	149		—		130				
6	TYPE	AM	PM	162		150		147				
7	TYPE	AM	PM	155		144		150				
8	TYPE	AM	PM	144		160		133				
9	TYPE	AM	PM	~~162~~								

Whenever I mention this problem of dry labbing at one of our patient-oriented educational conferences, a large majority of the 1500-plus participants start to laugh. My next comment is, "Those of you who laughed have done this before!" It is important to emphasize that people who falsify their results or who seem to consistently forget their logbooks are not bad people. It simply means that there are emotional barriers that have not yet been broken down. It is an important challenge to me as a diabetologist and to other caregivers to be able to develop a strong doctor-patient relationship so that the patient feels comfortable or is not afraid or ashamed to tell the truth (either did not test at all or changed the numbers). Part of the solution to this problem definitely lies with the attitude of the physician, certified diabetes educator (CDE), primary care physician, or any professional working with that person.

Home glucose monitoring and the knowledge to act on the results are the keys to freedom for people with diabetes. It allows you to have a more flexible lifestyle, while achieving tight glucose control at the same time. HGM and CGM makes you feel in control of your condition both physically and mentally. They allow you to take control of your diabetes. (See *Chapter 10* and *Chapter 12* for more details.)

Continuous Glucose Monitoring: Technology to Help Predict the Unpredictable

Continuous glucose monitoring (CGM) devices (discussed in detail in *Chapter 12*) have already revolutionized the way we treat diabetes, and the health insurance coverage of these devices, although not perfect by any means, has improved greatly. The JDRF (Juvenile Diabetes Research Foundation) study on CGM clearly showed that this technology can reduce the highs and lows (fluctuations), reduce the episodes of hypoglycemia, lower the A1C, and improve the quality of life of people living with type 1 diabetes of any age as long as they wore it pretty much 24/7. Other studies have also documented the benefits in insulin-using type 2 diabetes.

People living with diabetes have many day-to-day struggles, and this is especially true with type 1 and insulin-requiring type 2 diabetes. There are so many factors that go into insulin-dose decisions several times each day, 7 days a week, 12 months a year, year after year. Some of these factors include type and amount of food to be ingested, prior type and intensity of exercise, anticipated type and intensity of exercise, other illnesses and stresses, the blood glucose level at the time, and the trend of blood glucose levels preceding the current test (important information that too few people currently have). In addition, the way we are given insulin is not physiologic; subcutaneous insulin delivery can be inconsistent and lead to unpredictable blood glucose results.

Home glucose monitoring has been one of the more important advances in diabetes care, but it does have limitations. Even when people are testing frequently, they see only a partial snapshot of what is happening. We do not lack knowledge about how to treat the disease, but rather, we lack constant information about what our blood glucose levels are doing in order to effectively respond. CGM can now fill those wide and potentially dangerous gaps.

Like millions of Americans living with diabetes, I have struggled to control my blood glucose levels as best I could while avoiding the lows. Now that I have been using CGM for over 5 years, I feel it is the greatest advance in type 1 diabetes since the discovery of insulin. It is the rare person with type 1 diabetes that would not benefit greatly from it.

The challenge now is to get over the pretty dense patient and clinical inertia and get this technology into the hands of the people who could benefit the most from it. This will take a concerted effort to educate the people living with diabetes, the professional community, and the insurers. At the current time, several companies are working on CGM devices as discussed in detail in *Chapter 12.*

Summary

Knowledge is power… plain and simple. Knowing the basics of diabetes gives you a foundation to have an intelligent discussion with your health care provider and be assured that you are getting the best type of preventative, diagnostic, and therapeutic care for your type of diabetes. Although I know the basics fairly well, I experience and continue to deal with the same physical and emotional challenges that many of you experience living with diabetes 24/7. I know it is not an easy task to take control of your diabetes and to stay in control.

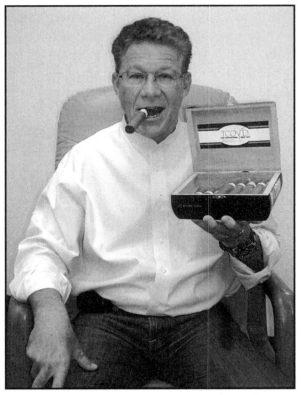

Showing off the boxes of TCOYD cigars gifted by Randall Brown… everything in moderation!

3

I Know What I'm Supposed to Do, So Why Am I Not Doing It?

by William H. Polonsky, PhD, CDE
and Susan J. Guzman, PhD

"Diabetes is easy." When you first developed diabetes, perhaps some of your friends, your family members, or even your health care providers told you that. After all, you just need to make some small changes in your everyday behavior. For example:
- Exercise regularly
- Check your blood sugars frequently
- Take your new medications and don't ever forget them
- See your health care provider regularly
- Make sure your blood sugars never get too high or too low
- Lose some weight (but not too much)
- Don't forget to check your feet regularly
- Pay attention to your blood pressure and cholesterol
- Pay attention to your portion sizes when you eat
- Make sure you are consuming the correct the amount and type of carbohydrates (remember that there are good carbohydrates and bad carbohydrates)
- Eat more fruits and vegetables
- Try to eat less of the bad fats (but remember to eat enough of the good types of fats)
- And on and on and on…

Don't worry if you start to feel confused, because you have a 10-minute appointment with your doctor sometime next month. Certainly you will get all of your concerns and questions addressed then. See, just like you were told, diabetes is easy. Right?

Of course, you know that's not the way it really is. Diabetes can be tough, even though friends, family, and even some health care providers may not realize this. Not surprisingly, many people with diabetes are struggling. Take Ralph, for example. He is a middle-aged man who has been living with type 2 diabetes for more than a decade. While he has always taken his diabetes medications regularly, he stopped checking his blood sugars several years ago. When asked why, Ralph explained,

"Trust me, whenever I check, it is always too high. So what's the point?" He started walking regularly after he was first diagnosed, but life has gotten busier and busier, and walking began to seem increasingly boring, so now Ralph hardly ever gets any exercise. He had made some healthy changes in how he eats, but he is only able to maintain those healthy habits until dinnertime. After dinner, Ralph starts to snack, and he keeps snacking until bedtime. This is not an uncommon problem; we call it the "werewolf syndrome." Diabetes "werewolves" are seemingly normal people who are able to follow a fairly diabetes-friendly way of eating, but only while the sun is up. When the moon rises in the sky, they are transformed. It is almost as if hair begins to sprout on their face, their eyes grow large, and God help any food that can't jump out of their path. Sound familiar?

Ralph was labeled by his physician as "in denial," but that was an insulting, inaccurate, and unhelpful diagnosis. Ralph certainly knew he had diabetes, and he had lots of thoughts and feelings about it. While he wanted to manage his diabetes effectively, he felt overwhelmed and defeated. Nothing seemed to work. He was angry and frustrated with himself, and he felt alone with his diabetes. He knew his wife and his kids cared about him, but they didn't understand diabetes and why he had become so discouraged. As a result, Ralph decided to just not think about diabetes anymore. So he was avoiding seeing his doctor (since she would be certain to remind him about his diabetes), was no longer checking his blood sugars (since that would make him think about diabetes), and was not talking about it with his family and friends (so they would not bring up the subject).

There are many people like Ralph. In a survey of more than 600 people with diabetes around the United States, my colleagues and I at the Behavioral Diabetes Institute (BDI) found that the majority had tough feelings about diabetes. For example, more than two thirds reported feeling at least somewhat hopeless about serious long-term complications, believing that there was nothing they could do to avoid them. More than half reported being at least somewhat angry, scared, or depressed about diabetes. Recent studies have also shown that most people are not taking perfect care of their diabetes... not even close. It is likely that the majority are struggling with following a diabetes-friendly way of eating, are not getting enough physical activity, and are not checking blood sugars frequently enough. Many are not taking their medications as prescribed. The result? Too many people never achieve the metabolic goals needed to stay healthy and avoid complications. Therefore, if you have ever felt down, discouraged, or aggravated about diabetes, know that these are very common feelings. If you don't think you're giving your diabetes the attention it needs, welcome to the club. You are not alone.

Why is managing diabetes so tough? A large survey conducted by BDI in collaboration with TCOYD found that health care providers commonly think the reason is that their patients don't have enough willpower or aren't scared enough about complications. The evidence, however, doesn't support these beliefs. In fact, almost no one is unmotivated to live a long, healthy life. But diabetes care, day in and day out, is tough. It can be a lot of work. It is tough to change one's habits. And diabetes is mostly invisible. After all, high blood sugars or high blood pressure don't really hurt, and they may not even be noticeable. Plus there are common, often unconscious obstacles that can dampen your enthusiasm to manage diabetes.

The Top Six Obstacles in Controlling Your Diabetes
1. Depression
People with diabetes are almost twice as likely to develop a serious problem with depression as people who don't have diabetes. And no one is quite sure why. One recent scientific review suggested that 20% or more of people with diabetes may be suffering from a clinically significant depressive disorder right now. Of course, everyone feels down or blue from time to time, but a clinically significant problem—such as the diagnosis of "major depressive disorder"—means that depression is actively interfering in your ability to function effectively in your life.

Some people with depression describe feelings of persistent sadness, while others report more irritability or even an "empty" or numb feeling. In addition to these mood changes, other worrisome signs of a possible depressive disorder are:
- Loss of interest in things or a diminished ability to experience pleasure (things that used to bring joy, such as friends, food, favorite activities, and sex, no longer do)
- Lasting fatigue (your "get up and go" has got up and went)
- Chronic sleeping problems
- Trouble concentrating
- Significant changes in appetite
- Suicidal thoughts or thoughts of giving up.

Depression can take the joy out of life, diminish your energy and motivation, and cause you to feel hopeless and worthless. There are many reasons why someone might get depression. Sometimes it may be related to diabetes, sometimes not. In either case, when you combine the two, it can lead to a downward spiral. Having diabetes puts you at greater risk for depression and having depression can make diabetes harder to manage.

One of our BDI program participants referred to the experience of depression and diabetes as the "deadly duo." Depression is especially worrisome in diabetes because it can interfere with your ability and your interest in following diabetes self-care recommendations. Exercise, for example, can seem a lot more difficult, or even impossible, when depression looms. When it is hard to get out of bed or you are struggling with your will to live, it is pretty hard to care about eating healthfully or checking blood glucose. Not surprisingly, depression is associated with poorer metabolic control (especially higher A1C levels), more frequent hospitalizations, higher rates of long-term complications, and even mortality.

2. *Harmful Beliefs*

How you think about diabetes has a big influence on how you feel and what you do. There are two common beliefs that can be problematic. They are problematic because they are just plain wrong. The first is "diabetes is no big deal." Perhaps a friend or even your health care provider told you this. You may have type 2 diabetes and all you know is that at least you don't have the "bad" kind (type 1). Perhaps you think that since you aren't taking any medication, or not too many different medications, or not using insulin, then your diabetes doesn't really need to be of great concern. Since long-term complications typically come on slowly over the course of years, it is seductive to think that you can start worrying about them sometime later. It is, therefore, easy to conclude that diabetes isn't that important, at least not right now. As one of my patients said, "Look, I promise you that I'll get serious about this disease, just as soon as something falls off."

The second belief is "diabetes is a death sentence." You have probably heard about the many long-term complications associated with diabetes. Maybe you have even been warned by a health care professional that you will suffer these bad outcomes if you don't start taking better care of yourself. Or perhaps you have known people who have been hit hard by the disease—losing their eyesight, ending up on dialysis, undergoing amputations, and more. Scary stuff. If you hear enough stories like these, it is easy to begin thinking that this will be your fate as well. Once you become convinced that complications are inevitable, that there is nothing you can do to stop these from occurring, who wouldn't get discouraged about their own diabetes care? If making major changes in your lifestyle and taking a variety of different medications aren't going to matter for you down the road, why would you bother?

For those who have type 2 diabetes, there are lots of other common misbeliefs that can cause you to feel guilt, shame, and discouragement about being diagnosed with diabetes, and these can get in the way of you taking action. For example, many people believe that getting type 2 diabetes is their own darned fault. But type 2 diabetes is—to a large degree—a genetic disease. When you have the right genes, certain factors (such as being overweight) can trigger diabetes. More and more Americans are becoming heavier and developing type 2 diabetes because most jobs now require little physical activity, life is more stressful, and too many foods tempt us that are high in calories, large in size, and much too convenient. There is, in other words, a powerful interaction between genes and the environment that leads to type 2 diabetes. Diabetes is not your fault, and there is a lot you can do about it. Want to know more about other common diabetes beliefs that can get in the way? Get the real facts by checking out BDI's free booklet *Don't Freak Out: 10 Things To Know When Diagnosed With Type 2 Diabetes* at *http:// behavioraldiabetesinstitute.org/downloads/Dont-Freak-Out-10-Things -To-Know.pdf*.

3. *Vague or Unreasonable Ideas About What to Do*

Even people who have been through comprehensive diabetes education programs may not be entirely clear about what they need to do to manage their diabetes. There is a lot to learn and a lot to do, and it can be confusing. Some people have overly demanding ideas about what needs to be done. Said one of our patients, "I know I am supposed to give up all of my favorite foods, eat perfectly, and never cheat." She believed that she needed to be "perfect" with her diabetes care, but since this was impossible to achieve, she ended up feeling like a failure every day. Other people have notions about what to do that are too vague or incomplete. Consider the following quotes from patients, "I was told I have to start eating healthy" and "I've gotta lose 10 pounds before my next doctor visit, which is tomorrow!" It is tough to be successful when you don't have a clear, concrete, and achievable plan.

Why do so many people end up being confused? This is embarrassing to admit, but often it is our fault, health care providers just like us. We get so enthusiastic about wanting to be helpful that sometimes we try to tell you everything all at once. Without meaning to do so, we may overwhelm you with facts, stories, and things to do. It can be hard to know where to start when your head is full of a zillion healthy changes you should make in your diet, new rules about foot care, physical activity, blood glucose monitoring, and the like.

4. Poor Social Support

If you are alone with diabetes, it is tougher to deal with the disease. When you have people in your life who are rooting for you, making and maintaining some of the tough changes that diabetes demands may become more doable. For example, trying to make diabetes-friendly changes in how you eat is easier when your family decides to join you in that endeavor. Making the time for regular exercise might be less difficult if your spouse volunteers to go with you.

But sometime friends or family members provide you with too much support, taking on the role of the "diabetes police." Sound familiar? The diabetes police are loved ones who have decided that God has deputized them to help you manage your diabetes, whether you like it or not. They frequently say things like "Should you be eating that?" "You seem upset, maybe you should check your blood sugar." "Y'know, you really should get some will power." "Gee, your numbers are high again. What did you do wrong this time?!" When friends and family act this way, they are usually coming from a place of love. They mean well, and they are trying to help—even though they are driving you crazy. The more they try and offer help in this manner, the more you may bristle. In fact, since most people don't like being nagged, there is a tendency to act out, to do the opposite of what has been suggested. What a mess!

5. Life Gets in the Way

Most of us live in a challenging environment for managing diabetes. If you have a lot of stress in your life, your diabetes care can suffer. If you are terribly busy, it can be hard to find the time to exercise or even to check your blood sugars. And most of us are terribly busy, with many competing demands on our time. Money is another big issue. Many people can't afford their medications, and many don't have enough money for health insurance. Perhaps the biggest culprit is the culture in which we live. In the United States, life is sedentary and food is served and sold in very large portions, both in restaurants and at home. And, as you know, these are not necessarily the healthiest foods in the world. Even though we may not notice it, portion sizes influence us, even if it doesn't taste so good. The bigger the portion on your plate, the more we eat. So Americans grow heavier and heavier as the years go by. This is not because we are gluttonous or lazy, but it is the insidious influence of the culture that surrounds us. However, this doesn't mean we are helpless. As discussed below, you can fight back.

6. Discouraging Results

Many of our patients have given voice to this problem. Here are some representative comments:

- "I did everything I was supposed to, and my blood sugars are still all over the place!"
- "I tried that new medication and I don't feel any better."
- "I've been walking regularly for two months now, but I haven't lost an ounce of weight!"
- "My A1C is finally at goal and now I am struggling with hypoglycemia!"

When you feel like you've put out your best efforts, and you still don't see the results you expect, it can be hard to stay enthused about your diabetes. Coping with errant blood glucose results is probably the most aggravating aspect of this problem. Many people, in fact, can start to develop an unusual relationship with their blood glucose meter. Their meter can start to influence how they feel. Blood glucose running too high or too low in the morning? Then you are a bad person, a failure. When you start letting your meter determine your self-worth as a human being, you may eventually start to hate your meter. And who wants to check their blood sugars then?

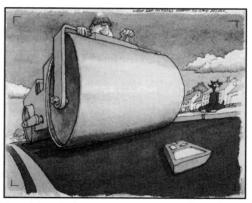

Your blood glucose meter readings yo-yo up and down... discouraged, your meter becomes your enemy!

Solutions to Consider

So diabetes is tough because there are a lot of obstacles that make it tough. But that doesn't mean there isn't something you can do about this! Here are six solutions to consider...

1. Fight Back Against Depression

If any of the symptoms of depression described above sound familiar, don't waste a moment. You can feel good again. There are a number of effective strategies for overcoming depression, so talk to your physician and find out what you can do. There is no need to blame yourself for your feelings (as if you aren't depressed enough). Depression is not the result of a "weak mind." In fact, your doctor can help you discover whether there might be a physical cause to your depression (certain medications may contribute to depression, for example).

There is solid scientific evidence that brief forms of counseling (especially one form in particular, known as "cognitive-behavioral therapy") can help many people with diabetes to recover from depression. It is also well established that commonly prescribed antidepressant medications can reverse depression in diabetes. In addition, remember that regular physical activity (like daily walking) is an antidepressant! All by itself, exercise will not be enough to cure a problem like major depression, but as one part of a comprehensive treatment plan, it can work wonders. Don't let depression get you down or keep you down. Take the first step today. To learn more about the depression and diabetes connection, please check out BDI's free booklet *Breaking Free from Depression and Diabetes: 10 Things You Need to Know and Do* at *http:// behavioraldiabetesinstitute.org/downloads/Breaking-Free-from-Depression-and-Diabetes.pdf.*

2. *Challenge Your Own Discouraging Beliefs*

The most important step you can take is to get educated about diabetes. And since you are reading this book right now, you have already gotten started! If you are feeling frightened and hopeless about diabetes, please remember this one fact: while poorly controlled diabetes is the leading cause of many serious problems (like blindness, nontraumatic amputations, kidney damage, and more), well-controlled diabetes is the leading cause of... nothing! With good care, odds are good that you can live a long, healthy life with diabetes.

Of course, no guarantees are possible, but the scientific evidence is overwhelming. Your risk of running into long-term complications of diabetes can be dramatically lowered when you are working closely with your doctor to keep your blood glucose, blood pressure, and cholesterol levels within a safe range. In fact, you may find that following a diabetes-friendly lifestyle that includes regular activity and a healthy way of eating can even extend your life. As one of our most famous physicians from the beginning of the 20th century, Sir William Osler, said: "To live a long and healthy life, develop a chronic disease and take good care of it."

And it would appear that more and more people are following this advice. Did you know that the world famous Joslin Diabetes Center in

Boston gives out medals each year to people who have been living well with diabetes for 50 years or longer? 50 years! And there are a lot more medal winners every year. In the past 20 years, the number of medals awarded each has more than tripled. Yes, diabetes is a serious disease, but you are not doomed. There is more and more good news about diabetes emerging as our knowledge and treatments are improving.

To learn more about other common discouraging beliefs about diabetes and strategies to fight back, check out BDI's booklet *The Emotional Side of Diabetes: 10 Things You Need to Know* at *http://behavior aldiabetesinstitute.org/downloads/brochure-Diabetes-10-Things-To-Know .pdf#zoom=100*.

3. Find Out How You Are Really Doing

Frustrated that you haven't seen positive results from your self-management efforts? Maybe it is time to reconsider how you measure success. For example, many people judge how well or how poorly they are doing with diabetes by how much medication they are taking. The more pills they are taking, the sicker they must be. And if insulin is needed, that must mean your diabetes is now very, very serious. When people think this way, discouragement is almost inevitable. Said one of my patients, for example, "This just isn't fair; I've been doing everything I was supposed to do, and now I have to start insulin?! Why have I even bothered trying?" But let's consider this carefully: the individual who takes no medication and has an A1C of 9.0% is at a much higher risk of developing complications than the person who is on multiple shots of insulin and has an A1C of 7.0%. In other words, it is the blood sugars that determine your risk, not the number or kind of medications being taken. And remember that no matter what you do, diabetes changes over the years and can get harder to handle, requiring more and different medications. This is not your fault, and it doesn't mean that your diabetes is now "worse."

Other common ways that people measure their diabetes success is by how well how they are eating, or how they are feeling, or whether or not they ever see a blood glucose level higher than, say, 200 mg/dL. But none of these are appropriate ways to judge how well or how poorly you are doing. In fact, you can drive yourself crazy this way!

So what to do? Find out about the major medical tests that can help you to really determine your diabetes health. The most important ones are those that measure your A1C level (a blood test typically done at your doctor's office which measures your average blood sugar level over the past 10 to 12 weeks), blood pressure, and cholesterol. When the results of these tests are in a safe range, you can be assured that you are doing well and your risk of complications is pretty darned low. You, not just your doctor, need to make sure you get these tests done regularly (blood pressure and cholesterol at least once yearly, A1C every 3 to 6 months). And you need to know the actual numerical results of these tests and what they mean. If your doctor tells you that you are "fine," that is not sufficient. As my friend and colleague, Dr. Richard Jackson, a well-known endocrinologist at Joslin Diabetes Center says, "Imagine going up to a bank teller and asking how much money you have in your account. The teller looks up your records and tells you, 'Not to worry, you are fine.'" Would you be satisfied with this response? Of course not. It is your money and your life. You need to know your numbers.

4. Develop a Sensible, Personalized, Action-Oriented Plan for Self-Management

To manage your diabetes more effectively tomorrow, just tomorrow, what exactly should you do? If you were going to make one positive change in your diabetes management over the next week, what would it be—and why? And what is stopping you from taking this step? These are not easy questions to answer, but they are critical. To succeed with diabetes, you need a plan and a reason for taking action.

Set a specific, small, short-term goal for action. If you just have a vague sense that you should be "exercising more" or "checking blood sugars more often," you might believe you are never doing enough. To start, pick one action that might have an impact on your improving your blood glucose. Be specific. For example, exactly how much exercise this week? Exactly what are you going to do? When? How often? Break this down into small steps. By clarifying your action plan, you will know exactly what to do and will be able to tell when you are successful.

As you think about what first steps you might take, make very sure that they are specific and are truly actions to start. Many people make this mistake of focusing on vague and unachievable actions, such as "I'm definitely going to get myself some will-power." Others commit the error of focusing on actions they want to stop, like "Starting tonight, I'm going to quit eating ice cream." But few people are successful in the long-term when their chief goal is to deprive themselves. Instead, if the goal is to give up ice cream, then consider what action you could start doing that will help you achieve that end. It doesn't have to be an enormous step, but it should be a first step and it should be very specific. For example, "When I get home tonight, I am going to throw away the ice cream in our freezer and have a snack of diet cherry Jello instead."

Plans are best when they are personally meaningful (you must have a good reason for wanting to take control of your diabetes, not just because your doctor thinks it is a good idea), when the action steps you have chosen are very specific, and when the steps chosen are achievable and reasonable (given the other stresses and priorities in your life). Don't try to change everything at once; the best approach is one small healthy step at a time. Work together with your doctor to help you choose a place to start that has potential for some real payoff with your diabetes. For more helpful examples and specific strategies, see Dr. Polonsky's book, *Diabetes Burnout: What to Do When You Can't Take It Anymore.*

5. Seek Out Rewarding Relationships

If you only have time to make one change, this is it! If at all possible, don't do diabetes alone. Reach out to the people in your life for the love and support you need. At a practical level, invite one or more of your loved ones to join you in making a healthy change. For example, you will be more successful at diabetes-friendly dietary changes if you can convince your family and/or friends to take those same healthy steps along with you. Regular physical activity is much easier when you have an exercise partner. Don't know anyone who might join you in, say, taking a walk around the park each morning? Then perhaps it is time to knock on a neighbor's door. Make a new friend, and help someone else to make a healthy change in their life as well. When you are looking for loving support, remember that the key is to be as specific as possible. Don't just ask your spouse to "be more supportive"; instead, explain that you would like him or her to—for instance—sit with you at the kitchen table every morning when you check your blood sugars.

As a way to start a conversation about this subject with someone in your life, BDI has developed the Diabetes Etiquette Card, developed especially for those people who don't have diabetes. When someone says something annoying to you about diabetes, you don't have to get angry. You can just calmly explain to them that they must not know the proper rules about how to behave, then hand them the etiquette card. It is a humorous way to initiate a serious conversation. The Diabetes Etiquette Card is a list of common "do's and don'ts." For example, etiquette point #4 is:

DO offer to join me in making healthy lifestyle changes. Not having to be alone with efforts to change, like starting an exercise program, is one of the most powerful ways that you can be helpful. After all, healthy lifestyle changes can benefit everyone!"

A downloadable version of this card can be found on our website (in English and Spanish), and there is a new version for parents of teens with type 1 diabetes): *http://behavioraldiabetesinstitute.org/downloads /Etiquette-Card.pdf#zoom=100.*

Also, consider attending a diabetes support group or joining an online forum. It is a powerful experience to connect with other people who are going through some of the same, or similar, experiences. Your doctor, local hospital, or local chapter of the American Diabetes Association may be able to suggest one in your area. You can check out BDI's list of the best online forums and resources at *http://behavioraldiabetes institute.org/resources-diabetes-information-website-links.html.*

6. *Do Something About Less-Than-Rewarding Relationships*

If your loved ones are acting like diabetes police, select a quiet, dispassionate moment to discuss this matter with them (or perhaps consider writing them a letter). Let them know that you understand they mean well, but they must realize that their nagging is not helpful. Remember, since they love you, odds are good that they will never stop trying to be helpful. Therefore, you must give them something to do instead. You might explain, for example, that always asking you "should you be eating that?" is not helpful, but if they could please remember to keep the refrigerator stocked with diet soda, that would be terrific. The Diabetes Etiquette Card, mentioned above, also addresses the common "don'ts" and can be helpful as a playful way to arrest the diabetes police in your life. Consider, for example, the first rule of diabetes etiquette:

> *DON'T offer unsolicited advice about my eating or other aspects of diabetes. You may mean well, but giving advice about someone's personal habits, especially when it is not requested, isn't very nice. Besides, many of the popularly held beliefs about diabetes ("you should just stop eating sugar") are out of date or just plain wrong.*

In Summary

Remember that living with diabetes is not necessarily so easy. Diabetes care is a job, and it is not a job you volunteered for! As we have described, there are many reasons why managing diabetes can be emotionally tough, but there are solutions as well. So don't give up. With effort and support, you can live well with diabetes. And for more information about the emotional side of diabetes, please visit us at the Behavioral Diabetes Institute, *www.behavioraldiabetes.org.*

4

The Diabetes Warranty Program, Sick-Day Rules, and the Scoop on Alcohol

Developing a Diabetes Warranty Program

One of the more powerful and simple tools that you can use to take control of your diabetes is to follow a diabetes warranty program. The concept is simple and is similar to the warranty program that accompanies a new automobile. If you follow the regularly scheduled maintenance program, your new or used car will run better and last longer. Following a diabetes warranty will also help you pick up problems early so that complications do not reach end-stage levels. I designed the diabetes warranty program in order to detect, as early as possible, any complications, such as eye, kidney, or nerve disease, that may arise over time. Remember that our first goal is to prevent the onset of any complications in the first place, but the next best thing is to be the first to know about them so that early and aggressive therapy can be started ASAP! The early stages of eye, kidney, nerve, and heart disease do not come with any symptoms, which make screening so important. If you follow the regularly scheduled maintenance program that is recommended by leaders in the field of diabetes, you will feel better and live a longer, healthier, and more productive life. Please try not to get overwhelmed with the list of things that us folks with diabetes need to do over time, as it can seem daunting. All of this "stuff" will become a normal part of your life, and you will be in better shape in the long run.

All people with diabetes need a maintenance record book that lists the recommended tests with dates and results (**Figure 4-1**). This information is vital, primarily to those of us with diabetes, and secondarily to our caregivers, in order to diagnose and track the common problems that can occur with diabetes. In many cases, your record will be more orderly and complete than the one in your medical chart. It is also not uncommon to change physicians or see specialists from different health care systems, so your record keeping takes on an even greater importance. The individual items in **Figure 4-1** will be discussed in the appropriate chapters throughout the book. Remember to keep updated and organized records. If you can, it would be very helpful to make a

Figure 4-1
Diabetes Warranty Program

What Should Be Done at *Every* Visit

	Date	Result	Normal Range or Goal
Weight			
Blood pressure			
Glycosylated hemoglobin[a] (know the normal range)			
Foot examination[b]			

What Tests/Examinations Should Be Done at Least *Every* Year

	Date	Result (recommendations)	Normal Range
Cholesterol levels (fasting):			
▪ Total cholesterol			
▪ Triglycerides			
▪ HDL			
▪ LDL			
Urine protein (microalbumin)			
Serum creatinine			
Thyroid function test (TSH)			
Eye examination (dilated)			
Dental examination			
Other tests/examinations (depending on individual needs):			
▪ Cardiologist (for heart disease)			
▪ Podiatrist (for foot problems)			
▪ Gastroenterologist (for stomach problems)			

a Glycosylated hemoglobin (A1C) is a long-term diabetes control factor (see *Chapter 1*).
b This may not be necessary, since you should examine your own feet as discussed in *Chapter 17*.

file on your computer so that you can easily update it and print it out for your health care visits and/or bring on a flash drive to input into the EMR (electronic medical records). As a physician who cares for people with diabetes, I love it when my patients keep good records of their medical problems, list of medications, other doctors they see, tests, etc. It helps me take better care of them.

How Often Should You Be Seen by Your Caregiver?

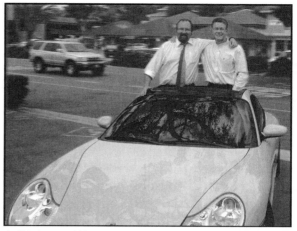

A *Diabetes Warranty Program* is like the warranty program that accompanies a new car. Famous artificial pancreas researcher, Dr. Howard Zisser, from the Sansum Clinic in Santa Barabra, California.

The official recommendations state that if you are currently on insulin, your physician should see you approximately every 3 to 4 months. If you are not on insulin, you should been seen approximately every 3 to 6 months. The frequency of visits obviously depends on how well or how poorly you are doing and whether you have taken control of your diabetes. For example, if your home glucose monitoring (HGM) values are consistently in the desirable ranges and your diabetes regimen is stable, you do not need to see your caregiver as often as someone who never tests their blood glucose levels at home and has no clue how he or she is doing. If you are really on top of your diabetes and know that you are doing well via HGM and/or continuous glucose monitoring (CGM) data, then in reality you may only need to be seen once a year, if you also have a primary care physician, in order to renew your prescriptions and to make sure all of the appropriate tests and exams are done according to your diabetes warranty program. I prefer at least every 6 months, even if you are doing well. Don't forget that you can stagger your medical visits between your primary care doctor and your diabetes health care provider (such as every 6 months for each, staggered so that you are seeing someone every 3 months).

When you visit your physician, be prepared to discuss the most important issues with which you have been struggling. **Table 4-1** lists some of the areas that you may want to discuss with your caregiver. There is obviously not enough time at any one visit to discuss all of these issues; however, you should decide which ones are the most important to you at the time of your visit. Please do not come in with a list so long that it freaks out your caregiver even before starting your visit. Also, mention to your doctor that you have a list of questions when he or she first walks in the room so that the limited time of your visit can be used to get to the issues most important to you. If you need new prescriptions, try to coordinate them so they can all be done at once with a 1-year supply of refills. I have to say that filling and renewing prescriptions is one of the biggest pains in the medical profession. The system is improving slowly with EMRs but is still very archaic in many health care systems. (see *Redefining the Diabetes Doctor Visit* in *Chapter 25*.)

Write Up Your Own Diabetes History Sheet and Keep It Updated

It is also helpful to have a basic information sheet about your medical history (**Figure 4-2**). Write up your own diabetes history sheet. Much of your medical history does not change and is easy to update periodically. You can then bring a copy of your medical history, along with your diabetes warranty program sheet, to any health care professional, such as your dentist, physician, diabetes educator, or pharmacist. It will also allow more time for other important issues during your appointment. I have listed my medical information in **Figure 4-2** as an example. As you can see, I spilled my guts telling all of my medical problems to the world!

Table 4-1

Potential Topics to Discuss With Your Caregiver

- Home glucose monitoring (HCG) results
- Continuous glucose monitoring (CGM) results
- Problems with hypoglycemia
- Medication questions
- Test or examination results and when necessary, options for therapy
- Pregnancy issues
- Exercise routine
- Meal planning
- Sexual dysfunction issues
- Immunization requirements (ie, yearly flu shot)
- Sick-day rules
- Any tests or examinations not completed that are recommended by your diabetes warranty program

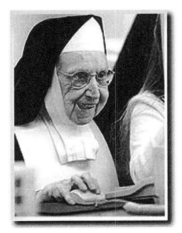

If an 80-year-old nun can be online, why can't prescription refill requests be made easier?

If you discover that a test or examination has not been done that is needed in order to comply with your diabetes warranty program, you should discuss this with your caregiver and request the test or examination. Phrase your comments and questions constructively and not too aggressively (for example, "Is it possible to please check my cholesterol levels next visit? My last values were done over a year ago, and I am concerned about them.") You must work with your caregiver in order to maintain your health and quality of life. Staying healthy is much easier when preventive measures are taken early, especially with diabetes. Most caregivers will be glad to help with your requests if they are appropriate and reasonable.

What Should Be Done at Your Office Visits?

The standards of care call for certain things to be done at your office visits, including measurement of your weight (I know this may be painful and embarrassing for some of you) and blood pressure (BP), a discussion of your HGM results, your CGM results (if appropriate), and laboratory values. You should have had your blood drawn a few days before your appointment, which makes the visit so much more meaningful. I get pretty frustrated with no recent lab results on my patients, and especially if there are no HGM or CGM data as well. A foot exam may also be in order, especially if you are experiencing a problem or have loss of sensation (neuropathy).

As is true with all official recommendations, certain items may not be as pertinent in your case. For example, if you examine your own feet and have no current problems, this part of your office visit is not necessary and not a good use of the limited time you have with your caregiver. In addition, if you have a BP device and take your own readings at home, these numbers are more meaningful than a sporadic measurement at the doctor's office. This is especially true if you have the "white coat" phenomenon—your BP goes up when you get it measured at the doctor's office.

Top Ten Tips on How to Make Your Doctor's Appointment a Success

Recommendations from Dr. Ian Blumer—diabetes specialist and advocate from Toronto, Canada (www.ourdiabetes.com)— and author of Chapter 27 in this book

Have you ever left a doctor's appointment feeling that the visit was not a resounding success? Maybe you felt that you spent too much time in the waiting (and waiting... and waiting...) room? Or maybe you had a

Figure 4-2

Sample Diabetes Medical History

Last updated	October 2012
Name	Steven V. Edelman
Date of birth	September 6, 1955
Date of diabetes diagnosis	1970 (15 years old)
Type of diabetes therapy	1. 1971-1976: One injection per day (NPH/Regular) 2. 1976-1982: Two or three injections per day 3. 1982-2000: Insulin pump (basal rate 0.7 units/hour), carbohydrate-to-insulin ratio (15:1), correction factor 1 unit rapid-acting will lower my blood glucose ~50 mg/dL 4. 2000-2008: The untethered regimen (75% of my basal requirements from Lantus and 25% via the insulin pump) 5. 2008-Present: Insulin pump (basal rate 0.6 units/hour from 7 AM to 3 AM and 0.75 units/hour from 3 AM to 7 AM. I also take 60 mcg of Symlin with every meal and use a continuous glucose monitor (CGM)
Incidence of hypoglycemia	Mild ones once or twice a week, not at any consistent time, with symptoms of light-headedness and dizziness when I get into my 50s; I no longer experience palpitations or getting sweaty
Other medical problems	1. 1979: Retinopathy diagnosed (received laser treatment of both eyes; Dr. Paul Tornambe is my ophthalmologist) 2. ~1985: Kidney disease diagnosed (see diabetes warranty sheet for most recent kidney tests; Dr. David Ward is my kidney doctor) 3. ~1985: High blood pressure diagnosed, take three different medications *(see Medications list below)* 4. ~1989: High cholesterol levels diagnosed *(see Medications list below)* 5. Gastroparesis and heartburn 6. The syndrome of limited joint mobility/trigger fingers
Recent hospitalizations	2010: Bike accident; taken to ER by ambulance and suffered a shoulder separation, two broken ribs, a contused back, and sprained ankle
Surgery or operations	1. 1997: Right middle trigger-finger repair 2. 1999: Left middle trigger-finger repair 3. 2000: Left knee surgery (ACL repair) 4. 2002: Left ring finger trigger-finger repair 5. 2003: Frozen shoulder treated with physical therapy 6. 2008: Right knee meniscus tear; underwent laporoscopy 7. 2009: Sinus surgery
Medications	1. Rapid-acting insulin analogue (Apidra, Humalog, or Novolog) in my pump or pen (~45 units/day) 2. Lantus (glargine) 20 units when not on my pump 3. Symlin (pramlintide) 60 mcg before each meal 4. Lozol (indapamide) 2.5 mg once a day

Continued

Figure 4-2

Sample Diabetes Medical History *(continued)*

Medications *(continued)*	5. Monopril (fosinopril) 20 mg twice a day 6. Norvasc (amlodipine) 5 mg once a day 7. Lipitor (atorvastatin) 40 mg once a day at bedtime 8. Aspirin 81 mg once a day (enteric coated) 9. Fibercon two tablets a day
Allergies	My dog
Important family history (heart disease, cancer, diabetes)	1. Great uncle (mother's side) and grandmother (father's side) had type 2 diabetes 2. Grandfather (mother's side) died of a heart attack at the age of 65 years 3. Several relatives on my father's side of the family died of stomach cancer 4. Uncle (mother's side) with Alzheimer's disease at the age of 67 years

question that never got answered? Or you felt rushed? Or you did not get part of you checked that should have been? If this rings a bell, then you have come to the right place, because here (with apologies to David Letterman) I present my Top Ten Tips to Make Your Next Family Doctor or Diabetes Specialist Appointment a Success.

Number 10: Think of your doctor as being your guidance counselor, not your school principal. Your doctor gives advice; that is all. You can choose to accept this advice or you can choose to reject it. Thank goodness we live in a society where the decision is yours! (But, of course, if you are rejecting your doctor's advice because you do not trust it, you need to ask yourself if it is time to change doctors.)

Number 9: Imagine, if you will, that you have your entire life's savings invested in the stock market. Every hard-earned dollar. Now imagine you call your broker and ask how your investments are doing. What would you think if your broker said to you, "They're fine!" and then hung up? Does "fine" mean you are making lots of money? Or does "fine" mean you are having an average rate of return? Or does it mean you have lost some money, but from your broker's perspective it could have been worse? Who knows? I sure wouldn't. So when your doctor checks your BP or your kidney urine test or your A1C, do not accept being told the result is "fine" or "good" or "okay" or some such thing. Make sure you find out the exact result. Ask if the result is above target. If it is, ask how you can work with your doctor to improve it. Your doctor will not be offended. Quite the opposite. In fact, your doctor will be thrilled to have such a keen partner with which to work toward attaining a common goal—keeping you healthy!

Number 8: If you have had a lab test and you do not subsequently receive a call from your doctor's office, do not for one moment conclude that "no news is good news." Maybe no news means that the result got lost in the mail, got accidentally thrown out, or went to the wrong doctor. (Just ask my wife, who is a physician and shares the name of three other doctors in Toronto; she regularly has their patients' results mistakenly sent to her!). I would suggest that when you see your doctor, you ask how you will find out your results. Can you call the office to get them? Should you book a follow-up appointment to review them? Can you have the lab or the office send you a copy of the results? (Heck, it's your body fluid after all!)

Number 7: If you are being prescribed a drug, be sure to ask your doctor some crucial things about the medicine. For example, why is it being prescribed, how will it help you, what possible side effects can be expected, and what should be done if side effects occur?

Number 6: Tired of waiting until you become covered in cobwebs in the "waiting room?" Try booking your appointment for the first slot of the day or the first slot in the afternoon. Dollars to donuts, your wait will be a lot less.

Number 5: Need more time with your doctor than you are getting? Feeling constantly rushed during appointments? Next time, when you book your appointment, ask the doctor's secretary to book you in for a longer time slot. If that does not work, ask for the last slot of the day. Most likely, if you are the last patient the doctor has to see that day, he or she will not feel as rushed (which means more time for you).

Number 4: Want to get preferred appointment times? Longer appointment times? Want to get squeezed into an already-full schedule? Then remember, the doctor's secretary is a VIP! So be sure to be extra nice. Nice helps. Trust me. Better yet, trust my secretary!

Number 3: Your doctor should be checking your feet regularly, but this important part of one's anatomy often gets overlooked at the time of routine appointments. Not any more! Because now as soon as you go into your doctor's examining room, you are going to take off your shoes and socks and present your beautiful (or not so beautiful as the case may be) tootsies to your doc for an examination. If you have no issues with your feet, a yearly exam is perfectly fine.

Number 2: Almost everyone with diabetes should be testing their blood glucose levels and keeping a written record of the values in a logbook. (On my website—*www.ourdiabetes.com*—you can find what I think is the most helpful format for keeping a log.) Doing this will help keep you on the up and up regarding your status and progress and will similarly help your doctor help you. So be sure to bring the logbook to each and every appointment with your family doctor and diabetes specialist (and diabetes nurse educator). And remember: Your logbook is not a report card! It should never be used to judge you or used in a punitive way. It is a tool to help you and your doctor monitor and adjust your therapy; nothing more, nothing less. On the subject of writing things down, I would also suggest that you write down any questions you have before you see your doctor, then pull them out of your pocket or purse at the beginning of your appointment to double check that you have had all your questions addressed. So many people end up remembering a question they had meant to ask only after they have left the office! I would also suggest that you write down your doctor's answers or bring a loved one or trusted friend with you to hear your doctor's replies. (You know what they say about two sets of ears, eh?)

Number 1: Now, as much as I hope that you have found the preceding nine tips helpful, I have saved the absolutely, positively, most important tip for last. Forget about waiting-room lineups, log books, guidance counselors, and secretary VIPs. No, when it comes to the truly essential, number-one tip for making your doctor's appointment a success it is this: Whatever you do, never honk or yell (or worse) at the guy that cut you off in the doctor's parking lot; he could be the guy wearing the rubber glove that you will be seeing in 5 minutes!

What Tests or Exams Should Be Done at Least Annually?

Certain tests and exams must be done every year in order to initiate aggressive therapy when needed to avoid the end-stage complications of diabetes (**Figure 4-1**). A yearly cholesterol panel, a test of how your kidneys have been affected by diabetes, and thyroid levels are a few of the important ones and are discussed in subsequent chapters. The yearly dilated eye exam is a must for all people with diabetes and, depending on your list of other medical problems, you may need to see a periodontist, cardiologist, podiatrist, stomach specialist, etc, on an annual or more frequent basis.

What Should Be Discussed With Your Caregiver?

Please do not go into your doctor's office with a list of questions that is half a mile long! This will put the usually hassled caregiver immediately on edge. Decide what issues listed in **Table 4-1** are the most important to you. Try to do your homework first and look up the topic of the question so that you can get the most out of your office visit. It is like going to an auto mechanic for a particular problem; if you know a little about cars and how they work, you will understand the explanation of what is wrong with your car a lot better. Please, do not wait until the end of your appointment time to mention that you have a list. Mention it early so that there is enough time allotted to discuss each issue during your visit.

Sick-Day Rules

Every person on this planet living with diabetes must know his or her sick-day rules. What exactly do I mean by sick-day rules? It is basically having a game plan on how to manage your diabetes when you are sick. Sick-day rules are especially important for people using insulin to treat their diabetes.

One of the most common situations is when someone gets the flu or a bad cold. The way not to handle it is to withhold your diabetes medication because your appetite is down and you are eating a lot less than normal. In times of illness or stress (emotional or physical), your body normally becomes resistant to the glucose-lowering effects of insulin and/or oral medications, thus increasing the medication requirements.

If you are on insulin and you become ill, the key is to do a lot of testing of your blood glucose levels (as often as every 2 or 3 hours) and know what to do with the results. For people taking rapid-acting insulin, such as Humalog (lispro), Novolog (aspart), or Apidra (glulisine), taking small-to-medium amounts of extra insulin throughout the day may be in order to keep the blood glucose level from climbing above 200 mg/dL. The amount of insulin needs to be individualized according to your sensitivity and normal amounts that you take when you are not sick (insulin therapy is discussed in *Chapter 8*).

If you have type 2 diabetes and are on oral medication only, your sick-day rules will probably not include insulin injections. Drink plenty of noncaloric fluids, test your blood glucose frequently (approximately 3 or 4 times a day), and please do not stop your medications without talking to your caregiver.

In certain circumstances when you have been really sick with vomiting, you may need to test a substance in your body called ketones, which indicates a more severe illness and calls for closer monitoring, aggressive insulin therapy, or a visit to the emergency room. Ketones can be measured by a strip that you dip into a urine sample or by a drop of blood on some home glucose meters using a different type of strip. They can also be measured in most laboratories and are a commonly ordered test in the emergency room.

Treatment of Hypoglycemia

On May 27, 2006, I attended a memorial service for Cyndee Fena. Cyndee was a friend, patient, and TCOYD volunteer. She was found dead in bed from severe hypoglycemia. She lived alone and was discovered by her neighbor. The paramedics documented a blood glucose level of 20 mg/dL. Cyndee had hypoglycemia unawareness and had been found unconscious from hypoglycemia in the past, but I could not convince her to back off on her control because she was determined to not become blind, lose a leg, or go on dialysis… complications she fought so hard to avoid all of her life. Unfortunately, this is not an uncommon scenario. Prevention and proper treatment are especially important for any person with diabetes taking oral medication and insulin. Hypoglycemia unawareness is discussed in more detail in one of the cases in *Chapter 13*).

Treatment of hypoglycemia is another "taking control" topic that is super important. For people on insulin or taking oral medications that can cause hypoglycemia, awareness of low blood glucose is crucial for early treatment and avoidance of having a seizure or passing out. Unfortunately, this happens too frequently while people are at work, caring for young children, or driving an automobile. The results can be disastrous. In addition, the proper treatment of hypoglycemia is important in order to bring your blood glucose back into the normal range swiftly without overshooting to the other extreme of hyperglycemia.

First of all, you must always carry something sweet with you if you are at risk for hypoglycemia. Many drug stores sell special glucose tablets to treat low blood glucose levels. My favorite glucose tablets come from a company called GlucoLift developed by one of my patients with diabetes (I love the orange cream flavor). There is also an excellent under-the-tongue gel that rapidly elevates the blood glucose level. You can buy a roll of Lifesavers or some type of hard candy that is mostly sugar with no fat, such as Skittles or Mentos. Candy bars with chocolate and fat, such as Snickers, Milky Way, and 3 Musketeers (my favorite), do not raise your blood glucose as quickly because they contain fat and protein, and have a ton of calories (240 for a regular-sized Snickers Bar). In comparison, 4 to 6 ounces of apple juice or a regular soda is approximately 100 calories and is excellent for treating acute low blood glucose reactions. The faster you raise your blood glucose to normal, the faster you will lose that incredible craving to eat and eat and eat.

What not to do at night (or any other time for that matter) is what I used to do all the time. I would wake up in a sweat and shaking like a leaf, go downstairs, and eat everything in the fridge… cookies, leftovers, peanut butter and jelly sandwiches, and a couple bowls of cold cereal (Trix are my favorite)! I would then go back to sleep and wake up a few hours later feeling terrible with a blood glucose level over 400 mg/dL. This is not to mention all of the excess calories that you can rack up. A huge handful of Oreo cookies is at least 300 to 400 calories with lots of saturated fat. When your blood glucose is low, your body signals to you to eat as much as possible and, if you do not pick the quick-acting foods, you will overdo it. I now keep small cartons or cans of apple juice or glucose tablets at my bedside so that I do not even have to go near the fridge! It should go without saying that if you are experiencing hypoglycemia on a regular basis, you should really try to figure out what adjustment in your treatment regimen is warranted.

Diabetes and Drinking… Can You Mix Them Responsibly?

When I was diagnosed with diabetes in 1970, all of the diabetes educational literature said that people with diabetes (PWD) should never, ever drink alcohol. I believe one of the main reasons PWD were told to avoid alcoholic beverages was because if you had alcohol on your breath and became hypoglycemic, you could mislead the person who might be attempting to help you, which would ultimately delay the treatment you might desperately need. Even today, many health care professionals tell their patients that they should not drink at all. If you have diabetes and like to consume alcoholic beverages on occasion, there are a few common sense things you should know. In the same manner as dealing with desserts and sugary foods, a PWD need not avoid them completely, but merely know how to deal with them in terms of keeping their glucose levels in an acceptable range.

What goes without saying? First, if you are underage, you must wait until you are 21 years of age to drink. Second, no one should drink and drive. In addition, testing your blood glucose level frequently or checking your continuous glucose monitor, if you have one, is extremely important. Knowing what your glucose level is during a night of drinking, eating, and dancing, for example, is essential in order to avoid any issues or problems.

Now that we have the obligatory suggestions out of the way, let's talk about drinking and diabetes. Excessive consumption of low calorie alcoholic drinks on an empty stomach can supposedly lead to hypoglycemia, however, I do not think this is a very common occurrence. A more typical scenario is an elevated glucose value when food is consumed concurrently and the alcoholic drink is on the sweeter side. The calorie and fat content of alcoholic drinks can vary greatly and affect your diabetes differently (see **Table 4-2**). On one end of the spectrum, we have sugary drinks like piña coladas, margaritas, and mojitos. They have tons of simple carbs and will jack up your glucose level pretty quickly, especially when you're munching on chips and bar food at the same time. Also, some of these sugary drinks, such as Baileys (yum!), have a high fat content as well. Drinks that have fewer calories and no fat are better suited for PWD. Beer, wine (white or red), and hard alcohols (vodka, scotch, whiskey, gin, etc) are examples. I'll bet you did not know that Guinness is the lowest calorie, regular beer on the market (see the *Edelman Report on Alcohol and Diabetes* by visiting our YouTube channel TCOYDtv). If you use mixers, try to stick with things like diet cranberry juice, diet tonic, diet ginger ale (great with bourbon) and club soda, or mineral water.

Like everything in life, moderation is the key. We all have our individual preferences for certain types of alcohol and tolerability for the amount we can consume responsibly. With that said, becoming intoxicated may be an occasional reality for some, so surround yourself with friends and family who know you have diabetes, get yourself to a safe place, test your blood sugar frequently, don't ever get behind the wheel

Table 4-2

Comparison of the Calorie and Fat Content in Alcoholic Beverages

	Serving Size (oz)	Total Calories	Carbohydrates (g)	Total Fat (g)
Vodka	1	64	0	0
Whiskey	1	56	0	0
White wine	3.5	84	2.7	0
Guinness draught	12	125	9.9	0
Stella Artois lager	11.2	154	6.3	0
Piña colada	6.8	526	61.3	16.9
Margarita on the rocks	12	250	22	0.17
Bailey's Irish Cream	1.3	94	7.4	5.8

of a car, and don't throw up on your friend's new carpet! Now, just to set the record straight, I am not an alcoholic, nor am I trying to be inappropriate by talking about getting drunk, but it can be a reality, so why not be prepared and discuss it straight up.

People with diabetes can pretty much enjoy any type of food or beverage that anyone else can, and drinking alcohol is no exception. When it comes to drinking and diabetes, we need to exercise some common sense rules, keep a close eye on our glucose levels, be in a safe environment, choose the drinks that minimally disrupt our glucose values, and practice moderation. Cheers!

Summary

In addition to following the diabetes warranty program, you must be knowledgeable about the available tests and be aware of the kinds of therapy that are available for any abnormality or problem. Knowing your results is one thing but then finding out what to do with them is another important next step. Be as prepared as possible for your health care visits so you can get the most out of those precious moments. Understanding how your body reacts to being sick or hypoglycemic is of vital importance. Lastly, drinking alcohol is a normal part of many of our lives, and you just have to be smart about it... cheers. This is what taking control of your diabetes is all about.

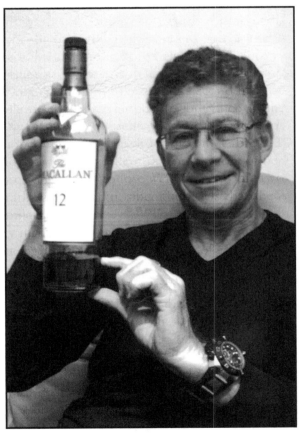

Drink alcohol in moderation... I just opened this bottle this morning!

5

If Eating in Moderation Is the Key, I Must Have the Wrong Lock!

by Lorena Drago, MS, RD, CDN, CDE

Introduction

These are the most common questions my patients ask after being diagnosed with diabetes: "*What can I eat now that I have diabetes?*" and "*How much can I eat?*" These are my answers:

- Eat foods that can help you keep your blood sugar (glucose) levels as close to the normal range as possible.
- Eat foods that can help you prevent and/or manage other common conditions associated with diabetes, such as high blood pressure and high cholesterol levels that increase your risk of heart disease. To accomplish these goals, eat nutrient-dense foods in the right amounts for you.
- Eat nutrient-dense foods most days of the week. Some examples of nutrient-dense foods are:
  - *Whole grains*: amaranth, barley, buckwheat, corn, millet, oats, quinoa, brown rice, rye, sorghum, teff, triticale, whole wheat, and wild rice. Reduction of cardiovascular disease and weight maintenance are some of the most common health benefits of whole grains.
  - *Fruits, vegetables, legumes, seeds*: sunflower, sesame, pumpkin, chia, flax, nuts.
  - *Lean animal protein foods*: poultry, beef, fish, eggs, healthy fats and oils (olive, avocado), and low-fat dairy food or dairy substitutes.

The amount of food you can eat depends on many factors: age, gender, activity level, weight, and medications. A good place to start is to know the amount of calories you need to maintain, lose, or gain weight.

How Many Calories Should I Eat?

Patients frequently ask, "*What foods can I eat?*" I need to know you a little better before I can answer this question. If you asked me what you could wear at a wedding, I could not give you a specific answer before I knew the time of the event, location, and even your favorite colors.

Get the picture now? However, most likely you will be able to eat at least 50% of the foods you eat now. They will also ask, *"How much can I eat?"* Probably not as much as you would like.

"How many calories do you need?" I use this rule of thumb:

- Adult women:
  - *Lose weight*: 1200-1500 calories/day
  - *Maintain weight*: 1500-1800 calories/day
  - *Underweight or are very active*: 1800-2200 calories/day
- Adult men:
  - *Lose weight*: 1500-1800 calories/day
  - *Maintain weight*: 1800-2200 calories/day
  - *Underweight or are very active*: 2200-2500 calories/day

These are just estimates. Consult with a registered dietitian to obtain your individualized calorie budget. To locate one near you, go online to *www.eatright.org*.

What does a 1500-calorie diet look like?

Breakfast

1 egg scrambled with ½ cup of raw spinach, ½ cup of chopped asparagus, and 1 tbsp of chopped red pepper cooked with 1 tsp of olive oil

2 slices of rye bread toast with ½ tbsp of cream cheese

Coffee with low-fat milk

Calories: ~ 340

Lunch

2 cups of arugula, ½ cup of grape tomatoes, ¼ cup shredded carrots, 4 oz of grilled chicken breast, 1 tbsp of dried cranberries, 1 tbsp of crumbled blue cheese, ½ oz of chopped walnuts, and 2 tbsp of balsamic vinaigrette with olive oil

1 glass of unsweetened iced tea

Calories: ~560

Snack

1 cup of mixed berries

Calories: 60

Dinner

3 oz of salmon with garlic and herbs, 1 cup of fettuccini al dente with broccoli rabe in olive oil and garlic.

Calories: ~550

Total calories: 1510

How do I calculate the calories in my food?

To get you started, these are some resources where you can find the calorie and nutrition information for many of the foods you eat:

1. American Diabetes Association—There are various calorie-counting books that list the calories and nutrition information of foods (*www.diabetes.org*). One popular book is *Diabetes Carbohydrate & Fat Gram Guide*, 4th edition (American Diabetes Association, 2010).
2. Online Resources:
   - *www.calorieking.com*
   - *www.nutritiondata.com*

Keeping track of the foods and beverages you consume each day will help you become more aware of the strengths and deficits in your diet.

1. Purchase a calorie-counting book, and start a food journal. Record everything you eat and drink, and total the amount of calories consumed at the end of the day.
2. Learn how to read and interpret the food label. One serving of cereal Brand A has 150 calories per serving. A serving is ⅔ cup. If you eat 2 cups, you will be eating 3 servings or 450 calories, and that doesn't even include milk.
3. *Measuring tools:* Find the carbohydrate and calorie composition of foods on the Nutriportion measuring cups. To order, visit *www.lorenadrago.com*.
4. Online food trackers, some of which have applications for your smart phones and tablets are:
   - *www.calorieking.com*
   - *www.myfitnessplan.com*
   - *www.sparkpeople.com*
   - *www.mycaloriecounter.com*
   - *www.choosemyplate.gov*.

How Much Should I Weigh?

Health professionals use a trendy term, body mass index (BMI), that measures your weight in proportion to your height. A BMI between 19 and 24 indicates a healthy weight. A BMI under 19 indicates that you are underweight and between 25 and 29 indicates that you are "Ruben-esque" (overweight). Obesity is categorized as a BMI over 30. Blood glucose, blood pressure, and cholesterol are harder to manage as the BMI increases.

What Is My BMI?

Refer to the BMI chart (**Table 5-1**). Find your height in inches and your weight in pounds. Look at the number at the top of the column where these two numbers intersect. That is your BMI.

What You Must Know First: Which Foods Raise Your Blood Glucose (Sugar) Levels the Most

Carbohydrate is one of the three nutrients that the body uses for ener-gy. Fat and protein are the other two remaining nutrients. Carbohydrate includes sugars, starches, and fibers. Foods that contain carbohydrate are broken down in the body into blood sugar or glucose. Manage your blood glucose levels by "budgeting" your carbohydrate. **Table 5-2** lists foods that have carbohydrates. If you eat more carbohydrates than your body can process, your blood glucose levels will be higher than desired. If you eat too little, your blood glucose levels may be lower than de-sired, especially if you take certain medications and/or insulin.

How do I know how much carbohydrate is in the food that I am go-ing to eat? Refer to **Table 5-3** to familiarize yourself with carbohydrate counting. The aforementioned calorie-counting resources also provide carbohydrate information. *Who eats ⅓ cup of rice?* One peanut? One potato chip? Unfathomable. One third cup of cooked rice has 15 grams of carbohydrate; ⅔ cup has 30 grams, and 1 cup has 45 grams. You can eat the quantity that fits your budget. Most "carbohydrate budgets" allow more than 15 grams per meal, so you can probably have a more realistic amount of rice on your plate.

How much carbohydrate can I eat? Are you a male? You can probably eat more. Are you inactive? You probably need to eat less (**Table 5-4**). When it comes to carbohydrates, *profile and discriminate*. Profile dubi-ous-looking carbohydrates and select those with high nutritional value. For example, a glass of soda and a glass of orange juice contain about the same amount of carbohydrate but they are *not* nutritionally equal.

Table 5-1
Body Mass Index Table

BMI	Normal						Overweight					Obese										Extreme Obesity															
	19	20	21	22	23	24	25	26	27	28	29	30	31	32	33	34	35	36	37	38	39	40	41	42	43	44	45	46	47	48	49	50	51	52	53	54
Height (inches)	Body Weight (pounds)																																			
58	91	96	100	105	110	115	119	124	129	134	138	143	148	153	158	162	167	172	177	181	186	191	196	201	205	210	215	220	224	229	234	239	244	248	253	258
59	94	99	104	109	114	119	124	128	133	138	143	148	153	158	163	168	173	178	183	188	193	198	203	208	212	217	222	227	232	237	242	247	252	257	262	267
60	97	102	107	112	118	123	128	133	138	143	148	153	158	163	168	174	179	184	189	194	199	204	209	215	220	225	230	235	240	245	250	255	261	266	271	276
61	100	106	111	116	122	127	132	137	143	148	153	158	164	169	174	180	185	190	195	201	206	211	217	222	227	232	238	243	248	254	259	264	269	275	280	285
62	104	109	115	120	126	131	136	142	147	153	158	164	169	175	180	186	191	196	202	207	213	218	224	229	235	240	246	251	256	262	267	273	278	284	289	295
63	107	113	118	124	130	135	141	146	152	158	163	169	175	180	186	191	197	203	208	214	220	225	231	237	242	248	254	259	265	270	276	282	287	293	299	304
64	110	116	122	128	134	140	145	151	157	163	169	174	180	186	192	197	204	209	215	221	227	232	238	244	250	256	262	267	273	279	285	291	296	302	308	314
65	114	120	126	132	138	144	150	156	162	168	174	180	186	192	198	204	210	216	222	228	234	240	246	252	258	264	270	276	282	288	294	300	306	312	318	324
66	118	124	130	136	142	148	155	161	167	173	179	186	192	198	204	210	216	223	229	235	241	247	253	260	266	272	278	284	291	297	303	309	315	322	328	334
67	121	127	134	140	146	153	159	166	172	178	185	191	198	204	211	217	223	230	236	242	249	255	261	268	274	280	287	293	299	306	312	319	325	331	338	344
68	125	131	138	144	151	158	164	171	177	184	190	197	203	210	216	223	230	236	243	249	256	262	269	276	282	289	295	302	308	315	322	328	335	341	348	354
69	128	135	142	149	155	162	169	176	182	189	196	203	209	216	223	230	236	243	250	257	263	270	277	284	291	297	304	311	318	324	331	338	345	351	358	365
70	132	139	146	153	160	167	174	181	188	195	202	209	216	222	229	236	243	250	257	264	271	278	285	292	299	306	313	320	327	334	341	348	355	362	369	376
71	136	143	150	157	165	172	179	186	193	200	208	215	222	229	236	243	250	257	265	272	279	286	293	301	308	315	322	329	338	343	351	358	365	372	379	386
72	140	147	154	162	169	177	184	191	199	206	213	221	228	235	242	250	258	265	272	279	287	294	302	309	316	324	331	338	346	353	361	368	375	383	390	397
73	144	151	159	166	174	182	189	197	204	212	219	227	235	242	250	257	265	272	280	288	295	302	310	318	325	333	340	348	355	363	371	378	386	393	401	408
74	148	155	163	171	179	186	194	202	210	218	225	233	241	249	256	264	272	280	287	295	303	311	319	326	334	342	350	358	365	373	381	389	396	404	412	420
75	152	160	168	176	184	192	200	208	216	224	232	240	248	256	264	272	279	287	295	303	311	319	327	335	343	351	359	367	375	383	391	399	407	415	423	431
76	156	164	172	180	189	197	205	213	221	230	238	246	254	263	271	279	287	295	304	312	320	328	336	344	353	361	369	377	385	394	402	410	418	426	435	443

Source: Adapted from Clinical Guidelines on the Identification, Evaluation, and Treatment of Overweight and Obesity in Adults: The Evidence Report. Available at www.nhlbi.nih.gov/guidelines/obesity/bmi_tbl.pdf.

Table 5-2

Foods With Carbohydrates

- All breads (and I mean *all*—even whole-wheat and 9-grain breads)
- Rolls, crackers, bagels, baguettes, breadsticks
- All cereals (cold and hot cereals, including "healthy" oatmeal)
- All beans (yes, healthy beans such as kidney beans, chick peas, black-eyed peas, etc)
- All starchy vegetables (white and sweet potatoes, green peas, and corn)
- All fruits (even fruits that are not sweet, such as grapefruit; and fruits in every form: juice, canned, frozen, and dried)
- All grains (from the exotic to the traditional: amaranth, barley, buckwheat, corn, emmer, granola, kammut, millet, oats, quinoa, rice, rye, sorghum, spelt, teff, triticale, wheat, wild rice) and foods made with these grains, such as pasta, tortillas, couscous, etc
- Milk and yogurt (whole milk, low-fat milk, and fat-free milk)
- Candy, baked goods, regular sodas, and beverages
- Seasonings and sauces: barbeque sauce, marinades, mayonnaise, ketchup, etc

Carbohydrate Counting in Action at Every Meal

Let's go over the following four steps to determine your carbohydrate budget:

1. Identify foods that have carbohydrates
2. Estimate the amount of foods with carbohydrates on your plate. Is it 1 cup? 2 cups?
3. Determine how much carbohydrate you can have in one meal. This is your carbohydrate budget.
4. Identify how you will modify this meal. Can you make healthier substitutions?

Deal or No Deal?

In all of the meal examples to follow, I have asked my patient detailed questions concerning food items typically eaten and preferred for any given meal. This helps to establish a routine eating pattern. Each patient's carbohydrate budget is based upon the individual's height, weight, blood glucose levels, and medical history.

Meal Deal #1

Joe's Breakfast (carbohydrate budget = 60 grams)

The Menu
1½ cups of cooked instant oatmeal made with water
½ cup of 2% milk
1 medium banana
Coffee with 2% milk (mostly dark)
Sugar substitute

Total amount of carbohydrate for breakfast
Oatmeal = 45 grams
Milk = 6 grams
Banana = 30 grams
Coffee = carb-free
Total carbs = 81 grams (21 grams over budget)

Meal Modifications
Joe loves oatmeal, so he is not confident that he can cut back on his usual breakfast portion. He is willing to eat half of the banana or skip it altogether. I would supplement Joe's modifications with the following recommendations:

- Use old-fashioned oatmeal or steel cut oats. Minimally processed foods are digested more slowly, resulting in a gradual and steady rise of blood glucose levels

Table 5-3
What Are Grams of Carbohydrate?

You are eating 15 grams of carbohydrate every time you eat *one* of the following foods:

- 1 slice of bread
- ½ cup cooked cereal
- ¾ cup cold cereal
- ½ cup starchy vegetable (corn, peas)
- ½ plantain – ½ cup cooked taro, cassava, or tannier
- ⅓ cup cooked rice, pasta
- ½ cup beans
- 1 small potato
- 1 small fruit
- 4 oz (½ small glass) juice
- 1 glass milk
- 6 oz plain yogurt

Carbohydrate bargains are ½ cup of cooked vegetable or 1 cup of raw vegetable. These have only 5 grams of carbohydrates!

Table 5-4
How Much Carbohydrate Can I Eat in One Meal?

	Grams of Carbs *(per meal)*	
	Woman	Man
You need to manage your weight…	50	60
You have a healthy weight…	60	75
You are very active…	75	75

- Switch to 1% or fat-free milk to reduce saturated fat (too much saturated fat may elevate risk of heart disease)
- Exchange banana for strawberries. Five medium-sized strawberries (2 oz) have about 5 grams of carbohydrates while a medium-sized (7 inches long) banana has about 30 grams

---

Meal Deal #2

Rosa Maria's Lunch (carbohydrate budget = 60 grams)

The Menu

4 oz salmon

½ cup beans

2 small flour tortillas

1 cup mixed green salad with tomatoes, peppers, cucumbers (Rosa tells me that she avoids carrots because they have a lot of sugar.)

2 to 3 tablespoons fat-free Ranch salad dressing

1 can diet soda

Total amount of carbohydrate for lunch

Beans = 15 grams

Tortillas = 30 grams

Ranch salad dressing = 16 grams

Total carbs = 61 grams

Meal Modifications

Rosa is eating within her carbohydrate budget. These are some food tips that will enhance the nutritional value of the meal.

Food Tips

- Beans have protein and carbohydrates. They are an excellent source of soluble fiber that can help manage cholesterol levels.
- Corn tortillas are a better choice than flour tortillas, since corn meal is a whole grain.
- Salad greens are a "carbohydrate bargain." Dark vegetables are excellent sources of vitamins A and C.
- Carrots and beets have a reputation for having "lots of sugar." Although they might have slightly more carbohydrates than a cucumber or a cup of spinach, they are still a carbohydrate bargain. A cup of cooked carrots has about 10 grams of carbohydrate. A cup of cooked rice has 45 grams. See the difference?

- Fat-free salad dressings have added carbohydrates. Two table-spoons of some fat-free Ranch dressings contain as much as 11 grams of carbohydrate. Remember to check the carbohydrate content of fat-free salad dressing on all labeling. A better salad dressing choice is olive oil and vinegar.

Meal Modifications

Rosa almost met her carbohydrate quota! However, she has learned that she can add carrots to her salad without breaking the carb bank, and she will check the labeling for carbohydrate content of all salad dressings and sauces.

Meal Deal #3

Tony's Dinner (carbohydrate budget = 75 grams)

The Interview: Tony loves to cook and enjoys fine wines. He cooks with a lot of garlic and uses olive oil in his recipes. I ask him to tell me what some of his favorite foods are.

The Menu
- 1 bowl (about 1½ cups) homemade minestrone
- ½ plate linguini and broccoli rabe prepared with garlic and olive oil
- Lemon shrimp prepared with olive oil, garlic, and parsley
- Italian bread (about 4 inches long)
- 1 glass (5 oz) Pinot Grigio

Carbohydrate Load of the Menu

Minestrone soup = about 20 grams
Linguini = 45 grams
Italian bread (1½ oz) = 21 grams
Total carbs = 86 grams (11 grams over budget)

Meal Modifications

Tony could reduce the amount of linguini to ²/₃ cup for a savings of 15 grams of carbohydrate, adding more broccoli rabe to compensate for the reduction in pasta. Reducing the amount of bread by half would save another 10 grams.

Food Tips

- When cutting back food portions, it is wiser to reduce the carbohydrate with the least "nutritional power." For example, minestrone with its beans and vegetables is more nutritious than Italian bread, so it makes more nutritional sense to reduce the bread rather than to reduce the soup.

■ Soups vary in their carbohydrate content. To make a low-carbohydrate soup, add more nonstarchy vegetables and less pasta, potatoes, or rice. Measure your foods until you become an expert in "eyeballing" portions. Wine does not count as a carbohydrate choice, and on an empty stomach, it may lower blood glucose levels.

Smart Tips for Every Day Eating

- *Do not bring home what you cannot control.* There are certain foods that have magnetic appeal. If you bring them home, you are going to eat more than just one portion. Mentos have an overwhelming magnetic effect for me. I seldom buy them. I have fooled myself too many times trying to convince myself that the next time would be different.

- *Buy the smallest portion available.* When I crave ice cream, I buy the smallest size available, which nowadays is not really that small. I have outsmarted the super-sized friendly servers, and ask them to give me a scoop the size of a lemon.

- *When eating out, wrap before you grab.* Your plate is on the table, and it is overflowing with spaghetti, chicken, and a miniscule vegetable. I know that there is way too much spaghetti. With the fork, I separate what looks like about 1 cup and push the rest to the side. All of a sudden I question whether I truly have the correct portion and I allow my fork to wander to the neatly stacked pile waiting to go home for another meal and slowly pull some of the noodles to my "eat now" pile. I outsmart my wandering fork by asking for a container before I even eat the first bite in order to avoid the temptation. Wrap before you grab.

- Are you too busy to prepare breakfast so you eat the wrong choices and end up feeling guilty? Identify the barriers—they could include:
  – Waking up late
  – Not having anything healthy to take on the run
  – Not being hungry early in the morning

Ask yourself what can realistically be changed. A possible plan of action could include:

- Setting the alarm earlier
- Preparing foods the evening before

- Preparing a breakfast kit and leaving it at work. It can include such things as oatmeal packages, nuts, dried fruits, fresh fruits, low-fat milk, whole-grain cold cereals, boiled eggs, ready-to-eat shakes or bars (ie, Glucerna)
- Eating breakfast on the go in the car: fruit, ready-to-eat shakes or bars (ie, Glucerna), dried fruit/nut combination, whole-grain bread

Are you eating too much at night? Try these:
- Do not leave leftovers; freeze food after eating to avoid temptation
- Eat a mint and/or brush your teeth after dinner
- Eat a snack mid afternoon to avoid overeating at dinner
- Wrap food in opaque containers to avoid temptation—out of sight, out of mind!
- *How do I know what is the right amount of carbohydrate for me?* Test your blood glucose levels 2 hours after the beginning of your meal for 1 week. If the numbers are consistently high, eat fewer foods with carbohydrates. If the numbers are consistently low, eat a little more. If your blood glucose levels are consistently above or below the recommended range, talk with your doctor or educator for help in achieving levels that remain more constant with your target range.
- *Can I save some carbohydrates from one meal and add them to another?* It is not a great practice to save, let's say, 50 grams from lunch so you can have 100 grams at dinner. Unfortunately, your body is not going to remember your midday sacrifice, and it will have to process a larger amount at dinner.
- *I thought that vegetables such as spinach and broccoli did not have any carbohydrates?* Nonstarchy vegetables have carbohydrates but at a "bargain carb price" compared with rice or pasta. One cup of spinach has 5 grams of carbohydrates. One cup of cooked rice has 45 grams of carbohydrates. Vegetables are a carbohydrate deal!

Protein: Beef, Pork, Poultry, Fish, Cheese, and Eggs—How Much Can I Eat?

I have talked extensively about carbohydrates, because carbohydrates impact blood glucose levels the most. I will now talk about two other important nutrients: protein and fat.

Protein foods seldom travel solo. They are often accompanied by fat. Beef, pork, goat, chicken, turkey, fish, eggs, and cheese are frequently consumed protein choices. Super-sizing protein and fats leads to added calories, which translates into weight gain and poor diabetes control. Because diabetes increases the risk of heart disease, it is important to manage blood glucose levels in addition to blood pressure and cholesterol levels.

Excessive amounts of saturated and hydrogenated fats (trans fats) increase blood cholesterol levels. Most animal protein sources, such as beef, chicken, pork, etc, contain saturated fat. Your best bet is to select leaner cuts most days of the week, reserving higher fat choices for occasional treats (**Figure 5-1**).

Figure 5-1
Protein Foods and Their Fat Partners

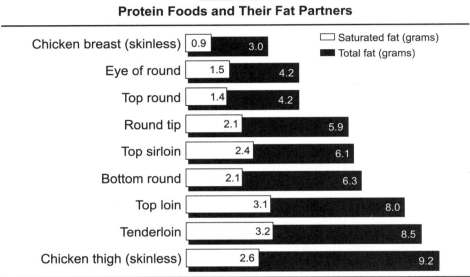

All values are based on 3-oz cooked servings of meat cuts.

Adapted from Michigan Beef Industry Commission. Available at www.mibeef.org /conleancuts.htm.

Lean Protein Foods
- Remove skin from chicken and turkey
- Trim all visible fats
- Select cheese with less than 2 grams of saturated fat per ounce
- Select lean cuts of meat

How much protein can I eat?

You probably have heard that the amount of a protein portion should not be bigger than the palm of your hand or a deck of cards. For most people, this holds true. The daily protein requirement for most people is between 0.8 to 1.0 g/kg of body weight (1 kg = 2.20 lb). A person who weighs 60 kilos (132.28 lb) would require between 48 to 60 g (~1.5 to 2 oz) of protein per day. A 3-ounce serving of cooked meat such as beef, chicken, or fish has approximately 21 g of protein. Legumes, grains, dairy, vegetables, and nuts also contain protein but in a lesser amount compared with animal protein sources.

Medium- and High-Fat Protein Foods

Medium-fat protein foods contain 7 grams of protein and 5 grams of fat per ounce. Some examples are:
- 1 oz ground beef (most cuts of beef, pork, lamb, or veal)
- 1 oz low-fat cheese
- 1 egg

High-fat protein foods contain 8 grams of fat per ounce. Some examples are:
- 1 oz pork sausage
- 1 oz spare ribs
- 1 oz cheese (American, Swiss, etc)
- 1 oz lunch meat
- 1 oz frankfurter or bratwurst

What do these numbers mean?

You can reach your fat quota very quickly if most of your protein foods come from the medium- and high-fat category.

If milk has carbohydrates, why is cheese listed as a protein food?

American, Swiss, cheddar and other hard cheeses do not have over 1 gram of carbohydrate per ounce. Cheese is a high-fat protein food. If you have cheese-dependency issues, minimize portions. Select low-fat cheese if you are unable to eat just one half ounce.

Lorena's Cheese Tip

I find Cabot's low-fat cheeses quite palatable. Grated cheese is always a welcome illusion. When I grate 1 ounce of cheese, it appears voluminous compared with a slice. I also mix and match. High-quality grated Romano or Parmesan cheese combined with sliced cheese will make grilled cheese go a long way. I place ½ oz of cheese on a slice of bread, then sprinkle 1 tablespoon of Romano cheese over the top.

Another trick is to heat a pan and place about 1 tablespoon of grated Romano or Asiago cheese on it. Let it melt and harden. This cracker-like piece of cheese can be added to salads for extra crunch and lots of taste with less fat. See **Table 5-5** for fat grams in 1 ounce of some common types of cheese.

Table 5-5

Fat Grams in 1 Ounce of Cheese

	Total Fat (grams)	Saturated Fat (grams)
American	7	4
Cheddar	9	6
Low-fat cheddar	2	1
Mozzarella	6	4
Low-fat mozzarella	4	3
Muenster	8	5
Provolone	8	5
Swiss	8	5
Cottage cheese (½ cup)	5	3

Fat: How Much Should I Eat Daily?

Limiting saturated fats and hydrogenated fats can lower your risk for cardiovascular complications. When using fats and oils, select monounsaturated fats, such as olive oil and avocado (**Table 5-6**).

Table 5-6

Daily Fat Budget

Calorie Budget	Total Fat (grams)	Saturated Fat (grams)
1200	40	9
1500	50	12
1800	60	14
2000	67	16
2200	73	22

Show Me the Food! (Do Not Show Me Fat Numbers)

I will use as an example Rebecca's daily budget:

- Calories: 1500
- Total fat: 50 grams
- Saturated fat: 12 grams

Let's take a look at two Meal Deals that are based on a daily fat budget of 1500 calories.

Meal Deal #4	Meal Deal #5
3 oz roasted chicken leg (with skin)	3 oz roasted chicken leg (skinless)
1 medium baked potato	1 medium baked potato
1 tablespoon sour cream	1 teaspoon sour cream
1 dinner roll	1 dinner roll
2 pats (teaspoons) of butter	1 teaspoon rosemary flavored olive oil
1 bowl of green salad	1 bowl of green salad
1 tablespoon Ranch salad dressing	2 teaspoons vinegar with 1 teaspoon olive oil
Calories = 609	Calories = 530
Carbohydrates = 54 grams	Carbohydrates = 54 grams
Total fat = 31 grams	Total fat = 19 grams
Saturated fat = 12 grams	Saturated fat = 5 grams

Meal Deal #4 will provide Rebecca with more than half of her daily fat allowance (31 grams) and all of her daily saturated fat allowance (12 grams), while Meal Deal #5 will provide her with less than half of her daily total fat and saturated fat allowances.

Food Tips

- A teaspoon of olive oil has the same amount of fat (5 grams) as a teaspoon of butter, but olive oil has less saturated fat than butter
- Select clear salad dressings. Creamy salad dressings have twice the fat and saturated fat compared with clear ones
- Omega-3 is a heart-healthy fat. Eat salmon, tuna, sardines, herring, and other fatty fishes a few times per week
- Alternate a high-fat meal with a very low-fat meal to achieve balance
- Select margarines that have less than 2 grams of saturated fat and less than 1 gram of trans fats

Cholesterol: How Many Eggs Can I Have Weekly?

The egg yolk has about 280 mg of dietary cholesterol. There are many brands of eggs that have a lower amount of cholesterol, some as low as 210 mg. The recommendation is not to exceed 300 mg of cholesterol daily. Reducing dietary cholesterol to less than 300 mg per day may result in a 3% to 5% reduction in your LDL (bad cholesterol) levels. Eggs should be consumed in context of the other foods in your diet. If your diet is usually low in dietary cholesterol, then you will be able to accommodate an egg yolk into your dietary cholesterol budget.

Eggs are not the only food with dietary cholesterol. Other foods with cholesterol include:

- Butter: 1 tablespoon = 30 mg
- Peanut butter: 2 tablespoons = 0 grams
- Broiled hamburger patty: 3 oz (75% lean/25% fat) = 76 mg
- Broiled hamburger patty: 3 oz (90% lean/10% fat) = 70 mg
- Broiled hamburger patty: 3 oz (95% lean/5% fat) = 65 mg
- Frankfurter (5 inches long): 1 = 24 grams
- Chocolate ice cream: 1 cup = 44 grams
- Whole milk: 8 oz = 24 grams
- Mozzarella cheese: 1 oz = 22 grams

Five Steps to Lower Your Cholesterol

1. Reduce weight (even a 10-lb loss can help lower your LDL cholesterol 5% to 8%).
2. Stay within your fat and saturated fat budget (see **Table 5-4**).
3. Eat very little trans fats (read the food labels, and select foods with "0" grams).
4. Eat more foods rich in soluble fiber (5 to 10 grams per day can help reduce your LDL cholesterol 3% to 5%):
   - Cooked oats: 1 cup = 4 grams
   - Cooked pearled barley: 1 cup = 6 grams
   - Cooked kidney beans: 1 cup = 6 grams
   - Strawberries: 1 cup (8 berries) = 3 grams
   - Cooked okra: 1 cup = 4 grams
   - Apple: 1 large = 3 grams.
5. Eat a handful of almonds or walnuts (about 23 pieces); nuts are healthy but "calorie-expensive," so if you add nuts to your diet, cut back on other foods to achieve "calorie balance."

Lowering Your Blood Pressure

Cutting back on salt is just one step up the ladder of blood pressure management. My advice is to continue taking your medications and check those numbers frequently. It is not uncommon to take more than one medication to control your blood pressure. Read more about controlling your blood pressure in *Chapter 14.*

You can also greatly assist the lowering of too-high blood pressure with the following lifestyle changes:

- Reduce weight until you achieve a level that is realistic for you (see **Table 5-1**)
- Try the DASH diet: A food-combination program that encourages the consumption of fruits, vegetables, and low-fat dairy while cutting back on saturated fat (DASH is an acronym for Dietary Approaches to Stop Hypertension [high blood pressure])
- Increase physical activity: don't squirm—just move, move, move about 30 minutes most days of the week
- Drink alcohol in moderation: That means men should have no more than two drinks and women no more than one drink per day
- Cut back on salt: Look at the sodium content on the food label (a low-sodium food has less than 140 mg of sodium per serving)

Frequently Asked Questions

1. *Which fruits have less sugar?* It depends on the serving size. A banana, a pear, a mango all have about 30 grams of carbohydrates; ¼ of a cantaloupe and 1¼ cup of strawberries each has about 15 grams of carbohydrates. *Remember:* All fruits have carbohydrates, which can raise blood glucose levels.
2. *Which foods cut fat?* The only foods that help you lose weight are those that remain uneaten on the plate. Low-calorie options, such as vegetables, allow you to eat more with fewer calories. Whole grains and beans are rich in fiber and increase satiety level. In general, eating less and moving more is the consistent—yet unexciting—message that still holds true to this day.
3. *Aren't nuts loaded with cholesterol?* Nuts have fats but they have no cholesterol. Only foods that are animal-based have cholesterol. Plant foods may have fat but no cholesterol.
4. *How much sugar can I have?* Let me clarify. There are naturally occurring sugars in foods with carbohydrates. The sugar listed on the food label is the sum of added sugars and naturally occurring sugars. To find out if the food has added sugar, look at the ingredient label. Common names for added sugars are brown sugar, high-fructose corn syrup, corn syrup, and maltose.

5. *Should I use butter or margarine?* Butter is high in saturated fat and low in trans fats. Margarine is lower in saturated fat yet high in trans fats. Look for spray/liquid margarines and avoid stick margarines. If you still prefer to use butter, try whipped butter, and use it sparingly.

6. *Should I take vitamins?* A multivitamin may be beneficial. Do not think, however, that a multivitamin will redeem you from a multitude of food sins!

7. *Should I eat sugar-free [fill in the blank]?* Sugar-free cookies and cakes contain slightly less carbohydrates than their regular counterparts. The sugar is replaced with sugar alcohols which have minimal impact on blood glucose levels. Nevertheless, they contain other carbohydrate sources, such as flour. Sugar-free is neither calorie-free nor carbohydrate-free. Proceed with caution and still count the carbohydrates.

8. *Can you give me low-carbohydrate options?* If you cringe at the thought of eating ⅓ cup of cooked rice or pasta, try jicama (Mexican potato), winter squashes, rutabaga, parsnips, or turnips.

Summary

1. Eat small portions except for nonstarchy vegetables.
2. Carbohydrates turn into glucose about 15 minutes after eating, and it is the nutrient that affects blood glucose levels the most.
3. Testing your blood glucose level will let you know if the meal plan is working for you.
4. Carbohydrates are found in all fruits, breads, cereals, starchy vegetables, pasta, rice, tortillas, potatoes, corn, crackers, milk, yogurt, and sweets.
5. Nonstarchy vegetables are carbohydrate bargains.
6. Protein and fats do not have much of an impact on blood glucose levels unless you super-size. Trim the fat from your meats and poultry, and select lean cuts. Use olive oil, avocado, and nuts in moderate amounts.
7. Read all food labels, and stay within your calorie, fat, saturated fat, trans fat, and sodium budgets.
8. Select foods high in soluble fiber.
9. Eat vegetables and fruits daily.
10. Get a diabetes coach—a health care professional who can help you put a plan into action that is realistic and makes sense to you!

6

If You Do Not Find Time for Exercise, You Will Have to Find Time for Disease!

by Sheri R. Colberg, PhD, FACSM

Introduction

Although exercise has long been one of the three cornerstones of diabetes management—along with diet and medications—it has generally been and continues to be the most overlooked and underutilized of the three. Why? My opinion, as an exercise physiologist and a person living with type 1 diabetes myself, is that people are less likely to exercise regularly because they just don't know enough about how, when, where, and why to fit physical activity into their daily lives. The reality of exercising with diabetes is that regardless of what type you have, being more active is just one more variable that you have to take into account when you're trying to take control of your blood glucose level. Whether you're just contemplating starting to exercise or you're already a regularly training athlete, by learning more about exercise, you

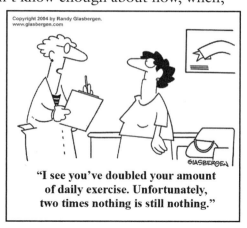

"I see you've doubled your amount of daily exercise. Unfortunately, two times nothing is still nothing."

will soon understand why it is so important to living well with diabetes and how to make it work best for you and your unique situation.

Why Exercise Is So Important to Your Health

Not only can regular exercise make you fitter, it can also help you lose weight (or at least not gain any more), keep you from regaining any weight that you do lose, enhance your mental health, decrease your blood pressure, and lower your risk of heart disease, cancer, other chronic health problems, and your chances of dying from any cause. What is more, people with diabetes experience similar or even greater health benefits from being active than the average nondiabetic person.

We already know for certain that people who exercise regularly really do live longer. A recent study looked at the effect of different levels of physical activity (ie, low, moderate, or high) on the total life expectancy of more than 5200 middle-aged and elderly people, most already older than 50 years. The study concluded that if you get in a vigorous workout almost daily (such as running 30 minutes 5 days a week), you can add nearly 4 years to your life. If you only engage in moderate exercise—the equivalent of walking instead of running for those 30 minutes—then you're likely to live 1.3 to 1.5 years longer for males and females, respectively, likely due to delaying the onset of heart disease, our nation's leading killer and a major cause of death and disability in people with diabetes.

I have to admit that when I first read about this study, I thought, "Doing moderate exercise 5 days a week will allow me to live only a year and a half longer?" To gain this extra time, you would have to walk moderately for at least 2.5 hours a week, 52 weeks a year, for most of your adult life (55 years beyond the age of 21, on average), meaning that you would end up spending over 7000 hours exercising, or about 300 24-hour days, in exchange for only 550 extra days. So, basically, you would have spent over half of your "extended" lifespan exercising the equivalent of 24 hours a day. I guess if you really enjoy exercising, that's not a bad thing (and there are some avid diabetic exercisers out there who wouldn't mind), but if you're like the majority of people, you're probably thinking that for no more than you gain, it's just not worth the extra effort.

Before you stay on that couch and vegetate some more, let me try to talk you out of it. What is likely much more important is that exercise can increase your health-related quality of life. Regular physical activity affects not only how long you live but also how long you live a healthy life. Being more active can give you more time in a healthy state, free from a host of chronic illnesses that can make it hard for you to really enjoy living. It can prevent your developing heart disease, regardless of any other risk factors you have… and just by having diabetes, you already have one strike against you. Even if you have not been diagnosed with heart disease, diabetes gives you the equivalent or greater risk of dying from a heart attack as someone without diabetes who has diagnosed heart disease. If exercising moderately can reduce your risk for dying even sooner from a heart attack because of diabetes, then you may have far more to gain from exercising than your nondiabetic friends and relatives.

Diabetes has the potential to rob you, on average, of more than 12 years of your life, not to mention that it can also dramatically reduce your quality of life for more than 20 of those lesser years. A lower quality of life can result from many physical ailments, but in people with poorly controlled diabetes, it often results from a compromised physical capacity, partial limb amputations, lesser mobility, chronic pain, blindness, and kidney dialysis, in addition to heart disease. What's the point of living longer if you aren't living well?

Maybe you've avoided exercising for years, and now you figure it's too late to start. If that's what you think, then you are just plain wrong (or maybe just misinformed)! It's never too soon to start following a healthy lifestyle, and it's never too late to start exercising. Even for people who are already middle-aged, exercising more can add years to their lives. Conversely, remaining sedentary is the most devastating thing you can do to your long-term health, longevity, and hope of avoiding or delaying the onset of chronic diseases and diabetic complications.

How Exercise Helps Improve Blood Glucose Control

Frequent, regular exercise is the key to good blood glucose control if you have any type of diabetes. The glucose-lowering effects of exercise are mainly due to a heightened sensitivity to insulin in exercised muscle, an effect that persists for no more than 1 to 2 days following the activity and that appears to be mostly related to the replenishment of stored carbohydrates (glycogen) in the muscles that you exercised. Thus in order to maximize exercise's positive effects on your blood glucose, you have to exercise regularly and use up as much glycogen as possible.

How does exercise help with blood glucose control? In the short term, any physical activity generally causes your muscle cells to take up more blood glucose, thus resulting in lower glucose during and following the activity. The only exception is really intense exercise (such as sprinting or heavy weight lifting), which can temporarily raise your blood glucose level. Following almost every type of physical activity, though, your muscle cells generally remain more sensitive to any insulin in your body (your own or injected insulin) for a period of time afterward—usually for anywhere from 30 minutes to 48 hours. This enhanced insulin action can result in your body requiring less insulin to process the foods that you eat, which in turn improves blood glucose control for most people with type 2 (or gestational) diabetes and oftentimes for type 1s and other insulin users as well. For type 1 exercisers, though, regular exercise will only improve their overall glycemic control if they also make appropriate changes to concurrently balance their insulin doses with their food intake and exercise.

It appears that exercise helps improve your blood glucose levels even if you lose little or no weight. In middle-aged men with prediabetes, an hour and a half of weekly exercise reduced their insulin resistance, whether or not they restricted their calorie intake or lost any weight. Furthermore, people with diabetes participating in studies conducted by the Pritikin Longevity Centers, who have followed diets that were

higher in fiber and complex carbohydrates and very low in refined sugar, cholesterol, fat, and salt, and engaged in 30 minutes or more of daily exercise have also experienced remarkable improvements in their diabetes control in only 3 weeks. For instance, almost 75% of people taking oral medications to control blood glucose levels were able to discontinue them, and close to 40% on insulin injec-

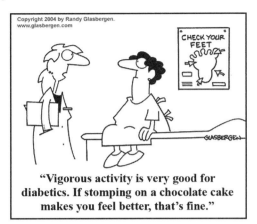

"Vigorous activity is very good for diabetics. If stomping on a chocolate cake makes you feel better, that's fine."

tions were also able to control their blood glucose levels without any extra insulin. Although modest weight loss resulted from their lifestyle changes, their post-program body fatness was far from ideal after only 3 weeks, and yet their diabetes control vastly improved.

If you have type 2 or gestational diabetes, daily or near daily activities are better for optimizing your blood glucose control and weight maintenance or loss. With type 1 diabetes, regular, predictable exercise makes your blood glucose easier to predict and manage effectively. With any type of diabetes, though, regular blood glucose monitoring will help you control your blood glucose when you participate in an exercise program, but it's easiest when your physical activity is consistent.

How to Be More Active

Luckily, becoming physically active doesn't require a daily trip to the gym or doing physical activities that you detest. It also doesn't mean that you have to be able to complete a marathon or a triathlon, although there are plenty of people with both type 1 and type 2 diabetes who do successfully complete and compete well in such events. It simply

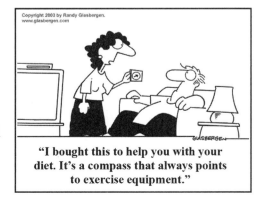

"I bought this to help you with your diet. It's a compass that always points to exercise equipment."

means that if nothing else, you will be able to go through your daily life without becoming unduly fatigued, even when doing such physical activities as walking up multiple flights of stairs, caring for your kids or playing with your grandkids, working, running errands, volunteering, or doing any other activities without resting. Remarkably, once you become more active, it is likely that you will have more energy throughout the day rather than less.

Getting started is simpler than you think. It's important that you realize that all physical activity you do during the day counts toward your daily total. Until recently, vigorous exercise was believed to be required for optimal health and fitness. While you may stand to gain more health benefits from harder workouts, we now know that almost any activity (including golfing, gardening, mowing the lawn, moderate walking, etc) done for 30 to 45 minutes per day is also beneficial to your health. Furthermore, lower-intensity exercises are beneficial even if you do them for only 10 minutes at a time. The latest research shows that we can all benefit by simply breaking up our sedentary time with any activity, even standing, from time to time. Start by standing up or walking around for 5 minutes after each hour that you spend doing something sedentary. If you do that every hour during a typical 8-hour workday, you can easily expend an extra 132 calories, lose body fat without trying, and keep your blood glucose levels under better control.

If you haven't been very active lately, you may need to see your doctor before you begin exercising more (**Table 6-1**). Medical clearance prior to relatively easy exercise (like brisk walking) is usually not necessary; however, if you plan

Table 6-1

You May Want to See Your Doctor First Before Starting Your Exercise If You...

- Are planning on participating in moderate to strenuous activities, more intense than brisk walking
- Are over 40 years old
- Are over 30 and have been diagnosed with type 1 diabetes for more than 15 years or type 2 for more than 10 years
- Know you have heart disease, a strong family history of heart disease, or high cholesterol or lipid levels
- Have poor circulation in your feet or legs (or lower-leg pain while walking)
- Have diabetic retinopathy (eye disease), nephropathy (kidney disease), or neuropathy (numbness, burning, tingling, or loss of sensation in your feet and/or dizziness when going from sitting to standing)
- Have not consistently been in good control of your blood glucose level
- Are a cigarette smoker

to do more vigorous exercise that raises your heart rate higher than you normally do, seeing your doctor beforehand is generally a good idea. The more risk factors that you have for heart disease, the greater your chance of having a cardiovascular problem during exercise, and simply knowing what you need to watch out for could be crucial to preventing more serious problems. For instance, if you have any symptoms like shortness of breath when you walk or pain in your lower legs, you may already have cardiovascular issues. It is usually still possible to exercise, but it pays to know what your safe limits are. In fact, regular moderate to vigorous activity can actually reduce your risk of a heart attack.

When it comes to being more active, if you're overweight, you may have special concerns about doing exercise routines. In particular, being overweight may make you acutely aware of your larger body size and self-conscious during certain activities or prevent you from wanting to participate at all. If you fit this profile, it is especially important for you to find activities that are enjoyable for you. For example, swimming or aquatic classes may be a viable alternative. Extra fat stored under your skin acts to insulate and keep you warmer in the pool. Also, the water serves to mostly hide your body, which may decrease any inhibition that you may feel when your figure is more plainly visible during other activities.

Your new goal is simply to be as physically active as possible to maximize your caloric expenditure and blood glucose use, and you don't necessarily have to join the nearest gym! Instead, just take the stairs instead of the elevator, park your car at the far end of the lot from where you're headed, walk in place during all the TV commercials, and then take the dog out for a walk. For motivation, you may want to invest in an inexpensive pedometer (step counter) and try to add at least 2000 steps a day (ie, the equivalent of about 1 mile) to your current activity level to start.

Other Important Physical Activities

Once you can simply start moving more throughout the day, you may feel more able to add in some other forms of more structured exercise while maintaining your new higher level of unstructured physical activity. These more-planned forms of exercise include aerobic, resistance, and flexibility training. While anyone can benefit from these activities, the strength and not just the endurance of your muscles will become more important as you age in maintaining your ability to care for yourself and to balance well enough to stay on your feet.

Structured Aerobic Exercise

The recommendation for everyone choosing to participate in more structured exercise programs is a minimum of 3 to 5 days per week of aerobic exercise (walking, jogging, cycling, swimming, rowing, etc), done for 30 minutes or more. When you begin a program of planned exercise, start out slowly, exercising a minimum of 3 days a week for 15 to 30 minutes a day, and gradually work up to doing longer daily workouts or more days per week. The federal exercise guidelines (2008) recommend engaging in moderate amounts of near daily, aerobic physical activity consisting of 30 minutes of moderate activities (like brisk walking) for 150 minutes per week or shorter sessions of more intense exercise, including jogging or playing basketball for 15 to 20 minutes at least 3 days per week (75 minutes total for each week), or a combination thereof. Running, tennis, and aerobic dance classes are examples of higher-impact forms of cardiovascular workouts, while lower-impact aerobic exercises include mild walking, swimming, cycling, tai chi, and the like. Moderate walking, though, is much more sustainable over a lifetime than many other activities, making it one of the best "medicines" for both the prevention and treatment of type 2 diabetes and for maintenance of your overall health. You can also make your workouts more taxing simply by adding faster intervals in them occasionally, like temporarily picking up your walking speed between two mailboxes or doing a hill profile on an exercise conditioning machine. Some recent research shows that the blood glucose benefits may be similar whether you exercise moderately every day for 30 minutes or engage in 60 minutes every other day (resulting in the same total exercise "dose"), but try never to let more than 2 days pass without engaging in some type of physical activity or your insulin action will start to decrease.

Ideally, your chosen activities should be ones that allow you to move your whole body over the greatest distance possible to maximize your energy expenditure, especially if your weight is a continuing issue. However, although both walking and jogging fall into this category of activities, most overweight adults will find jogging and running either too difficult or simply not enjoyable. As an alternative, you can trick yourself into walking more, simply by incorporating it into other activities—such as walking farther than you need to when you go shopping. Walking can be the gateway to more vigorous exercise (not necessarily running, though) and can further increase your overall health benefits. As a bonus, your self-confidence may improve once you start a walking program, which may lead you to start including additional physical activities in your life. You might even want to try out ballroom dancing, cycling, low-impact aerobics classes, or other forms of aerobic exercise.

Resistance Training

Strength or resistance training is imperative to maintain the amount of muscle you currently have, to gain more, and to prevent loss of muscle and strength as you age. Resistance training is just as important as—and possibly even more so than—aerobic exercise for diabetes control as well. Such training can increase your body's insulin sensitivity, along with lowering your risk for thinning bones and loss of muscle mass with aging. The current recommendation is to train 2 to 3 nonconsecutive days per week and include all the major muscle groups of your body. Some examples of strength exercises are biceps curls, triceps curls, overhead press, bench press, leg press, lunges, calf raises, and abdominal crunches.

If you are a novice at resistance work, you can start out with lighter weights, flexible resistance bands, or items that you find around the house (like water bottles or soup cans held in your hands) to complete one to two sets of 12 to 15 repetitions ("reps") on each exercise. When two to three sets of 15 reps are easy for you to do, make your workouts progressive by adding a little weight or resistance to each exercise and drop the number of reps back to 12. If all you can manage to fit into your schedule is one set once a week, don't despair—you'll still experience some strength gains!

When you have completed this elementary stage of your weight program for 6 to 8 weeks, you should be able to handle heavier weights and perform fewer reps per set. It appears far less important, however, to focus on how much weight you lift than to make sure that you are lifting any. By way of example, a study on postmenopausal women showed that both high-load (heavy weights, low reps) and high-repetition (lighter weights, more reps) resistance training were effective in increasing muscular strength and size, indicating that even easy resistance training is beneficial for older women. Likewise, muscular endurance and strength improved similarly in older adults doing only one set of twelve resistance exercises at either 50% of their one-repetition maximum (the maximal amount they could lift one time) for 13 repetitions or 80% for 8 repetitions, which they did three times weekly for 6 months.

You can choose either resistance-training regimen and have similar gains. For variety, you may even decide to have easy days where you do more reps with lighter weights and hard days when you lift heavier weights fewer times, depending on how motivated you feel. The only resistance-training principles you must follow are to work a particular area of your body (ie, upper body) no more frequently than every other day; to equally train muscles with opposite actions on a joint, such as the biceps and triceps muscles of your upper arm or the quadriceps and hamstring muscles of your thigh; and to breathe in and out smoothly while lifting (no breath holding).

Combined Aerobic and Resistance Training

Some recent studies have looked at the benefits of engaging in combined training and found that doing both is likely better for improving your overall blood glucose control than either one alone, even if you expend the same exact number of calories during combined training. If your blood glucose levels normally drop during aerobic activities, you may also lower your risk of exercise-induced hypoglycemia by doing resistance training first, followed by an aerobic workout. Similarly, if resistance training by itself tends to make your blood glucose levels rise, you can do aerobic training afterwards—or at least an aerobic cool-down—to help bring them back down.

Not enough research has looked at whether you should always do both types on the same or alternate training days, so for now feel free to add both into your weekly regimen however works best for you. Personally, I find it easiest to alternate my aerobic activities (doing different ones on successive days, but most days of the week) and adding resistance training in with my aerobic workouts 2 days a week, thereby varying my routine so that I have harder and easier days to keep my motivation higher and overuse injury risk lower.

Flexibility Training

Working on your flexibility also helps prevent injuries and is doubly important for anyone with diabetes. Everyone is becoming less flexible over time; some loss of flexibility is to be expected. However, poor diabetes control by itself can speed up this loss of flexibility by causing glucose to bind to joint structures (collagen and the like), making them more brittle and less flexible. A loss of flexibility leads to a reduced range of motion for your joints, an increased likelihood of orthopedic injuries, and a greater risk of developing some of the joint-related problems often associated with diabetes, such as diabetic "frozen shoulder," tendinitis, trigger finger, carpal tunnel syndrome, and others.

It is recommended that you work on your flexibility a minimum of 2 to 3 days per week, but I recommend engaging in some static or dynamic stretching before and/or after any exercise session or any other time that your muscles start to tighten up as well. It doesn't appear to matter when you stretch, as long as you do it, but it's usually easier to do once you've warmed up a little. Also include stretching exercises a minimum of 2 days per week to maximize strength gains and minimize the loss of flexibility caused by aging and accelerated by diabetes.

Balance Training

Just when you thought you were done, here's one more activity to add in your weekly routine: balance training. We all start losing some of our natural balance once we reach the age of 40, but having diabetes can accelerate your loss and increase your risk of falling. If you lose any of the feeling in your feet, that can alter the way you walk (your gait) and increase your risk, and having autonomic neuropathy that makes you dizzy when you stand up also raises your risk. The good news is that doing balance training can be as simple as practicing standing on one leg at a time. Resistance training that works the lower body or the core muscles improves your ability to balance while standing and walking. In addition, flexibility exercises that work the full range of motion around your joints can improve balance, as well as some alternative activities like tai chi and yoga. Even taking up dancing at any age can help you stay on your feet.

Risks and Precautions Associated With Exercise

Of course, although the benefits are immense, physical activity is not completely risk free. Both diabetes regimens and any potential complications can decrease your ability to exercise safely and optimally. To get the most out of your physical activities, it is important to know the risks and precautions and to take the steps necessary to minimize them.

Hypoglycemia

The greatest risk associated with exercise is the possibility of developing hypoglycemia, usually defined as a blood glucose level less than 65 mg/dL. As you know, insulin causes your muscles and fat cells to take up blood glucose. However, muscle contractions by themselves increase uptake of blood glucose through a separate mechanism without insulin. When you're exercising, your muscles are actually taking up glucose due both to contractions and to insulin circulating in your bloodstream.

Symptoms of hypoglycemia are varied but include shakiness, sudden fatigue, irritability, mental confusion, inability to do simple math, elevated heart rate, sweating, dizziness or light-headedness, poor physical coordination, and visual spots. If you experience hypoglycemia, treat it immediately with small amounts (5 to 10 grams) of readily absorbed carbohydrates, such as glucose tablets, hard candy, regular soft drinks (4 ounces), or sports drinks (8 ounces). Rest 5 to 10 minutes before rechecking your glucose level. Consume the same amount of carbohydrate again only if your symptoms have not begun resolving. Do not overtreat it by eating too much, though, or you'll end up battling a high blood glucose level instead.

Your training state is important in accurately predicting your glycemic response to an activity and lowering your risk of developing hypoglycemia. Becoming more trained increases the proportion of fat your body uses for similar low- or moderate-intensity activity done after training. Using a greater proportion of fat spares both your muscle glycogen and your blood glucose and allows you to more easily control your blood glucose level during physical activities. You will likely find that your blood glucose level drops less when you do the same activities after training for several weeks.

Insulin Use and Hypoglycemia Risk

If you normally take insulin (whether you have type 1 or type 2 diabetes), whatever insulin you have injected through a syringe, infused with an insulin pump, or inhaled, may raise your insulin blood level and elevate your risk of low blood glucose during or following an activity. For most people with type 2 diabetes not using insulin, this risk is minimal. For insulin users, the risk is much higher, and they will have to either eat extra carbohydrates, lower their pre-exercise insulin doses, or both to compensate and prevent lows. Generally, when no more than basal levels of insulin are circulating in your body during exercise, your physiologic response will be more normal, more like that of someone who doesn't have diabetes. If you exercise when your insulin levels are peaking or higher, however, you'll have an increased risk of hypoglycemia.

Oral Diabetic Medications and Hypoglycemia Risk

Use of certain oral diabetic medications may also increase your hypoglycemic risk associated with exercise. Some of the sulfonylureas increase your risk of developing hypoglycemia. For instance, Diabinese (chlorpropamide) and Orinase (tolbutamide) cause insulin release from the pancreas and somewhat decrease insulin resistance, but typically have a longer duration (up to 72 hours) and, therefore, can potentially cause your glucose levels to go too low during and/or following exercise. Amaryl (glimepiride), DiaBeta (glyburide), Micronase (glyburide), and Glucotrol (glipizide) generally don't last as long and carry a smaller risk; of these, DiaBeta and Micronase carry the greatest risk due to their slightly longer duration (24 hours versus only 12 to 16 hours for the others). You will have to frequently monitor your glucose when exercising if you take any of the sulfonylureas that stay in your system longer and, when your exercise becomes regular enough, you may need to check with your doctor about lowering your doses of these medications if you are frequently experiencing hypoglycemia during or following exercise.

Other medications usually have less of an effect on exercise. Insulin sensitizers, such as Avandia (rosiglitazone) and Actos (pioglitazone) mainly affect the action of insulin at rest, so the risk of these medications causing exercise hypoglycemia is almost nonexistent. Similarly, Glucophage (metformin) is unlikely to cause exercise lows. Prandin (repaglinide) or Starlix (nateglinide) only potentially increase your risk of a low blood glucose level if taken immediately before prolonged exercise as they increase insulin levels only temporarily when taken with meals. Medications that slow down the absorption of carbohydrates (Precose [acarbose] and Glyset [miglitol]) would not directly affect your exercise blood glucose, but could slightly delay your treatment of low blood glucose, as could either of the newer injectable medications, Symlin (pramlintide) and Byetta (exenatide). Finally, the newest medications that mimic bodily peptides (ie, incretin mimetics) or increase concentrations of peptides that prevent degradation of natural insulin-stimulating enzymes may keep insulin circulating in your blood longer and slow how quickly you digest your food, but are unlikely to cause exercise-related hypoglycemia. Byetta and Bydureon (exenatide) are two such medications, along with Victoza (liraglutide) and others. If you plan on exercising, it would behoove you to not take any of these latter medications within 2 hours of when you are going to start being active, just in case you need to treat a low blood glucose.

Hyperglycemia

Technically, any blood glucose level in excess of 125 mg/dL qualifies as hyperglycemia, but your exercise responses will likely be normal up until your glucose level is twice as high or higher, or above 250 mg/dL. Although very uncommon in type 2 diabetes, ketosis (ie, acidosis detected by ketones in the bloodstream and urine) may develop in people with limited or no insulin production. If it does, you should not exercise until you get rid of the ketones as they indicate that your body is insulin deficient, which will likely cause your blood glucose level to rise even more if you exercise. If you're somewhat hyperglycemic right after eating and you took an insulin injection (maybe just not a high enough dose), though, your blood glucose will likely still decrease during extended exercise because enough insulin will be in your body during the activity. Use caution when exercising with blood glucose levels over 300 mg/dL without ketones.

Dehydration

If you're exercising with any elevation in your blood glucose level, take care to drink enough water as it will be easier for you to become dehydrated. Elevated glucose can increase your water loss through excessive urination, and your risk of losing extra fluids is greater with poorly controlled diabetes. Exercising itself compounds the risk by increasing sweating (thus loss of water), which can rapidly compound a dehydrated state. Since exercising during hot weather can be especially dangerous for older individuals who may not release heat as effectively as younger adults, adequate fluid replacement and frequent rest are needed. Being better trained and fitter also makes you less likely to overheat during activities.

Interestingly, despite the emphasis on proper hydration, it appears that you're more likely to harm yourself with excessive fluid intake than with dehydration during exercise. If you drink too much of anything during exercise, you increase your risk of diluting the sodium content of your blood, potentially causing a medical condition known as water intoxication and putting you at risk for seizures, coma, and even death. While adequate hydration prior to exercise with fluids consumed early (17 ounces of fluid taken 2 hours before exercise) is recommended, in order to avoid overhydrating, it is more prudent to start drinking only when you actually feel thirsty. The only exception is in people with poorly controlled diabetes, since they may have an elevated thirst threshold (meaning that they don't feel thirsty as quickly, even when dehydrated). If that applies to you, start drinking small amounts of water as soon as you start sweating.

Orthopedic Injuries and Arthritis

Simply by having diabetes, you already have a high risk of both joint-related injuries and overuse problems like tendinitis. You may, therefore, find that adopting a more moderate exercise like walking rather than a more vigorous one like running makes more sense since you'll have less potential for joint trauma with the former type of exercise. The best defense is to prevent all of these injuries with good diabetes control, flexibility exercises that help emphasize and maintain a full range of motion around your joints, and moderate amounts of exercise training.

Arthritis is also more common in people with type 2 diabetes due to the extra body weight most of them are carrying around. Lower extremity joints (the hip, knee, and ankle) are most often affected, and, when present, osteoarthritis can severely limit your ability to exercise. However, exercise is an effective means of managing arthritis, even the more severe rheumatoid type. Get started with some basic range-of-motion exercises to increase your joint mobility, and then move on to specific resistance work. If you have arthritic knees or hips, walking may be uncomfortable or painful. Your best option is to try non–weight-bearing activities, such as walking in a pool (with or without a flotation belt around your waist), aqua aerobics, lap swimming, recumbent stationary cycling, upper-body exercises, seated aerobic workouts, chair dancing, and resistance training activities.

Exercising With Diabetic Complications

Finally, there are some exercise risks that may arise if you have certain diabetes-related complications. If you have had diabetes for a number of years, it is likely that you may develop some complications, particularly if your blood glucose control is less than optimal. You can still exercise (and you should!), but you will have to take any health problems into account to exercise as safely and effectively as possible.

Peripheral Neuropathy and Peripheral Artery Disease

If you have lost some of the feeling in your feet due to nerve damage (neuropathy), as long as you do not have any unhealed ulcers on the bottom of your feet, you can participate safely in most activities. If you're having problems with blisters or irritation with walking or other weight-bearing activities, you can always consider switching to ones like swimming or stationary cycling to minimize potential trauma to your feet. If you experience pain in your lower legs when moving around, a symptom of peripheral artery disease, walking may actually be good for you. A recent study showed that people may actually experience symptom relief and lesser decline in their ability to walk when they participate in walking at least 3 days a week, either in a supervised exercise program or on their own. In either case, to protect your feet, choose athletic shoes with silica gel or air midsoles (the middle section of the shoe that provides the most stability and shock absorption), as well as polyester or cotton-polyester socks to prevent the formation of blisters and to keep your feet dry during physical activities. You or someone else (if you are not able to) should check your feet daily for signs of trauma and treat them aggressively. Use a mirror to see the bottom of your feet if it is hard for you to check them otherwise.

Autonomic Neuropathy

If you have damage to your central nervous system known as autonomic neuropathy, this complication may make it harder for you to change your body position without experiencing light-headedness or fainting. You're also more likely to overheat and become dehydrated. If it affects your ability to digest food quickly (known as gastroparesis), any carbohydrate you eat may be more slowly absorbed, and hypoglycemia during exercise can become more severe as a result. It may cause an elevated heart rate at rest, but a lower heart rate than normal during exercise. Thus avoid making rapid changes in movement that may result in fainting and spend more time warming up and cooling down. Drink extra fluids, avoid being continuously active for long periods during hotter weather, and eat only smaller meals and snacks before exercise. Last, monitor your exercise by some means other than your heart rate alone (such as your perceived exertion, or how hard you feel like you're working out).

Diabetic Eye Disease

While exercise itself has not been shown to accelerate proliferative diabetic eye disease (retinopathy), certain precautions may be needed to prevent intraocular hemorrhages or retinal tears. If your eye disease is only mild or moderate with no active bleeds, you should simply avoid activities that dramatically increase the blood pressure inside your eyes, such as heavy weight lifting or activities during which your head is lower than your heart. If your retinopathy is moderate to severe, avoid all jumping, jarring, or breath-holding activities as they increase the pressure inside your eyes and can cause more bleeding and increase your risk of blindness, retinal tears, or retinal detachment. If you have an active retinal hemorrhage or notice sudden, dramatic changes in your sight, stop any activity you are doing immediately and check with your ophthalmologist before resuming your exercise.

Kidney Disease

Intense or prolonged exercise would not usually be recommended for you if you have severe kidney disease, but only because your exercise capacity is likely to be limited. Light to moderate exercise is fine, and even patients requiring dialysis can exercise during treatment sessions with no ill effects. If you are undergoing dialysis, exercise would only be advised against if the levels of certain substances in your blood (hematocrit, calcium, or potassium) become unbalanced as a result of the treatments.

Cardiovascular Disease

If you have diagnosed heart disease, you can still participate in most forms of exercise. In fact, resistance training is now recommended for everyone (in addition to aerobic activities), even for people who have had a heart attack or stroke. Be aware that a heart attack can potentially have symptoms other than pain localized in your chest, such as pain that radiates down one arm or shoulder or your neck or that feels like bad heartburn. If you experience any unusual pain or other symptoms during or following exercise, get checked out by your doctor as soon as possible. Diabetes can also potentially cause you to experience silent ischemia, a reduction in blood flow to the heart muscle through the coronary blood vessels that is painless and symptom free. If you ever experience a sudden, unexplained change in your ability to exercise, without any other symptoms, immediately stop exercising and consult your physician as soon as you can to rule out silent ischemia.

When in doubt, follow the exercise guidelines published by the American Diabetes Association with regard to exercising with diabetic complications (**Table 6**-**2**). Always include proper warm-up and cool-down periods (3 to 5 minutes of a lower intensity activity before and after your planned exercise session) to ease the cardiovascular transition and minimize your risks.

Special Exercise Concerns for Insulin Users

Once you learn how your body responds to different types of exercise and what type of regimen changes you need (particularly if you take insulin), you can effectively control your blood glucose. Many insulin users (with both type 1 and type 2 diabetes) employ a combination of short- or rapid- and long-acting insulins (varying by time to peak action and total duration) given 1 to 4 (or more) times daily. Others receive a continuous infusion of insulin through an insulin pump, which deliv-

Table 6-2

Precautions for Exercising With Diabetes and/or Its Complications

- Have a blood glucose meter accessible to check your glucose level before, possibly during, and/or after exercise, or if you have any symptoms of low blood glucose
- Immediately treat any hypoglycemia during or following exercise with quickly absorbed carbohydrates like glucose tablets, dextrose-based candy, or regular soft drinks
- Inform your exercise partners about your diabetes, and show them how to give you glucose or another carbohydrate should you need assistance
- Stay properly hydrated with frequent intake of small amounts of cool water
- Consult with your physician prior to exercising with any of the following conditions:
  - Proliferative retinopathy or current retinal hemorrhage (diabetic eye diseases)
  - Neuropathy (nerve damage), either peripheral or autonomic
  - Foot injuries (including ulcers)
  - High blood pressure
  - Serious illness or infection
- Seek immediate medical attention for chest pain or any pain that radiates down your arm, jaw, or neck and for serious indigestion, any of which may indicate a lack of blood to your heart and a possible heart attack
- If you have high blood pressure, avoid activities that cause it to go up dramatically, such as heavy weight training, head-down exercises, and anything requiring breathholding
- Wear proper footwear, and check your feet daily for signs of trauma, such as blisters, redness, or other irritation
- Immediately stop exercising if you experience bleeding into your eyes caused by unstable proliferative retinopathy
- Wear a diabetes Medic Alert bracelet or necklace with your physician's name and contact information on it

ers self-programmed basal amounts of insulin and boluses for food via a subcutaneous catheter. The insulin regimen that you use, along with the type, duration, intensity, and timing of exercise you choose to do, will determine what changes you will need to maintain control over your blood glucose.

When only minimal levels of insulin are circulating during exercise, your body's metabolic responses will be closer to normal. If you choose to exercise during peak times of injected insulin, however, you will experience an increased risk for hypoglycemia unless you cut back your insulin doses, eat extra carbohydrates, or do a combination of both. The more common basal insulins used now, Lantus (glargine) and Levemir (detemir), are designed to last 12 to 24 hours and provide only basal insulin coverage, making a separate dose of rapid-acting insulin (such as Humalog [lispro], Novolog [aspart], or Apidra [glulisine]) needed to provide enough insulin for meals and snacks. If you give some rapid-acting insulin and exercise within 1 to 2 hours, you are much more likely to experience low blood glucose compared with a Lantus or Levemir user with no insulin peaks. Alternately, if you use an insulin pump, you can lower your risk of lows by either disconnecting your pump or reducing your programmed basal rates before, during, and/or after physical activity.

A multitude of other variables affecting insulin action can confound your glycemic response to exercise as well. For instance, prebreakfast exercise is less likely to make your blood glucose level drop than the same activity done later in the day (even just after breakfast) because in the morning before you eat, your body has higher levels of hormones (eg, cortisol) that make you more insulin resistant. Thus early-morning exercise usually requires fewer changes in your diabetic regimen. Exercising in the late evening can cause you to develop hypoglycemia during your sleep, but it still can be done safely if you take the proper precautions (eg, eating a bedtime snack and/or lowering bedtime insulin dose).

Moreover, your glucose response can be altered by the type, intensity, and duration of the activity; your starting blood glucose level, when you last ate or took any insulin (and how much), whether the activity is a new or unusual one, if you exercised recently, and many more factors that experience and trial and error can help you figure out. Keep in mind that during higher-intensity, prolonged activities such as moderate-paced running (or faster), carbohydrate is almost exclusively your muscles' fuel of choice, and depletion of both muscle glycogen and blood glucose is inevitable if you exercise at that level for long. For shorter-duration and more-intense activities, carbohydrate supplementation alone can work effectively for glycemic control, but for more prolonged exercise sessions, you will likely need to reduce your insulin doses as well.

If you consume some carbohydrate or even a balance of carbohydrate, protein, and fat within 30 minutes after exhaustive exercise, your muscles will restore their muscle glycogen more rapidly, and you will be less likely to experience late-onset hypoglycemia that can occur up to 24 hours after exercise. Your insulin sensitivity is generally heightened immediately after a workout, and during that time, you don't need much insulin to take up glucose into your muscles for glycogen replacement. Good blood glucose control during this period is essential, though, for optimal glycogen replacement.

To learn your body's unique response to different exercise situations, you will need to go through some trial and error to find the best way to handle your diabetes for each one, and you will need to test your blood glucose level more frequently until you can establish a glycemic pattern. Even becoming more trained doing each unique activity will change your body's use of blood glucose and likely result in smaller drops in your glucose than before you trained. For additional exercise guidelines and regimen-change advice, please consult my book, *Diabetic Athlete's Handbook: Your Guide to Peak Performance* (Human Kinetics Publishers, 2009). It covers diabetes regimen changes and gives real-life athlete examples for more than 100 recreational physical activities and sports.

Maintaining Exercise for Life

The inspiration to make a change in your daily routine can come in many forms. If motivation is your biggest problem, make a game out of trying to count your daily steps. Even instructing sedentary, overweight women to walk 10,000 steps per day (monitored by a pedometer, or step counter) is more effective in increasing their daily exercise than asking them to walk 30 minutes on most days of the week. If nothing else, keeping track of your steps should at least help you become more conscious of how active you are (or aren't) and remind you to add in more steps and movement whenever and wherever you can.

Many people also complain all of the time about being too tired to exercise. What you may not realize, though, is that your lack of exercise is probably most responsible for making you feel tired. Even normally active individuals who take a few weeks off from their usual activities begin to feel more sluggish, lethargic, and unmotivated to exercise. The best thing to do is to start moving more, and you will likely begin to feel more energized and motivated to continue exercising.

If you still need more motivation to keep going, try any of the following: Put your more structured activities down on your calendar, keep track of your progress (using online tracking tools if that is motivating for you); reward yourself for meeting your goals; recruit an exercise buddy or two to join in the fun; find ways to distract yourself during workouts to make the time pass more quickly; and keep your physical activities convenient, enjoyable, and varied to prevent excuses to avoid doing it. More importantly, don't start out working too hard, or you will likely either decide to quit or injure yourself. If you do fall off the exercise wagon, get back on it as soon as you can, but start back slowly.

Conclusions

Undoubtedly, exercise conveys certain risks and challenges for diabetic individuals, such as the risk of exercise-induced hypoglycemia. However, physical activity is an integral part of taking control of your diabetes, whether you're a beginning exerciser or an elite athlete. Anyone with diabetes can follow some basic exercise strategies to best control blood glucose levels and to exercise safely and effectively. Just keep in mind that you do not have to be an exercise fanatic to reap the benefits of increased physical activity. Adding just a little activity to your daily routine can have major health benefits. Experts suggest that even 15 to 30 minutes of walking each day is probably enough to gain substantial health benefits. Get up and get moving in every way that you can every day, even if that just includes standing more and taking more daily steps. If you're already a regular exerciser, then you are likely reaping maximal health benefits from your activities and should continue to do so by staying active.

For more information on getting and staying more physically active and living well with diabetes, please read *The 7 Step Diabetes Fitness Plan: Living Well and Being Fit with Diabetes, No Matter Your Weight* (Marlowe & Company, 2005). If you're already an exercise enthusiast, and particularly if you are an insulin user, consult *Diabetic Athlete's Handbook: Your Guide to Peak Performance* (Human Kinetics, 2009) for regimen changes and real athlete examples for over 100 sports and recreational physical activities. For additional inspiration about living long and well with diabetes—and how physical activity plays a key role—check out our book, *50 Secrets of the Longest Living People With Diabetes* (Marlowe & Company, 2007) by myself and Dr. Edelman. Most of all, just get up and get moving to secure your good health for the rest of your life.

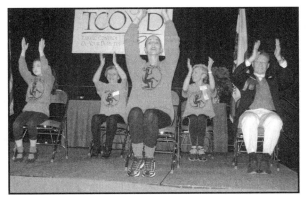

Chair dancing led by Jody Stolove.

7

Glucose-Lowering Medications for Type 2 Diabetes

Oral Agents and the Incretins

Introduction

Prior to 1995, there was only one type of oral medication for people with type 2 diabetes: the sulfonylureas (SFUs). This meant that people with type 2 diabetes had the option of either SFUs or insulin, or both, to control their blood glucose levels. Sulfonylureas lose their effectiveness over time, and since no one likes to take injections and it was easier for the caregivers to prescribe pills instead of an insulin regimen, many people with type 2 diabetes lived with poor glucose control for many years. Commonly, it was only when the blood glucose level became extremely high, into the 300- to 400-mg/dL range, that insulin therapy was initiated to finally bring down the toxic and harming glucose levels. With the advent of multiple new oral medications, this situation is improving. The progress has been painstakingly slow because some caregivers do not know about the advances made in this area, and much of the public is ignorant as well, which is why patient education and self-advocacy are so important. The bottom line is that if you have type 2 diabetes, you need to know what new therapeutic advances have been made and are available right now. If you think that any of the medications you read about in this chapter may be good for you, please discuss it with your caregiver.

We now have lots of choices! Since 1994, several new types of oral medications for people with type 2 diabetes are available, with many more under development. These oral agents can be given together and/or with insulin to more effectively control the glucose level throughout the day. Since many of these oral agents have not been on the market for an extended period of time, it is of utmost importance that you become knowledgeable about all of them, and determine if one or more of them would be helpful to you. Oral diabetes medications are generally not intended for people with type 1 diabetes or for women who are pregnant and/or are breastfeeding.

Oral Agents for Type 2 Diabetes

There are now eight major classes or types of oral medications for people with type 2 diabetes:

1. Sulfonylureas (insulin secretagogues)—stimulate pancreatic insulin production
2. Nonsulfonylurea insulin secretagogues—same as SFUs, but have a different chemical structure
3. Biguanides—inhibit the excess glucose production by the liver
4. Carbohydrate absorption inhibitors—retard carbohydrate absorption in the intestine
5. Insulin sensitizers (chemical name: thiazolidinediones)—increase the body's sensitivity to insulin action
6. DPP-4 inhibitors or incretin enhancers—enhance action of incretins (explained in detail later in this chapter)
7. Bile acid sequestrants (mechanism of action is not known, but they originally were developed as a lipid-lowering medication)
8. Dopamine receptor agonists (restore the dopaminergic activity, which is important for the glucose and lipid levels).

As you will learn, these eight types of diabetes medications work in different ways and many can be used in combination with each other to attain desirable glycemic control. In fact, many of them now come together in combination pills.

Sulfonylureas (Insulin Secretagogues)

Sulfonylureas, or SFUs, have been around for a long time. For decades, these were the only oral medications available for people with type 2 diabetes. They were the workhorses of the 70s, 80s, and early 90s. There are many different SFUs on the market today, and they all work primarily by stimulating the pancreas to secrete more insulin. As discussed in *Chapter 2*, type 2 diabetes is a condition in which the insulin secreted from the pancreas does not work well (insulin resistance) and/or there is not enough (relative insulin deficiency). Even though the tissues of the body are resistant to the glucose-lowering effects of insulin, if the insulin level becomes high enough in the blood from taking SFUs, the glucose levels will eventually start to fall. The various SFUs on the market are listed in **Table 7-1**, along with the recommended dosage range, including how often they should be taken per day (depending on the duration of action). The only SFU that requires extra caution, especially if you are elderly, is Diabinese (chlorpropamide), because it tends to stay in your system for up to 3 days even

Table 7-1

Prescribing Information for Sulfonylureas

Generic Name	Trade Name	Daily Dose Range (mg)	Recommended Frequency
Older Sulfonylureas			
Acetohexamide	Dymelor	250 to 3000	Twice
Chlorpropamide	Diabinese	100 to 800	Once or twice
Tolazamide	Tolinase	100 to 1000	Once or twice
Tolbutamide	Orinase	500 to 3000	Once to three times
Newer Sulfonylureas			
Glipizide	Glucotrol	2.5 to 40	Once or twice
Glipizide (extended release)	Glucotrol XL	5 to 20	Once
Glyburide	DiaBeta	1.25 to 20	Once or twice
	Glynase PresTab	0.75 to 12	Once or twice
	Micronase	1.25 to 20	Once or twice
Glimepiride	Amaryl	1 to 8	Once

after it is discontinued. If you become ill and cannot eat, you will have the tendency to have low blood glucose for a prolonged period of time despite stopping the medication.

The SFUs are effective in bringing down the blood glucose values and are generally well tolerated by people with diabetes. However, they do have some shortfalls (**Table 7-2**). One of the main problems with the SFUs is that they lose effectiveness over time, on average after about 5 years of use; however, the response is different from individual to individual. The results of the ADOPT (A Diabetes Outcome Progression Trial) published in 2007 clearly demonstrate that SFUs fail to maintain con-

Table 7-2

Benefits and Shortfalls of Sulfonylureas

Benefits

- Effective at quickly lowering the blood glucose levels (at least initially)
- Well tolerated by people with diabetes (few side effects)

Disadvantages

- Lose effectiveness over time, requiring combination therapy with other pills, incretins, and/or insulin
- Weight gain (normally just a few pounds) after the sulfonylurea is initiated
- Hypoglycemia, especially with strenuous exercise or a missed meal(s)

trol over time compared with other oral medications such as metformin and rosiglitazone (**Figure 7-1**). Some researchers believe it is because the SFUs work by continuing to make the pancreas work overtime, eventually leading to exhaustion and reduced insulin secretion capacity over time. If the pancreas is exhausted, it cannot put out any more insulin, and you will not be responsive to SFUs anymore. Thus blood glucose goes out of control. When a person's blood glucose value starts rising while being treated with an SFU, it is usually necessary to add another oral medication or initiate an incretin agent or insulin therapy to get the diabetes under control.

Figure 7-1
ADOPT: First to Fail Study

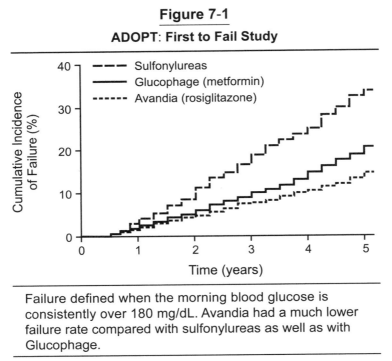

Failure defined when the morning blood glucose is consistently over 180 mg/dL. Avandia had a much lower failure rate compared with sulfonylureas as well as with Glucophage.

DREAM Investigators. *Lancet.* 2006;368:1096-1105.

A second shortfall is that SFUs commonly cause 5 to 10 pounds of weight gain, most likely because of the way they work. When insulin levels go up, either due to insulin secretagogues or insulin injections, the body weight also has a tendency to go up.

A third shortfall is that SFUs can cause low blood glucose (hypoglycemia), especially after strenuous exercise, if you miss a meal, or if you lose weight. It must be remembered that hypoglycemia is not a severe problem in the majority of cases and is normally recognized early and easily treated. If you are a person whose diabetes has been recently diagnosed (less than a few years ago) or if you have near normal blood glucose levels, you might be at a higher risk for hypoglycemia on SFUs than someone who has had diabetes much longer with poor control.

Hypoglycemia is discussed in *Chapter 3* and *Chapter 13*; however, the main symptoms of hypoglycemia are shaking, sweating, palpitations (feeling your heart beating over your chest area), and confusion. If you think your blood glucose is getting too low, you should drink or eat something sweet, such as 4 to 8 ounces of fruit juice, regular soda, four to six Lifesavers, or one of the many forms of glucose tablets that are sold over the counter in pharmacies. You should always carry something sweet, such as a pocket-sized container of glucose tablets, and keep similar items in your car, place of work, and/or school. It may also be important to tell your family members and coworkers about helping you (if necessary) during a low blood glucose episode.

Try to test your blood glucose level before treating yourself with sugar to make sure that your symptoms are in fact due to hypoglycemia. This helps you and your caregiver to properly adjust your medication. You should call your doctor if you have low blood glucose reactions frequently, especially if it happens without a ready explanation, such as a missed meal or strenuous activity.

Nonsulfonylurea Insulin Secretagogues

Prandin (repaglinide) and Starlix (nateglinide) work in a fashion similar to the SFUs; namely, by stimulating the pancreas to secrete more insulin. The difference is that they work faster than SFUs and are taken before each meal. Prandin and Starlix have a completely different chemical structure than the SFUs and have been described as non-SFU insulin secretagogues. The word secretagogue is used because it explains how the SFUs, Prandin, and Starlix work by stimulating the pancreas to secrete insulin. Since Prandin and Starlix cause rapid bursts of insulin secretion when taken, it may be helpful to people with irregular eating habits (take it only when you eat). Because both Prandin and Starlix cause an elevation of the insulin levels, they can cause hypoglycemia and weight gain in a similar fashion as the SFUs. These side effects are minimized by the fact that the effect of stimulating insulin secretion wears off quickly after the meal. This rapid-on and rapid-off action results in better blood glucose levels after eating and less delayed hypoglycemia or low blood sugar several hours after your meal or during exercise. In general, Prandin and Starlix should not be used with other SFUs, but they can be used safely with other oral agents. See **Table 7-3** for dosing information.

Table 7-3
Prescribing Information for Nonsulfonylurea Insulin Secretagogues

Generic Name	Trade Name	Daily Dose Range (mg)	Recommended Frequency
Nateglinide	Starlix	120 to 360	Two to four times a day with each meal
Repaglinide	Prandin	0.5 to 16	Two to four times a day with each meal

Biguanides

Glucophage (metformin) has been available in the United States since 1994 and is the only biguanide on the US market. However, Glucophage has been used around the world for over 32 years. Glucophage is now recommended as the first drug of choice for people with newly diagnosed type 2 diabetes unless there is a contraindication to it. In fact, it is also recommended to be started immediately upon diagnosis along with lifestyle modification.

Glucophage is an effective medication that works mainly by preventing the liver from producing too much glucose. In the normal nondiabetic state, one of the important jobs of the liver is to produce just enough glucose to keep the body functioning normally. However, in people with diabetes, the liver inappropriately overproduces glucose, mainly at night. This overproduction of glucose at night leads to elevated blood glucose levels, especially in the morning. This is one reason Glucophage especially improves the fasting or prebreakfast blood glucose value as well as at other times. Glucophage is now available in an extended-release formula (Glucophage XR) and in combination with other oral medications (see *Combination Oral Medications for Type 2 Diabetes* later in this chapter). Both the extended-release and combination pills make your daily medication regimen a little easier and simpler (**Table 7-4**).

The benefits and shortfalls of Glucophage are listed in **Table 7-5**. Glucophage is effective in lowering glucose values and has made a major impact in this country as the first new oral drug for diabetes to become available in over 40 years after the introduction of the SFUs in the 1950s. Glucophage does not stimulate the pancreas to secrete insulin, and this explains why there is no weight gain or problems with hypoglycemia. Weight gain and hypoglycemia are observed with SFUs, Prandin, Starlix, and insulin. In addition, Glucophage may also improve your cholesterol and triglyceride levels as well as other cardiovascular

Table 7-4

Prescribing Information for Biguanides

Generic Name	Trade Name	Daily Dose Range (mg)	Recommended Frequency
Metformin	Fortamet	500 to 2500	Once
	Glucophage	1000 to 2550	Twice to three times
	Glucophage XR	500 to 2000	Once
	Glumetza	1000 to 2000	Once

risk factors, which is an important advantage since heart disease is such a big problem in people with type 2 diabetes. Glucophage has recently been shown to reduce certain types of cancer, including breast.

Shortfalls of Biguanides

Glucophage is generally well accepted by patients, although it may cause mild stomach upset or loose stools when initiating therapy. If any symptoms occur, they usually do so in the first few weeks after starting the medication. In order to avoid stomach problems, I recommend starting with the lowest dose 500 mg (1 tablet) with dinner for 1 week. If no problems are present after the first week, you may increase the dose to 500 mg 2 times a day

Table 7-5

Benefits and Shortfalls of Biguanides

Benefits

- Effective in lowering glucose levels
- Does not cause weight gain
- Does not cause hypoglycemia or low blood glucose
- Improves cholesterol levels

Shortfalls

- May cause stomach upset (loose stools or diarrhea), especially when starting therapy
- Must be cautious if kidney disease is present
- Must temporarily stop treatment with Glucophage if you become seriously ill or require an x-ray study using dye (*see text*)

with breakfast and dinner, only with the advice of your caregiver. Your health care provider will adjust your dose further according to the level of improvement seen in your blood glucose values.

Glucophage generally is a safe medication. However, it is important to have your kidney function tested before you begin taking Glucophage in order to avoid an uncommon but serious and potentially fatal problem called lactic acidosis. Testing your kidneys involves a nonfasting blood test called the serum creatinine, which must be 1.5 mg/dL or lower in men and 1.4 mg/dL or lower in women in order to take

Glucophage safely. If you are older than 80 years or if your serum creatinine is borderline high, it is recommended that you perform a urine collection so that your doctor can get a more sensitive measurement of your kidney function, called the creatinine clearance or GFR (glomerular filtration rate). Creatinine is a substance that comes from muscle; levels of creatinine increase in the blood and filter into the urine in excess when kidney disease is present. If your kidney function is borderline, you should have repeat kidney tests at least every 6 to 12 months while being treated with Glucophage. I would also encourage you to track and keep good records of your kidney function. It is important to understand that metformin or Glucophage is not harmful in any way to your kidneys. However, metformin is cleared from the body by the kidney and if the kidneys are not working well, the levels of metformin in your blood can elevate and cause lactic acidosis.

It is also important to remind your doctor(s) that you are taking Glucophage if you become severely ill at home, are hospitalized, or if you are going to have a radiographic (x-ray) test for which you will be receiving a dye (colored fluid). Glucophage should be temporarily halted in these situations and restarted when the acute illness or test is over and normal kidney function resumes.

Carbohydrate Absorption Inhibitors

Precose (acarbose) and Glyset (miglitol) are the two drugs in this class currently available in the United States (**Table 7-6**). They work mainly by delaying the absorption of carbohydrates after meals, thus blunting the rapid rise in blood glucose that is usually observed after eating. In a similar fashion to Starlix and Prandin, Precose and Glyset are postprandial drugs (prandial = meal). Postmeal hyperglycemia contributes to the absolute level of the glycosylated hemoglobin (or A1C) value and, over the long term, the prevalence of diabetic complications.

Precose and Glyset are safe medications that one may take with no concerns about kidney or liver disease. Precose and Glyset do not stimulate the pancreas to secrete insulin, so there is no weight gain and

Table 7-6

Prescribing Information for Carbohydrate Absorption Inhibitors

Generic Name	Trade Name	Daily Dose Range (mg)	Recommended Frequency
Acarbose	Precose	50 to 300	First bite of each meal
Miglitol	Glyset	50 to 150	First bite of each meal

no problems with hypoglycemia. Their benefits and shortfalls are listed in **Table 7-7**.

Shortfalls of Carbohydrate Absorption Inhibitors

Precose and Glyset may cause excess gas (flatulence) or mild stomach upset. These side effects tend to occur when you first begin therapy. The side effects can be minimized by starting with a low dose and increasing the dose very slowly ("start low, go slow, and no blow"). Instructions for initiating therapy with Precose and Glyset are listed in **Table 7-8**.

Insulin Sensitizers (Thiazolidinediones)

Insulin sensitizers (Avandia [rosiglitazone] and Actos [pioglitazone]) represent an important class of oral medications for the treatment of type 2 diabetes. They are also called TZDs, which is short for... are you ready for this... thiazolidinediones (thia-zo-la-deen-dions)! It took me 2 years to get the pronunciation of this word correct. The United States was the first country to approve the first TZD, Rezulin (troglitazone), in 1996; however, it was removed from the market due to a low incidence of severe liver damage. TZDs, or insulin sensitizers, work mainly by reducing insulin resistance. One of the earliest and main defects observed in type 2 diabetes is insulin resistance. Basically, the problem is that the body is resistant to the normal glucose-lowering effects of insulin. The end result is that the blood glucose rises because the insulin cannot do its job of getting the glucose out of the bloodstream and into the cells of the body for energy. TZDs allow the insulin that is present in the body, either secreted by the pancreas or injected by a needle, to work more effectively to lower the blood glucose levels. Avandia (rosiglitazone) and Actos (pioglitzone) are the two available insulin sensitizers. Rosiglitazone is not being actively used or marketed because of suggestions that it may cause heart disease; however, no de-

Table 7-7

Benefits and Shortfalls of Carbohydrate Absorption Inhibitors

Benefits

- Very safe medications
- Do not cause weight gain
- Do not cause hypoglycemia or low blood glucose
- Can be used with all other oral agents and/or insulin currently available

Shortfalls

- May not lower glucose levels and glycosylated hemoglobin (or A1C) as much as other medications
- May cause stomach upset and/or gas, especially when starting the drug; must titrate the dose slowly (start with a small dose and slowly increase it over time)

Table 7-8

Instructions on How to Start Precose or Glyset: Start Low and Go Slow![a,b]

Step 1:	Start with 25 mg at breakfast only for 1 to 2 weeks
Step 2:	Take 25 mg with breakfast and dinner for 1 to 2 weeks
Step 3:	Take 25 mg with breakfast, lunch, and dinner for 1 to 2 weeks
Step 4:	Take 50 mg with breakfast and 25 mg with lunch and dinner for 1 to 2 weeks
Step 5:	Take 50 mg with breakfast and dinner and 25 mg with lunch for 1 to 2 weeks
Step 6:	Take 50 mg with breakfast, lunch, and dinner

[a] Do not increase the dose further unless you have discussed this with your caregiver. If, at any step, you have bothersome gas or stomach pain, do not go to the next step; stay at the current step or revert to a previous step until your symptoms improve. Then continue with the steps as listed. Last, it is extremely important to take Precose and Glyset at the beginning of your meal(s). They will not work to lower your blood glucose if you take them more than 10 minutes before you eat. The maximum dosage of Precose is 100 mg 3 times a day, which is equivalent in efficacy or effectiveness to Glyset 50 mg 3 times a day.

[b] Take Precose and Glyset with the first bite of each meal.

finitive information shows that it does. The TZDs have been around for about 10 years and are available worldwide.

Actos is easy to take because it may be taken only once a day at any time that is convenient (**Table 7-9**). In addition, TZDs are well tolerated with few side effects. In a similar fashion to Glucophage, Glyset, and Precose, TZDs do not stimulate the pancreas; therefore, hypoglycemia is not a problem and there is better long-term effectiveness by resting the pancreas compared with the SFUs and Glucophage (see previous discussion on the ADOPT and **Figure 7-1**). TZDs have also been shown to improve abnormal cholesterol and triglyceride levels

Table 7-9

Prescribing Information for Insulin Sensitizers (Thiazolidinediones)

Generic Name	Trade Name	Daily Dosage Range (mg/day)	Recommended Frequency
Pioglitazone	Actos	15 to 45	Once a day
Rosiglitazone	Avandia	2 to 8	Once a day

and blood pressure. TZDs have additional effects that may help keep the heart and cardiovascular system healthy (such as reducing inflammation and the tendency of the blood to be too thick), thus reducing the risk of blood clots. The benefits and shortfalls of Actos are listed in **Table 7-10**.

Shortfalls of the Insulin Sensitizers

The TZDs in general are very safe and well-tolerated medications. Actos (pioglitazone) is the only TZD currently being used in the United States. Avandia (rosiglitazone) is not being used because of the concern that it may cause heart disease. Although this side effect has never been proven, the FDA has taken the cautious side and limited its use. Most people who were taking Avandia have been switched to Actos.

The most common side effects of the TZDs are fluid retention, commonly presenting as edema or swelling of your ankles, and weight gain. The vast majority of people who take Actos do perfectly fine with no problems whatsoever; however, a small percentage (4% to 8%) will have some fluid retention. For some, the ankle edema is very mild and the benefits of improved glucose con-

Table 7-10

Benefits and Shortfalls of Insulin Sensitizers (Thiazolidinediones)

Benefits

- Easy to take (only once a day) at any time that is convenient
- Well tolerated by people with diabetes
- Do not cause hypoglycemia or low blood glucose
- Improve the abnormal cholesterol and triglyceride levels
- May improve the blood pressure and other cardiovascular risk factors
- Slows down the progressive nature of type 2 diabetes

Shortfalls

- May cause fluid retention or swelling (ankle edema)
- Can cause weight gain
- May take several weeks to see the full benefit
- May precipitate a condition called congestive heart failure if you already have a weak heart
- May increase the risk of osteoporosis and bone fractures in women
- Has been associated with a possible risk of bladder cancer (definitely not proven, but need to mention it here to be complete)

trol far outweigh this side effect. However, some individuals may have significant swelling and the medication must be discontinued (the swelling goes away after stopping or reducing the medication). If you have a condition called congestive heart failure, you are not a candidate for an insulin sensitizer since the fluid retention may make your heart failure worse, and this is especially true if you are also on SFUs and/or insulin.

Like all medications, there have been other side effects associated with Actos, such as bone fractures in women and bladder cancer, so it is very important to discuss this with your caregiver. It really comes down to the risk-benefit ratio, and the decision to use Actos (or any drug for that matter) should be individualized.

The typical weight gain that is observed with Actos in clinical studies is about 5 to 10 pounds; however, there are many variables that may affect potential weight gain. Some individuals do not gain any weight at all and others, who are on insulin and/or SFUs, may gain more weight. Once again, in my opinion, this is a small price to pay for improving blood glucose control and in turn, reducing the complications of diabetes. It is important to know that because of the way the insulin sensitizers work (mechanism of action), it may take several weeks for you to observe any improvement in your blood glucose level. Your caregiver will decide the correct dose for you according to your glucose values.

DPP-4 Inhibitors or Incretin Enhancers

Januvia (sitagliptin), Onglyza (saxagliptin), and Tradjenta (linagliptin) are members of a relatively new class of oral medications for type 2 diabetes called the DPP-4 inhibitors or incretin enhancers (see *The New Incretin Hormones* section that follows for a detailed description of incretins). In order to understand how these new drugs work, I need to review how our bodies regulate glucose control. In addition to insulin, our bodies release a relatively newly discovered group of hormones called incretins, such as GLP-1 and GIP. These are abbreviations for long medical words. In any case, these hormones called incretins are normally released from the gut in response to the ingestion of food, and they work to lower glucose levels by stimulating insulin release and by inhibiting glucagon, which is a good thing since glucagon works in an opposing manner to insulin and raises glucose levels. In addition, these incretin hormones have been shown to reduce appetite. In people with type 2 diabetes, the GLP-1 and GIP incretin hormone levels are below normal. Once these incretin hormones are released, they are rapidly inactivated in the gut by an enzyme called DPP-4. Here is where Januvia, Onglyza, and Tradjenta come in.

Januvia, Onglyza, and Tradjenta work by inhibiting the enzyme (DPP-4) that rapidly breaks down GLP-1 and GIP, hence delaying these hormones from being degraded and prolonging their action so they can continue working to keep the blood glucose from going up, especially after eating. This is why they are called DPP-4 inhibitors. These three DPP-4 inhibitors can also automatically sense when your blood glucose level is getting near the normal range so that they can shut off their own actions to avoid hypoglycemia. In addition, neither Januvia, Onglyza, nor Tradjenta cause weight gain or fluid retention. In general, the DPP-4s can be used with other oral agents and especially with metformin. The use of DPP-4 inhibitors in clinical practice around the world has been tremendous, mainly because these medications come in a pill, only need to be taken once a day, and have basically no side effects. The drugs in this class of compounds are fairly similar, but there are some differences among the individual drugs as listed in **Table 7-11**.

Table 7-11
Prescribing Information for DPP-4 Inhibitors or Incretin Enhancers

Generic Name	Trade Name	Daily Dosage Range (mg)	Recommended Frequency
Linagliptin	Tradjenta	5	Once; no adjustment needed for kidney function
Linagliptin/ metformin	Jentadueto	2.5/500	Twice with meals
Saxagliptin	Onglyza	5	Once; adjust for kidney function
Saxagliptin/ metformin XR	Kombiglyze XR	5/500	Once with evening meal
Sitagliptin	Januvia	100	Once; adjust for kidney function
Sitagliptin/ metformin	Janumet	50/500	Twice with meals

Bile Acid Sequestrants (Colesevelam or Welchol)

Bile acid sequestrants such as Welchol (generic name is colesevelam) were originally developed to lower cholesterol levels and are discussed in *Chapter 14* on preventing heart disease. It is the only drug officially approved by the FDA for the treatment of both diabetes and elevated cholesterol levels.

Welchol is not absorbed into the bloodstream. It works in the intestines, where it binds to bile acids. Bile is a fluid that is produced by the liver. It is released into the intestine through the bile duct as part of digestion. Bile contains substances called bile acids, which the liver makes from cholesterol in the blood. Bile acids aid the digestion of fats consumed in the diet. Following digestion, the bile acids are reabsorbed into the bloodstream and are then returned to the liver.

Welchol binds to the bile acids in the intestine and prevents them from being reabsorbed into the bloodstream. Instead, they pass through the intestine with the Welchol and are excreted in the feces. This triggers the liver to produce more bile acids from the cholesterol in the blood, which lowers the level of cholesterol in the blood. I know this is complicated! No one really knows exactly how Welchol lowers glucose levels, but it was observed during the initial cholesterol-lowering studies, then eventually approved for the treatment of type 2 diabetes.

Welchol can safely be combined with other oral agents, insulin, and incretin mimetics. Please see **Table 7-12** for the prescribing guidelines. Welchol is the ideal oral medication for individuals with both type 2 diabetes that is not under control and concomitant hyperlipidemia.

Table 7-12

Prescribing Information for Bile Acid Sequestrants

Generic Name	Trade Name	Daily Dosage Range (mg)	Recommended Frequency
Colesevelam	Welchol	Tablets: six 625-mg tablets once daily or three 625-mg tablets twice daily Oral suspension: one 3.75 g packet once daily or one 1.875 g packet twice daily (mix with ½ to 1 cup [4-8 oz] of water, fruit juice, or diet soft drink)	Once or twice daily with meal and liquid Once or twice daily with meals; should not be taken in its dry form

Dopamine Receptor Agonists (Cycloset [bromocriptine])

I know there are a lot of complicated medical terms in this chapter and especially describing the details of this new medication, so please bear with me. Cycloset (generic name bromocriptine) was recently approved by the FDA as an adjunct to diet and exercise to improve glycemic control in adults with type 2 diabetes.

The mechanism by which Cycloset improves glycemic control is not well understood. It is thought that brain activity (dopaminergic tone) in the morning may be important in regulation of fuel metabolism, including glucose and lipid or cholesterol metabolism. This naturally occurring brain function can be mimicked by morning administration of the quick-release bromocriptine formulation called Cycloset. Cycloset does lower the A1C in modest amounts and seems to work well with other oral medications. It has also shown to be safe for the heart and possibly have some positive impact on heart health (heart attacks and strokes).

Cycloset is generally well tolerated with a low incidence of nausea, fatigue, and headaches lasting about 14 days that were more likely to occur during the initial titration. The administration of Cycloset is time-sensitive. It should be taken once daily with food within 2 hours after waking in the morning. The initial dose is 1 tablet (0.8 mg) daily and increased weekly by 1 tablet until the maximal tolerated daily dose of 1.6 to 4.8 mg is achieved (**Table 7-13**).

Table 7-13
Prescribing Information for Dopamine Receptor Agonists

Generic Name	Trade Name	Daily Dosage Range (mg)	Recommended Frequency
Bromocriptine mesylate	Cycloset	Initial dose is 0.8 mg and increased by one tablet/week until a maximum daily dose of 4.8 mg or the maximum tolerated daily dose is reached)	Once within 2 hours after awakening

Combination Oral Medications for Type 2 Diabetes

Combination oral medications for type 2 diabetes are becoming very popular for several reasons. Swallowing one pill that contains two effective medications that work well together is simpler than taking two different pills separately. Combo pills also allow for a single copay, which may be helpful to folks on a limited income. The number of combination medications continue to grow and will expand as the number of new classes of oral agents increase. **Table 7-14** is an up-to-date list of combination medications.

The New Incretin Hormones: GLP-1, Byetta (Exenatide), Bydureon (Once Weekly Exenatide), and Victoza (Liraglutide)

What the heck is an incretin hormone? In medical school when I was training to be a diabetes specialist, the only hormone responsible for

Table 7-14

Prescribing Information for Combination Oral Drugs

Generic Name	Trade Name	Daily Dosage Range (mg)	Recommended Frequency
Glipizide/ metformin	Metaglip	2.5/250 to 20/2000	Twice with meals
Glyburide/ metformin	Glucovance	1.25/250 to 20/2000	Twice with meals
Linagliptin/ metformin	Jentadueto	2.5/500	Twice with meals
Pioglitazone/ glimepiride	Duetact	30/2 to 30/4	Once
Pioglitazone/ metformin	Actoplus Met	15/500 to 45/2550	Twice with meals
Pioglitazone/ metformin XR	Actoplus Met XR	15/1000	Once
Repaglinide/ metformin	Prandimet	1/500	Twice to four times with meals
Rosiglitazone/ glimepiride	Avandaryl	4/1 to 8/4	Once
Rosiglitazone/ metformin	Avandamet	2/500 to 8/2000	Twice with meals
Sitagliptin/ metformin	Janumet	50/500 to 50/1000	Twice with meals
Saxagliptin/ metformin XR	Kombiglyze XR	5/500	Once with evening meal

glucose control was thought to be insulin, which comes from the pancreas. In fact, most endocrinologists like myself believed that the world revolved around the pancreas and that it was the most important organ in the human body (if you are a guy, the second most important organ!). Well, a whole new class of hormones called the incretins was recently discovered to be super important in controlling blood glucose and body weight and that they come not from the pancreas, but rather from cells of the gut or intestines.

There are a whole bunch of incretin hormones; however, one of the more important ones is called GLP-1 (glucagonlike peptide-1). GLP-1 is normally released from the gut upon ingestion of food and its main action is to prevent the abnormal rise in glucose levels after eating.

GLP-1 performs many important functions in the body, which are listed below and shown in **Figure 7-2**.

1. GLP-1, when released from the gut after eating, causes the pancreas to secrete insulin, which helps to prevent blood glucose levels from rising excessively after eating.

2. GLP-1, when released from the gut after eating, causes the pancreas to decrease the secretion of glucagon, which is a good thing because glucagon leads to glucose production and elevation of glucose values. In people who do not have type 2 diabetes, glucagon goes down after eating; in people with type 2 diabetes, it inappropriately goes up and GLP-1 prevents this rise.

3. GLP-1 helps to regulate the peristaltic contractions of the stomach, which turns out to be pretty important in regulating glucose values throughout the day and especially after meals. When food goes into the stomach, it is broken down by digestive enzymes but the nutrients are not absorbed and thus do not raise the glucose levels. It is only when the broken-down nutrients leave the

Figure 7-2
GLP-1 Effects in Humans

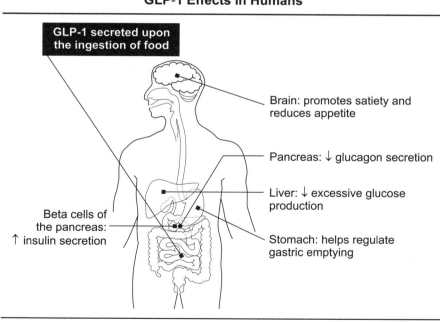

Adapted from Flint A, et al. *J Clin Invest.* 1998;101:515-520; Larsson H, et al. *Acta Physiol Scand.* 1997;160:413-422; Nauck MA, et al. *Diabetologia.* 1996;39;1546-1553; and Drucker DJ. *Diabetes.* 1998;47:159-169.

stomach and enter the intestine or gut that they get absorbed and contribute to postmeal hyperglycemia. In people who do not have diabetes, the peristaltic contractions of the stomach slow down when the blood glucose level is approaching the upper limit of normal (about 140 mg/dL) in an attempt to prevent the glucose level from rising above normal. Conversely, when the glucose level approaches the lower limit of normal (about 60 mg/dL), the peristaltic contractions of the stomach speed up, dumping nutrients faster into the gut for absorption, in an effort to prevent hypoglycemia. It turns out that in people with diabetes, the peristaltic contractions of the stomach are too fast and that by replacing GLP-1, the stomach motility is slowed down to the normal rate.

4. GLP-1 also has a significant effect to induce satiety, reduce the appetite, and lead to weight loss. This last effect of significant weight loss, in addition to improving the glucose control, is a unique combination of effects not seen with other medications for type 2 diabetes with the exception of Symlin, which will be discussed in *Chapter 8*. GLP-1, when released into the circulation after eating, travels to the appetite and satiety centers in the brain, and weight loss has been a consistent finding in every clinical study conducted in people with type 2 diabetes. By the way, satiety is a term to describe the feeling of being satisfied when eating. It turns out that when people with type 2 diabetes take synthetic human GLP-1 before sitting down to a meal, they eat approximately 20% to 24% fewer calories since they experience satiety and reduced hunger. The DPP-4 inhibitors (Januvia, Onglyza, and Tradjenta) described previously are classified as incretin enhancers, because they allow the naturally occurring incretins that are released from the body to hang around longer. The incretin mimetics described next are incretinlike hormones that raise the levels much higher, leading to weight loss and greater A1C reductions compared with the DPP-4 agents.

Incretin Mimetics: Byetta, Bydureon, and Victoza

With all these great effects, why not put incretins into the drinking water for people with type 2 diabetes? GLP-1 and other incretin hormones are a peptidelike insulin and need to be injected, which is not the problem. The problem is that GLP-1 is rapidly deactivated by an enzyme called DPP-4, which is found throughout the body. Once GLP-1 and other incretins are released from the gut upon ingestion of food, it is deactivated by DPP-4 within 90 seconds. Hence, the only way to give GLP-1 and take advantage of its benefits is to give it continuously intravenously or via some type of pump. This makes giving GLP-1 impractical. Scientists at Amylin and NovoNordisk pharmaceuticals have developed ways of altering the natural GLP-1 molecule just enough to have the same effects clinically but be resistant to the rapid inactivating effects of the enzyme that breaks it down.

How was Byetta developed? Believe it or not, a substance called exenatide was accidentally discovered in the saliva of the Gila monster (a venomous lizard found in Arizona that is on the endangered species list) that mimics the action of GLP-1 almost exactly, but it is different in one important way. Exenatide (chemical name), also called Byetta (trade name), was different enough that it did not get rapidly inactivated like GLP-1. Byetta can be given twice a day before the two main meals of the day and has all of the beneficial effects of GLP-1. Bydureon, also called once-weekly exenatide, is the first once-weekly medication developed for type 2 diabetes.

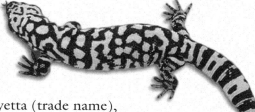

Bydureon is basically exenatide embedded into a substance that is similar to liquid absorbable suture material (biodegradable microspheres). Surgeons use absorbable sutures to stitch tissues together deeper down below the skin line that dissolve slowly over time. After Bydureon is initiated for the first time (given once a week), it takes 6 to 7 weeks to reach a steady level in the body. Because the levels of exenatide are raised so slowly over several weeks, the incidence of nausea is much lower than seen with Byetta. In addition, the administration of this long-acting form of Byetta leads to the presence of exenatide in the blood stream 24/7 compared with the regular Byetta (two peaks before the two main meals), and it is more effective at lowering the blood glucose levels and A1C values. Both lead to equivalent weight loss.

Bydureon must be mixed with the biodegradable microspheres just prior to injection, so it comes in a kit or tray. The needle used to inject Bydureon has to be slightly wider, not longer, since the liquid absorbable suture material is thicker than water, for example. For experienced Bydureon users, it takes just a few minutes to prepare and take the weekly injection.

Victoza is very similar to human GLP-1 as well but is made resistant to inactivation by the DPP-4 enzyme by altering its structure to allow for it to be given once a day at any time that is convenient. It uses the same technology, binding to a protein in the body called albumin, as the long-acting insulin detemir that Novo Nordisk produces. Victoza does not have to be mixed and has similar viscosity as insulin, so it can be given with the thinnest needles that get put on the Victoza pen.

The majority of people who are started on Byetta, Bydureon, and Victoza have no side effects at all. The most common side effect that occurs in a minority of patients is nausea. The nausea is usually mild and goes away over time. As mentioned above, the longer-acting incretin mimetics such as Victoza, and especially Bydureon, have the lowest rates of nausea. In rare cases, the nausea precludes the continued use of these medications. These incretin mimetics do not cause hypoglycemia but if used with medications that can cause hypoglycemia such as SFUs or insulin, then of course hypoglycemia is possible. The educational material given to the prescribers says that the SFU dose may need to be reduced or stopped when using Byetta, Bydureon, or Victoza. It is not uncommon that hypoglycemia may occur as the patient loses weight on Byetta, Bydureon, and Victoza and becomes more sensitive to his or her other diabetes medications. The prescribing information for these incretin mimetics is given in **Table 7-15**; benefits and shortfalls are listed in **Table 7-16**.

Table 7-15
Prescribing Information for Incretin Mimetics

Generic Name	Trade Name	Daily Dosage Range	Recommended Frequency
Exenatide	Byetta	5 mcg for first month, followed by 10 mcg thereafter	Twice a day with two largest meals of the day
Exenatide (extended release)	Bydureon	2 mg	Once weekly
Liraglutide	Victoza	0.6 mg for the first dose, then increase to 1.2 mg; if blood glucose levels are not at goal, increase to 1.8 mg	Once at any time of the day

Incretins In Development

Intarcia is developing a new product called ITCA 650 which is an injection-free GLP-1 therapy for type 2 diabetes. ITCA 650 combines the well-established advantages of a proven GLP-1 receptor agonist (exenatide) with a novel delivery system that allows patients to passively receive up to a full year of treatment from a single administration. Intarcia's proprietary technology provides continuous delivery of exenatide, which is the same GLP-1 used for Byetta and Bydureon discussed above, from a matchstick-size osmotic mini-pump that is placed just beneath the skin, in a few minutes in the physician's office, by a physician, physician's assistant, or a nurse practitioner (*see photo*). This novel delivery eliminates the need for self-injection, ensures 100% adherence, and based on early clinical results appears to hold great potential to improve the degree and durability of glucose control and weight effects compared with other oral and injection therapies.

Lixisenatide is another GLP-1 agonist or incretin in development for the treatment of people with type 2 diabetes. Lixisenatide is being developed by Sanofi, the makers of Lantus and Apidra, and mimics the naturally occurring GLP-1 that is released within minutes of eating a meal in a similar fashion as that of Byetta, Bydureon, and Victoza. It also suppresses the inappropriate glucagon secretion and stimulates insu-

Table 7-16

Benefits and Shortfalls of Incretin Mimetics

Benefits

- Significant and sustained weight loss while the blood glucose level is improving
- Reduced appetite
- Does not cause hypoglycemia
- No need to initiate or increase home glucose monitoring frequency

Shortfalls

- Can cause mild nausea when intiating therapy
- Has been associated with pancreatitis (inflammation of the pancreas). No direct cause-and-affect relationship has been proven
- Has been associated with a rare form of thyroid cancer, however, no direct cause-and-affect relationship has been proven

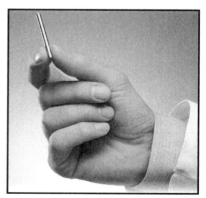

The ITCA 650 currently under development by Intarcia Therapeutics, Inc.

The photo was given with permission from Jamie Blose and Intarcia.

lin secretion after meals. Studies are ongoing in order to get this medication approved for use.

FDA Guidelines on Using Combinations of Oral Medications, Incretin Hormones, and Insulin Together

It is important to be aware that some of the combinations of medications discussed in this chapter are not FDA approved yet. The FDA will officially approve a drug or combination of medications to be used together once an official study has been done, usually conducted by the drug company that makes one of the medications to be combined, with the data submitted to the FDA for review. It is impossible for new drugs to immediately be approved with indications for use in combination with all other diabetes medications because there are too many combinations now, and it would take too long. Eventually, most effective combinations are studied and formally approved by the FDA. It is not unusual for practicing physicians with lots of clinical experience to use medications in combination "off label" before the FDA formally approves their use in this way.

General Guidelines for Taking Diabetes Medications Alone or Together

There are many variables that should be considered before any diabetes medication is chosen. There is no one perfect regimen that should be used for everyone. **Table 7-17** lists some of the variables that should be considered when choosing a medication to help control your diabetes.

Now that there are eight different classes of oral medication, incretin hormones, plus insulin (discussed in *Chapter 7*) for treating type 2 diabetes, and because we can mix and match them safely, there are many different regimens that are now possible. You have many options to choose from for the agent(s) that best fits your personal needs. There are

Table 7-17

Variables to Consider When Choosing an Oral Medication

- Are you overweight?
- Do you have abnormal cholesterol levels?
- How is your kidney function?
- How is your liver function?
- Do you have problems with your heart, such as congestive heart failure?
- Do you have osteoporosis?
- How good are you about taking pills regularly?
- Are you prone to having hypoglycemia?
- Do you already have a sensitive stomach?
- What does your health care plan provide for?

many ways to design a successful treatment regimen for people with type 2 diabetes. A perfect regimen is one that helps you achieve normal or near-normal glucose levels, avoiding bothersome side effects, and does not disrupt your lifestyle to a significant degree. General guidelines for a successful treatment program are listed in **Table 7-18** and discussed below.

First and foremost, there is no oral agent(s), incretin hormone, or insulin that will control your blood glucose level if you are not following some type of dietary program. You can't just eat anything you want at anytime and expect a good blood glucose level. I don't expect a perfect diet from anyone, but there has to be some regularity in the types and amounts of food that you ingest.

Attaining blood glucose control with only one oral medication (monotherapy) is most successful when the diagnosis of diabetes has been made recently (within the past few years). Because of the natural history of diabetes as discussed in *Chapter 2*, when the

Table 7-18

General Guidelines for a Successful Treatment Program

- A minimal amount of dietary discretion is required
- The earlier the treatment, the better
- The chance of good glucose control on one oral medication (monotherapy) in part depends on how long the diabetes has been present
- When one oral medication alone is not controlling the blood glucose level, addition (not substitution) of another oral agent is the rule rather than the exception
- Consider the addition of an incretin mimetic because of their beneficial effects on A1C reduction and weight loss
- Consider the addition of bedtime insulin to your regimen if the fasting or prebreakfast glucose value remains excessively high on the oral agent(s)
- Do not hesitate, or wait too long, to switch to an injectable medication such as insulin and/or incretin mimetics if the oral medication(s) is not controlling your blood glucose level.

pancreas becomes exhausted, the likelihood that any single oral agent will control blood glucose values is slim to none. As times goes on, the chances increase that you will need more than one oral medication, incretin hormone, and/or insulin to control your blood glucose level.

Another rule of thumb that I promote to caregivers is that when one oral medication (no matter which type) is not controlling the glucose value, it is recommended that another oral agent or incretin hormone be added to, and not substituted for, the initial drug.

Finally, it is important not to wait too long before initiating insulin if the pills and/or an incretin hormone are not working to control glucose levels. The longer you have diabetes and the higher your blood glucose value, the greater the likelihood that the oral medications will not work well enough and that you will require insulin therapy to achieve control. In certain situations, adding a single bedtime injection of a long-acting insulin to the day-time oral medication(s) and/or an incretin hormone may be quite effective and will be discussed further in *Chapter 8.*

Treatment Algorithm

Figure 7-3 is a treatment algorithm that I developed with my good friend and colleague, Dr. Robert Henry. It was originally printed in a book written for caregivers and has been modified for this book. It is a general treatment plan designed to help guide practicing physicians, nurse practitioners, and physician assistants in making therapeutic decisions for their patients. It is important to remember that these are simply guidelines and that every patient's care must be approached on an individual basis.

Case Presentations

Case #1: Monotherapy (You Are Lucky if Your Diabetes Is Diagnosed Early)

David is a 56-year-old business executive who was told he had "a touch of diabetes" during a yearly routine physical. David felt good and had no symptoms of diabetes, such as excessive thirst or urination. His mother and one brother have type 2 diabetes and weight problems, just as David does. The only other major medical condition that

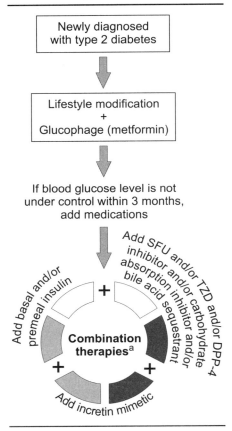

Figure 7-3

Treatment Algorithm for Type 2 Diabetes

Key: DPP-4, dipeptidyl peptidase 4 [inhibitor], SFU, sulfonylurea; TZD, thiazolidinedione.

a If the combination of several oral and/or injectable medications does not control your blood glucose level, you may need a more intensive insulin regimen. See your diabetes specialist.

David has is high blood pressure (hypertension), which is being treated with an ACE inhibitor. The only abnormal lab results were a fasting (first test in the morning) glucose value of 134 mg/dL and an elevated triglyceride level of 247 mg/dL. His A1C was 7.4% (normal 4% to 6%). According to the most recent American Diabetes Association recommendations, David was started immediately on Glucophage (metformin), as well as lifestyle modifications.

Discussion—David was lucky to have his diabetes diagnosed early before his condition deteriorated to the point of having symptoms. The early diagnosis increases the chance that his diabetes can be controlled with diet and exercise alone and/or with only one medication. David now needs to be educated about diabetes (he should already have been knowledgeable since both his mother and his brother have the same kind of diabetes), as well as getting on a realistic diet and exercise regimen that he can follow. He should also be educated in home glucose monitoring periodically before breakfast and after a large meal. If after 3 months his blood glucose value is not in the desired range (premeal level below 120 mg/dL and postmeal value below 160-180 mg/dL), starting a second oral medication or an incretin mimetic (such as Bydureon or Victoza) would be appropriate. One of these two incretin mimetics would be a good choice because of the weight loss that occurs in addition to glucose control. TZDs (Actos), a DPP-4 inhibitor (Januvia, Onglyza, or Tradjenta), a bile acid sequestrant (Welchol), or a dopamine receptor agonist (Cycloset) would also be appropriate choices.

The choice of the medication should depend on David and his caregiver's preferences. Some factors that should go into the decision of which drug to choose are the presence of liver or kidney dysfunction, abnormal cholesterol levels, and obesity. In this particular situation, I would be cautious with SFUs and TZDs because David already has a weight problem, and I do not want to expose him to the risk of hypoglycemia or low blood glucose. I agree with the choice of an ACE inhibitor for his blood pressure and would suggest that David get a home blood pressure measuring device. His cholesterol levels should be checked after his blood glucose value has improved. Sometimes, this is all that is needed to control the cholesterol levels; however, a cholesterol-lowering medication is often needed to aggressively lower the values to normal.

Case #2: Combination Therapy (Do I Really Have to Take All of These Meds?)

Mary is a 64-year-old, obese (220 pounds) woman who has had type 2 diabetes for the past 14 years. She has been treated with an SFU for the past 10 years. Her glucose control for the past 3 or 4 years has not been good. Her most recent A1C is over 9.5% (normal range is 4% to 6%, with a goal of 7% or less). In addition, both her premeal and postmeal glucose values are excessively high (above 200 mg/dL). She is afraid of "the needle" and does not want to start insulin. In addition, Mary was recently diagnosed with early diabetic eye disease (retinopathy) and nerve disease (neuropathy).

Discussion—Unfortunately, Mary's story is a common one. The SFU has lost its effectiveness over time and her blood glucose levels have been excessively high for years. As a result, she is developing the classic complications of diabetes. She has several different therapeutic options at this point because of the availability of the newer oral medications. Even though Mary's glucose value is not under control, the SFU is probably working to some degree to keep her blood glucose from really going through the roof. This is why I would now add a second oral medication to her regimen. The choice of the second medication could be any of the ones discussed in this chapter but once again, the choice would depend on the many different variables that go into making a decision as mentioned in Case #1 and outlined in **Table 7-17**. Bydureon or Victoza would also be an excellent option because of her need to improve her glucose control and to lose weight. The only two that I would not use are Starlix and Prandin, since the SFUs that she is already taking work in a similar fashion.

Other options for Mary include adding an injection of Lantus, Levemir, or NPH insulin at night or adding an injection of Humalog Mix 75/25, Humalog Mix 50/50, or Novolog Mix 70/30 before dinner. Stopping the SFU and going to a full insulin regimen is a viable and effective option. Combination therapy with oral medications and insulin are discussed in more detail in *Chapter 8*.

Case #3: Adding Oral Medications to Your Insulin Regimen

Mike is a 52-year-old, very obese (270 pounds) male with the diagnosis of type 2 diabetes for the past 12 years. Seven years ago, he was taken off of SFUs and started on a full insulin regimen because of poor glucose control. Mike is now taking 55 units of premixed insulin twice a day, before breakfast and dinner. His A1C is 11%. He is frustrated with his diabetes control and his weight problem.

Discussion—Mike's exasperating situation is also very common. There are many people with insulin-requiring type 2 diabetes with inadequate control despite being on large doses of insulin (over 100 units per day). In this scenario, I would recommend adding an oral agent to his insulin regimen, with the main goal being to reduce his A1C and blood glucose value. One choice would be an insulin sensitizer such as Actos, since these drugs work to lower insulin resistance and will allow the insulin that is present to do its job better. However, caution must be used when using TZDs and insulin together, especially because of weight gain but also for the possibility of fluid retention. Glucophage and a DPP-4 inhibitor would also be beneficial in this situation. Symlin is also a consideration (discussed in *Chapter 8*). Don't forget that he may also need a higher dose of insulin. Your choice will be determined by the variables listed in **Table 7-17**.

When the blood glucose value starts to fall after an oral medication is added, you will need to eventually lower your insulin dose by 20% to 25% if your premeal level is consistently below 120 mg/dL and/or your postmeal level drops well below 140 mg/dL. Do not make these changes on your own.

Summary

There are now eight different classes of oral medications and a new category of important hormones called incretins for the treatment of type 2 diabetes. All people with type 2 diabetes should be knowledgeable about the old and new diabetes medications available. Whether you are newly diagnosed and only on a diet and exercise program or have had diabetes for a long time and are now taking insulin, you may be a good candidate for a newer oral medication and/or an incretin mimetic (Bydureon or Victoza) now or in the near future. Each medication has its benefits and shortfalls, and there are many different variables that help determine the best one for your situation.

Early diagnosis and aggressive treatment are important for long-term success. In addition, when one oral agent is not effective in controlling your blood glucose, addition—not substitution—of another medication is the rule rather than the exception. The addition of a basal insulin to daytime medication(s), discussed in detail in the *Chapter 8*, is an easy and valuable tool for achieving glucose control in certain individuals, and there should be no delay in proceeding to a full insulin regimen when the oral medications alone cannot control the glucose levels.

There is no one perfect treatment plan for everybody. You need to work with your doctor to design the best regimen that fits your needs and your lifestyle. Having a good knowledge base regarding the available medications is crucial for you to take control of your diabetes.

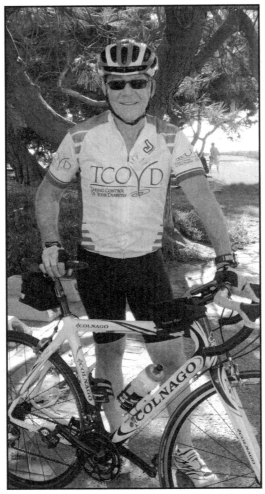

Steve Edelman modeling the new TCOYD biking jersey.

8

Insulin Therapy Must Be Custom Fit for You

Insulin 101, Newer Designer Insulins, and Symlin

by Steven V. Edelman, MD and
Jeremy Pettus, MD

Introduction

Like Dr. Edelman, I was diagnosed with type 1 diabetes at the age of 15. I was started on Regular and NPH insulin, which were the only available options. I had to mix the two together in a syringe and would inject myself twice a day. I also had a blood glucose meter that required a huge dollop of blood and took over a minute to give you result (and a lot of the time it would give you an error that it needed more blood!). I was on this regimen forever because I thought it worked for me and didn't really know what else was out there. Then I met Dr Edelman. After about 10 minutes of listening to his rant about me living in a cave, he started to tell me about all the new insulins and Symlin. Now I use Lantus once a day at nighttime and take Humalog with meals via an insulin pen. I have also started using Symlin and a continuous glucose monitor as well. All these changes have made a *huge* difference in my life. I find I have more freedom with my daily life, have less hypoglycemia, and generally spend less time dealing with my diabetes. The point of my story is that with some basic knowledge and awareness of what is available, you may be able to make some changes to your diabetic/insulin regimen that can impact your life significantly. Whether you are just starting insulin or have been on it for years, there are some important and basic concepts you need to know to be a successful user. So let's get started.

Every single person you know uses insulin, whether it comes from their own pancreas or from an injection. Insulin therapy needs to be individualized to custom-fit the lifestyle of each and every individual who uses insulin to control their diabetes. It is unrealistic to drastically change lifelong daily habits to conform to a rigid and inflexible insulin regimen. Most medical textbooks usually discuss only two or three of the most commonly used insulin regimens, and this is what most physicians prescribe for their patients. However, there are many ways to design an insulin regimen that will successfully control your blood glucose throughout the day without disrupting your lifestyle. The information in this chapter will help you design or modify your insulin regimen, working with your caregiver, to better fit your personal needs and daily habits.

Don't Fear the Needle!

Before we start talking about the nitty-gritty of using insulin, first we need to talk about getting over the fear of starting in the first place. Patients *and* doctors often put off starting insulin for far too long. So let's look at some of the reasons people resist starting insulin. This can be a huge issue for people with type 2 diabetes. For people with type 1 diabetes, it is do or die! We have no choice but at least you can seek out the best needles and insulin regimen.

1. *It's going to hurt.* I hear you. Nobody likes the idea of injecting anything, especially every single day. The good news is that insulin needles have come a long way and are essentially pain-free these days. The original syringes (back when insulin was discovered in the early 1920s) were made of glass, the needles required sharpening with a grindstone, and both had to be disinfected every day. This type of insulin delivery was used well past the 1920s. Today we have plastic, disposable syringes and sophisticated insulin pens with needle tips that are extremely thin and short. I'm not lying when I tell you that these newer needles are basically pain-free.

2. *A second misconception for people with type 2 diabetes is that starting insulin means that their diabetes is getting worse.* For many patients (and some doctors), starting insulin means the end of the line for your diabetes. It is mistakenly interpreted to mean a sense of failure in that you were not able to get your blood glucose under control with pills and lifestyle changes. But here is the truth: as type 2 diabetes progresses, the pancreas is not able to keep up with insulin demands, and you will likely need insulin over time. In other words, you are not alone. This is what we call the natural history (normal progression) of the disease and is not a failure on your part. The important thing to remember is that insulin is another tool to get your control where it needs to be. If you use it well, it will serve you well.

3. *I don't want to have hypoglycemia or low blood sugar.* Insulin lowers your blood sugar, and with any medication that lowers your blood sugar, there is always an increased risk of hypoglycemia. This is something you will need to be aware of and work with your health

care provider to fine tune your insulin dosing to help avoid low blood sugar. You should always carry something with you when you are out and about that can raise your blood sugar should you experience hypoglyemia. This can be some sugar snacks or juice. I find that every person with diabetes has their own "go to" treat to get their blood sugar up. Check out the chapter on hypoglycemia for additional tips and tricks.

4. *Insulin regimens are too complicated.* This is one that I sympathize with the most. When I was diagnosed with type 1 diabetes, I had several days in the hospital of intensive teaching to get me up to speed on all the ins and outs of insulin therapy. Most people with type 2 diabetes are started on insulin in a 10-minute office visit, and that just isn't enough time! When you start taking insulin, your health care provider may want you to start checking your blood sugar more often, start counting carbs, be an expert on injecting insulin, and on and on. This can be overwhelming. The health care field realizes this and is always looking for ways to simplify starting insulin. Just remember that all patients find this somewhat daunting but if you take it one step at a time, you can definitely do it. Some caregivers have diabetes educators or nurses that can help instruct you on how to inject insulin so you won't be thrown out of the office with just a prescription and not a clue on how to start (you can always ask to see a CDE or certified diabetes educator). Also, health care providers generally like to start with just one injection a day (type 2 diabetes only) to get patients used to the whole process and go up from there. Remember, nobody expects you to be an expert at this right out of the gate, but with some time and education, you will be off and running. Don't be afraid to ask questions!

5. *The bottom line.* Insulin has been around for almost 100 years now and is the diabetic medication with which the medical field has the most experience. Also, this is a hormone your body makes and needs to survive. In that sense, you could look at insulin therapy as the most "natural" way to control your diabetes. The rest of this chapter will be dedicated to explaining the different types of insulins and their use.

Important General Considerations

The sophistication of the normal human pancreas, including the way it keeps the glucose level in the normal range throughout the day, is incredible. The pancreas of a nondiabetic individual can detect minute changes in blood glucose on a second-to-second basis and respond immediately. This is why a nondiabetic person will have a blood glucose level between 70 and 120 mg/dL at all times no matter if he/she eats five hot fudge sundaes in a 2-hour period or fasts for 48 hours. It is no wonder that blood glucose levels bounce around all over the place in PWD and who must take insulin, even when we try to do "all the right things" at correct times. Even with all our knowledge and "state-of-the-art" insulin formulations, we still cannot compete with the sophistication of the normal pancreas. We are trying to replace the intricate function of the normal pancreas with a few injections of insulin per day or with an insulin pump, and this is a very difficult task.

With this in mind, there are a few important concepts that you need to know. The human pancreas is secreting a small amount of insulin at all times to provide a baseline or basal rate. Without this small basal rate of insulin, our blood sugars would go through the roof. It may only be a small amount of insulin, but it is very important. Then at mealtimes, the pancreas secretes a large amount (or bolus) of insulin to help utilize the energy our food gives us. So when we have to start injecting insulin, we need to replace both a *basal* insulin rate as well as mealtime insulin. People with type 1 diabetes will need a basal/bolus regimen. For folks with type 2 diabetes, the regimen will range from a basal insulin at night plus pills during the day (discussed later in this chapter under *Combination Therapy*) to a type 1ish regimen of basal and bolus insulin. You will hear these terms *basal* and *bolus* over and over, and it is important that you understand what they mean. In general, the types of insulin we use will either be a long-acting type to serve as a basal therapy or a short-acting type that serves as a bolus therapy. Time and time again, I have met PWD that say they are on different insulins but don't know which is which or what they are doing. If that is the case, it means you could easily mix them up. It is important to know the time course of action of the insulins you take and when to look out for hypoglycemia.

The time course of action (pharmacokinetics) of the various types of insulin is listed in **Table 8-1** and shown graphically in **Figure 8-1** so you can see what each insulin is doing. It is important to know when a particular insulin starts to work, has its peak action, and how long it stays in your system. This information is not only needed to design an individualized insulin regimen, but it is also crucial to determine the best times to perform home glucose monitoring. In addition, it is important to know the time course of action of the insulin you are taking to help avoid hypoglycemia, or low blood glucose, especially during exercise. The last important issue is that the time course of action of the

Table 8-1

Time Course of Action of Insulin Preparations[a]

Insulin Preparation	Starts to Work	Peak Effect	Stays in Your System
Mealtime Insulins			
Short-Acting			
Regular	30 min	2-3 hr	6-8 hr
Rapid-Acting			
Apidra (glulisine)[b] Humalog (lispro)[b] Novolog (aspart)[b]	Minutes	1-3 hr	3-5 hr
Basal Insulins			
Intermediate-Acting			
NPH (isophane)	2-3 hr	6-8 hr	16-20 hr
Long-Acting			
Lantus (glargine)[b]	1-2 hr	Peakless	24 hr
Levemir (detemir)[b]	0.8-2 hr	Relatively flat	Up to 24 hr
Premixed Insulin Formulations[c]			
Humulin 70/30, 50/50 70% (50%) NPH-like/ 30% (50%) human insulin	30 min	2 peaks: 2-3 hr and 6-8 hr	16-20 hr
Humalog Mix 75/25, 50/50[b] 75% (50%) NPH-like/ 25% (50%) lispro	Minutes	2 peaks: ~1 hr and 6-8 hr	16-20 hr
Novolog Mix 70/30[b] 70% NPH-like/30% aspart	10-29 min	2 peaks: 1 hr and 4 hr	Up to 24 hr
U-500	30-90 min[d]	3-4 hr[d]	6-8 hr[d]

Abbreviation: NPH, neutral protamine Hagedorn [insulin].

[a] This table summarizes the typical time course of action (pharmacokinetics) of various insulin preparations. Values are highly variable among individuals, depending on the site and depth of injection, local tissue blood flow, skin temperature, and exercise.
[b] The insulin analogues more closely mimic insulin secretion in a person without diabetes, therefore they are more effective.
[c] Mixtures of short- and intermediate-acting insulins.
[d] U-500 has a very variable time course of action but in general, the reserach shows it acts somewhere in betewen the older Regular and NPH insulins.

Figure 8-1

Peak Action of Insulin Compared
With Peak Rise in Glucose After Eating

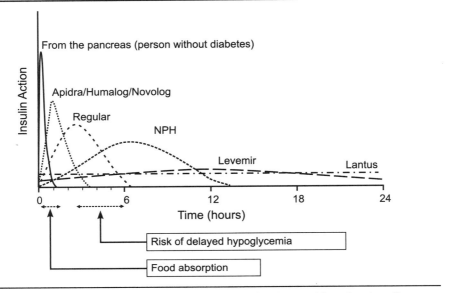

The time course of action (pharmacokinetics) for the rapid-acting insulin analogues (Apidra [glulisine], Humalog [lispro], Novolog [aspart]) is not as fast as insulin from the pancreas of a individual that does not have diabetes, but it is much more physiologic than the older Regular insulin preparation. Also shown is the time course of action of the intermediate-acting insulin (NPH [isophane]) and long-acting insulins Lantus (glargine) and Levemir (determir).

various insulins can vary from person to person and from day to day in the same person. It has been estimated that the variation in response to injected insulin on a day-to-day basis can account for up to 50% of the variability in glucose readings throughout the day. In addition, the way we give insulin to ourselves is very nonphysiologic and contributes to the wide swings in blood glucose levels that commonly occur on a daily basis.

When we give ourselves insulin, it is injected into the subcutaneous tissue, which is the layer of fat just below the skin. The insulin then has to travel through this fatty tissue in order to be absorbed into the bloodstream and this can take a very long time. The insulin that is released from a normally functioning pancreas of a nondiabetic individual goes directly into the bloodstream (intravenous), and that is why it works within seconds to minutes. It is imperative that one be familiar with the pharmacokinetics (time course of action) of the various types of insulin. Take a minute to look at **Table 8-1** and **Figure 8-1** to see the effects of the insulin you may be on.

The Different Types of Insulin
Mealtime Insulins

When we eat, our bodies are suddenly given a ton of energy as the nutrients are broken down in our stomach and absorbed in our intestines. The normal healthy pancreas reacts by meeting that demand with a bolus of insulin. To mimic that phenomenon in people with diabetes (PWD), mealtime insulins are injected just before meals to give our body the insulin they need. When I (JP) was diagnosed with type 1 diabetes in 1995 and when Dr Steve was diagnosed in 1970 , the only mealtime insulin was regular insulin and it was called "fast-acting." But if you look at **Table 8-1**, you can see that regular insulin takes at least 30 minutes to even start acting and doesn't reach peak effect for 2 to 3 hours. I personally found that it would sometimes take up to an hour to start working. This meant that at times, I would have to take an injection and wait an hour or so before eating. Thankfully, since I was diagnosed, three rapid-acting analogues have become available: Apidra (glulisine), Humalog (lispro), and Novolog (aspart). These newer analogues start working much faster and don't hang around in your system as long. These rapid-acting analogues have truly revolutionized diabetic insulin therapy and taken an important step toward making our mealtime insulins work more like our own pancreas: rapid on and rapid off.

As mentioned earlier, the route of delivery of injected insulin is different from the route of delivery of insulin by the pancreas and, as a result, injected insulin works slowly. The older Regular insulin, when given subcutaneously, peaks much later than the actual peaking of glucose in your blood after meals, leading to wide swings in the blood glucose values throughout the day. In other words, there is not enough insulin around when you need it (just after meals) and too much insulin around later when you do not need it (3 to 6 hours after eating). The new rapid-acting insulin analogues have one structural change on the insulin molecule (for you chemists out there… an amino acid substitution). This change allows the insulin analogue to be absorbed much more quickly into the bloodstream compared with the older Regular insulin. The end result is a much better match between the peak action of insulin and the peak rise in blood glucose after eating (**Figure 8-1**). When the peak action of insulin better coincides with the absorption of food, not only are the postmeal blood glucose values lower, there is also a significant reduction in the incidence of delayed hypoglycemia. The older Regular insulin peaks long after the food is absorbed, when you are not eating anymore or when you may be exercising. Some tips for using rapid-acting insulin analogues are listed in **Table 8-2**. I do not prescribe the older Regular insulin anymore because of the benefits of rapid-acting insulin analogues. If you are on the older Regular insulin and doing fine (no problems with frequent hypoglycemic reactions, elevated glucose levels after eating, or wide swings in your values), there is no need to change. We do not have to fix what is not broken!

Long-Acting Basal Insulin Analogues

As I mentioned before, the human pancreas secretes a small amount of basal insulin at all times. Two insulin formulations, Lantus and Levemir, were created to mimic this basal dose. Lantus (insulin glargine) was the first long-acting peakless basal insulin analogue. By altering the structure (changing the amino acid sequences), Lantus lasts for 24 hours without a peak. A true basal insulin ideally should not have a dramatic peak (**Figure 8-1**). Peaking of insulin should be under your control when you are able to eat or purposefully treat a high blood glucose level as with Apidra, Humalog, or Novolog. Lantus is an excellent alternative for PWD who require or can benefit from a steady basal level of insulin in a very similar fashion to the basal rate of an insulin pump described in *Chapter 9*.

Levemir (insulin detemir) is the newest long-acting basal insulin analogue. Levemir is made to last a long time because it is bound to albumin, a protein in our bodies that also hangs around for a long time. Levemir has been studied in people with both type 1 and insulin-requir-

Table 8-2

Tips for Using Rapid-Acting Insulin Analogues

- Take your dose about 15 minutes before your meal, unless your glucose value is excessively high (taking your insulin well before your meal, if your glucose is high, will prevent you from going excessively high right after eating)
- You may need a small dose of insulin for every snack. This may not have been necessary with the older Regular insulin because it hangs around in your system for 4 to 6 hours
- Make sure you have an adequate long-acting insulin dosing schedule to cover you in between widely spaced meals, periods of fasting, and during the night, when the rapid-acting insulin will have left your system
- It is convenient and wise to use an insulin pen and carry it with you at all times

ing type 2 diabetes who require basal insulin with or without the use of rapid-acting insulin analogues (**Figure 8-1**).

The use of Lantus and Levemir has also led to a lower incidence of hypoglycemia or low blood glucose in the night, which is a great advantage to these long-acting basal insulins. Lantus and Levemir both have a more predictable time course of action compared with older basal insulins, leading to reduced unpredictable swings in blood glucose levels on a day-to-day basis. Because of their chemical properties, it is not recommended that Lantus or Levemir be mixed with other types of insulin. They must be taken alone in a syringe or via a Lantus or Levemir insulin pen. Lantus or Levemir at night or twice a day with a rapid-acting analogue at mealtimes is the "poor man's" insulin pump!

The role of a basal insulin is to keep your blood glucose in the near-normal range between meals and overnight. If your dose of basal insulin is correct, your numbers will not change at all when you are fasting. In fact, this is how you can test to see if your basal rate is adjusted appropriately. To test how your basal rate is working during the daytime, fast most of the day and test your glucose level every 2 hours or so. If your basal dose is adjusted properly, your blood sugar will stay steady (not rise or fall) when you are not eating or sleeping. This is an important concept to keep in mind. The role of a basal insulin is *not* to lower your blood sugar but to give you just enough insulin to keep your blood sugar *even*. If your blood sugar is 250 mg/dL when you go to sleep and 250 when you wake up, that means your basal dose is perfect. It also means you have to figure out why it was 250 mg/dL when you went to bed! Usually it means that you aren't giving yourself enough mealtime insulin at dinner.

To test how your basal dose is working overnight, eat an early dinner and test your glucose level at bedtime, at 3 AM, and again upon awakening. Better yet, the use of a continuous glucose monitoring device would be ideal to see how your basal rate is working as they measure glucose values every 5 minutes throughout the night and day (see *Chapter 12*). In normal individuals, the pancreas secretes a little amount of insulin all of the time, even if the person is not eating a thing all day and night. We try to mimic that normal physiologic insulin secretion with a basal insulin or an insulin pump.

Intermediate-Acting Insulin and Mixed Formulations: Primarily for People With Type 2 Diabetes

If you take a look again at **Figure 8-1**, you will see that there is a clear distinction between the mealtime insulins (Regular and Apidra/

Humalog/Novolog) and the basal insulins (Levemir and Lantus). You might also notice that NPH doesn't seem to fit into either category. Well, good noticing, because it doesn't! NPH is an older insulin formulation and really in its own category: intermediate in action. The peak effect is around 6 to 8 hours, and this late peaking can be utilized to give coverage during the day or overnight. When NPH is combined with a rapid-acting insulin, you will get two distinct peaks. For example, taking NPH along with one of the rapid-acting analogues in the morning before breakfast would have the following effect:

1. The rapid-acting insulin would start working immediately and give you enough insulin for your breakfast.
2. The NPH dose would peak right around lunchtime, meaning you don't need to take more mealtime insulin for lunch.

This same technique can be done before dinner to provide you with immediate insulin for dinner and then some insulin coverage overnight. In a nutshell, this whole regimen can let you get away with two insulin injections a day instead of three or four. A subset of people with type 2 diabetes find this useful. Additionally, premixed formulations are available called 70/30 or 75/25 (70% to 75% NPH and 25% to 30% rapid-acting insulin) to help simplify combining the two insulins. The downsides are that NPH can cause more hypoglycemia and gives you less flexibility with timing of meals. If you take a dose in the morning, missing lunch can cause hypoglycemia and eating a large lunch can cause hyperglycemia. Additionally, taking a dose before dinner can lead to hypoglycemia at night around 1 to 2 AM when it is peaking. When compared with the true basal insulins of Lantus and Levemir, NPH has been shown to have more episodes of hypoglycemia. You can limit nighttime hypoglycemia by moving your NPH dose (taking it separately from the rapid-acting, which is given at dinner time) to bedtime, but this obviously would require an additional injection. Check out case #2 at the end of this chapter for more information on this type of insulin dosing. This is what we call a "split-mixed" insulin regimen and when used properly, it can work well for certain individuals. None the less, despite the issues described above with premixed insulins, many folks with type 2 diabetes do well on it. Premixed insulins are really not for people with type 1 diabetes.

U-500 Insulin

U-500 insulin is being used more and more these days, typically in overweight folks with type 2 diabetes taking over 100 units of insulin at a time. The typical U-100 insulin syringe only holds 100 units of the

U-100 insulin (this is the concentration of insulin on the market in the United States), so it is really impractical to take two injections at one time, and for someone on a multiple daily injection regimen the number of injections per day gets too onerous. U-500 is 5 times more concentrated as the normal U-100 insulin. So if someone is on 100 units of Regular insulin and is switched over to U-500 insulin, he would draw up 20 units of U-500 into a U-100 syringe (there are no U-500 syringes) for the equivalent dose. It turns out from multiple clinical studies that U-500 seems to work better than the equivalent dose of U-100 because of the smaller size of the depo (amount of fluid in one area) under the skin after injection and better absorption into the blood stream. The time course of action is very variable but somewhere between the older Regular insulin and NPH. It is typically given before each meal and not with any other basal insulin, however when folks are this insulin resistant, individualization of the oral and injectable medications is key and there are no set rules. If you are on over 100 units of insulin at a time then ask your caregiver about U-500.

Ultra Rapid-Acting Inhaled Insulin

Technosphere® Insulin, or Afrezza, is an inhaled insulin product currently in clinical development waiting for FDA approval (MannKind Corporation, Valencia, CA). The time course of action of Afrezza is different from rapid-acting insulin analogues, such as Humalog or Novolog. It has a more rapid onset of blood glucose–lowering action and has a shorter duration of glucose-lowering activity. These results more closely mimic the normal insulin release profile seen in healthy individuals. In addition, in patients with type 2 diabetes, it suppresses the body's own production of glucose made by the liver after a meal faster than rapid-acting insulin analogues. Patients taking Afrezza also had a lower rate of hypoglycemia and less weight gain than those treated with other insulins,

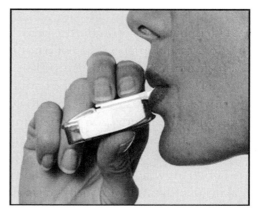

Afrezza is discreet and easy to use, has one inhalation per cartridge, requires minimal training for use, and reduces patient effort for insulin delivery.

Photo supplied by Alfred Mann, Founder of MannKind.

which in part is due to its rapid on-off time course of action. The safety of Afrezza has been extensively studied in a clinical program involving more than 5600 patients. The most common side effects observed have been hypoglycemia and cough. The cough occurred in 32% of patients but tended to be mild and occurred within minutes of inhaling the medication. The cough usually went away over time and rarely led patients to stop the medication. A slight reduction in pulmonary function was noted. It was nonprogressive and resolved after discontinuation of Afrezza.

More Physiologic Prandial or Premeal Insulin: Hyaluronidase (Hylenex)

A substance called Hylenex (rHuPH20) used at the site of injection along with insulin analogues has demonstrated the ability to make prandial or before-meal insulin more physiologic by accelerating dispersion and absorption of the insulin. Hylenex recombination, which is not yet available and is awaiting FDA approval, has made analog insulin more closely resemble the faster-on, faster-off profile of a nondiabetic individual. Studies have shown that the addition of rHuPH20 to an analog regimen (Apidra, Novolog or Humalog) has reduced post-meal excursions by up to 60% when compared with analog alone. In addition to showing reduced post-meal excursions, the co-formulation of rHuPH20 with analog insulin also demonstrated a reduction in hypoglycemia, which is what you expect for a rapid-on and rapid-off insulin. Use of Hylenex recombinant pretreatment in controlled pump studies has reduced the variability of insulin time course of action over 3 days of infusion set life by up to 80%.

Ultralong-Acting Basal Insuliln: Insulin Degludec (Tresiba)

Insulin degludec (Tresiba) is an ultralong-acting new generation basal insulin analog that was developed by NovoNordisk and which is currently in phase 3 clinical development (waiting to hear from the FDA). Degludec has a much longer duration of action than current basal insulin formulations, with a duration of action of more than 42 hours in adults. It has the potential to broaden the options for current diabetes treatment with a flexible 3-times-a-week dosing regimen that can be administered at any time of the day, however, it will be recommended to be given as once-daily dosing. These characteristics will facilitate the integration of insulin therapy with daily activities and potentially improve adherence and acceptance of basal insulin treatment. Degludec also demonstrated in clinical trials that because of its really flat time course of action, it had a very low rate of nocturnal hypoglycemia and acted very consistently from day to day.

Symlin: Another Important Hormone That Partners With Insulin

At one time, insulin was thought of as the only important hormone from the pancreas that helped to control the blood glucose levels throughout the day. Well, in 1987, another hormone called amylin was discovered that came from the exact same cells in the pancreas that produced, stored, and secreted insulin. It was also discovered that type 1 diabetics have a complete deficiency of amylin (we don't make any at all), and type 2 diabetics have a relative deficiency (they still make some but not enough). Hence, the San Diego–based company called Amylin was created by visionary Ted Greene, and what followed was a challenging 18-year scientific trek to understand the relationship of this natural partner hormone to insulin and its role in the management of diabetes. The scientists at Amylin produced an analogue of amylin called pramlintide (sort of like Humalog is an analogue of regular insulin) and the marketing name is Symlin. Symlin is currently approved by the FDA for people with type 1 diabetes and type 2 diabetes who use mealtime insulin and have not achieved glycemic control.

To make a long story short, amylin was discovered to have at least three main important functions in healthy nondiabetic humans to keep the blood glucose level in a very narrow and normal range after meals and throughout the day. When amylin is released from the pancreas at mealtimes along with insulin, its three main functions are:

1. To induce satiety (the feeling of being satisfied with meals), reduce the appetite, and help to limit or stop overeating. Every study to date has demonstrated significant weight loss with Symlin.
2. To prevent the release of glucagon (another hormone from the pancreas), which is a good thing because glucagon raises blood glucose.
3. To control how fast the stomach propels food down the gastrointestinal track, limiting the rise in glucose levels after eating.

All three of these mechanisms work primarily to control how high blood glucose rises after meals (postmeal or postprandial glucose levels). In clinical trials, patients treated with Symlin lowered their A1C, lost weight, and were able to lower their total insulin dose. A win, win, win in my book. **Figure 8-2** shows blood glucose levels in people with type

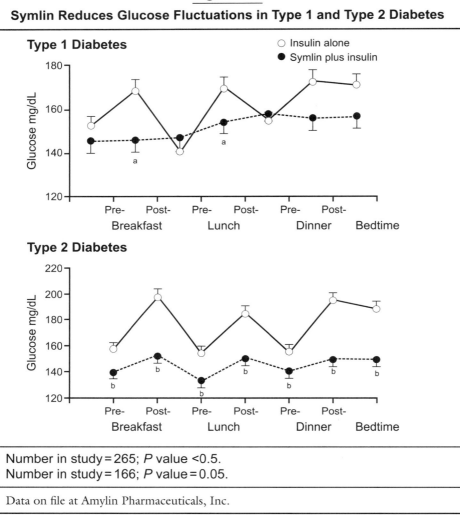

Figure 8-2

Symlin Reduces Glucose Fluctuations in Type 1 and Type 2 Diabetes

Type 1 Diabetes

○ Insulin alone
● Symlin plus insulin

(Glucose mg/dL)

a Number in study = 265; P value <0.5.
b Number in study = 166; P value = 0.05.

Data on file at Amylin Pharmaceuticals, Inc.

1 and insulin-using type 2 diabetes who were on insulin alone or on both insulin and Symlin at mealtimes. As you can see, the fasting values (before breakfast) are reduced; however, the big difference is the flattening of the postmeal glucose values and the daily glucose fluctuations. **Table 8-3** lists the benefits of using Symlin, and I put them in my order of importance.

Because Symlin can effectively act to reduce the amount of food ingested and the dose of insulin needed, it is important to follow the titration schedule suggested when initiating Symlin (**Figure 8-3**). In the early clinical studies, insulin was not reduced, which caused a high rate of hypoglycemia. Reducing the dose of insulin when starting Symlin has helped address this problem. The dose of premeal insulin (Apidra, Humalog, Novolog, Regular, inhaled [when it becomes available, and premixed insulins) should be reduced by about 50% in order to prevent hypoglycemia or low blood glucose. The reduction may be excessive and the dose of insulin may need to be adjusted upward according to your home or continuous glucose monitoring results.

Nausea is a side effect when initiating Symlin therapy. This is why the titration schedule shown in **Figure 8-3** starts off with a low dose and is gradually increased

Table 8-3

Benefits of Symlin in People With Type 1 and Insulin-Using Type 2 Diabetes

1. Less daily fluctuations in blood glucose throughout the day
2. Reduction of the postmeal glucose level, allowing for consumption of meals with a decent amount of carbohydrates
3. Reduction of the fasting glucose level (first thing in the morning before breakfast)
4. Lowering the A1C level
5. Controls hunger and leads to weight loss
6. Reduction of the amount of insulin needed (especially the premeal rapid-acting insulin dose)

over time. It turns out that people with type 1 diabetes are more sensitive to Symlin in terms of nausea so the titration is slower and final dose is lower compared with those in people with type 2 diabetes. Symlin is injected exclusively via a pen with predetermined doses. The type 2 pen has doses of 60 mcg and 120 mcg while the type 1 pen has 15-, 30-, 45-, and 60-mcg doses to make titration easy. The product was available in a vial and syringe form in the past, but this was discontinued in 2011. For more information, please visit *www.symlin.com.*

Dr Edelman was involved in a lot of the early clinical trials for Symlin, so he really is an expert on the subject. When I first met him, he told me about some of the benefits so I thought I would give it a shot. Two years later, I am a happier diabetic. It has helped me control my daily fluctuations of glucose levels and really flatten out my postmeal glucose value. I have lost a noticeable amount of weight, and my A1C improved. My dose of rapid-acting insulin has been reduced by about 30% and I don't feel that I have any more hypoglycemic reactions. Now that I have a CGM, I can really appreciate how well Symlin works to control my glucose level after meals and throughout the day.

With the help of Dr Edelman, I have collected a list of a few tips for successful Symlin use:

Figure 8-3

Initiation and Titration Schedule for Symlin (pramlintide)

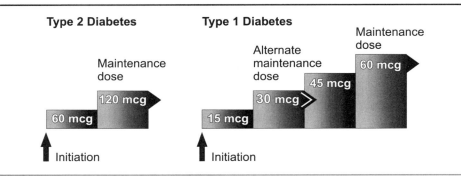

- Symlin should be administered immediately before major meals or snacks
- It is recommended that mealtime insulin dose be initially reduced by 50% upon initiation of Symlin
- Symlin should be initiated at a dose of 60 micrograms (mcg) in patients with type 2 diabetes and 15 mcg in patients with type 1 diabetes
- The dose of Symlin should be increased every 3 to 7 days (as tolerated, based on nausea) until the maintenance dose is reached. Patients with type 2 diabetes require one Symlin dose titration to reach a maintenance dose of 120 mcg with major meals. Patients with type 1 diabetes require three Symlin dose titrations (in 15-mcg increments) to reach a maintenance dose of 60 mcg with major meals.
- If nausea occurs and persists at a given dose, Symlin should be reduced to the previous dose
- Once a maintenance dose of Symlin is reached, insulin adjustments should be made, based on the individual patient's self-monitoring of blood gucose and treatment goals

Symlin (pramlintide) prescribing information, 2005.

1. Take your dose of Symlin at the beginning of the main part of your meal.
2. Consider taking your dose of rapid-acting insulin near the end of the meal when you have seen exactly how much you have eaten.
3. If on an insulin pump, give your bolus over 2 hours (extended-wave bolus).
4. If you have not experienced the satiety and appetite effect, discuss increasing your dose of Symlin past the current recommended dose with your caregiver.

When a company such as Amylin conducts a study and presents the results to the FDA, the final recommended dose must be the dose that was used in those studies. It is not uncommon to discover better ways to use a drug once it is released for public use. Always check with your caregiver when making dose adjustments of any medication.

Although Symlin leads to weight loss, it is not officially approved by the FDA as a medication for weight control at the current time. Clinical studies are currently under way to see if Symlin can be helpful as a weight loss agent in overweight people with or without diabetes.

Figuring Out How Much Insulin You Need With Each Meal: "Guesstimating" and Carbohydrate Counting

If you take mealtime insulin, you need to know how much insulin to give with each meal. So how do you determine your dose? The latest diabetes eating fashion is to count the carbohydrates and use a carbo-hydrate-to-insulin ratio to figure out how much rapid-acting insulin to take for the meal you are about to consume… or inhale, if you are a rapid eater! A typical carbohydrate-to-insulin ratio for someone with type 1 diabetes may be 15:1 (for every 15 grams of carbohydrate consumed, 1 unit of rapid-acting insulin should be given). For example, if someone with a ratio of 15:1 is about to eat 90 grams of carbohydrate, the dose of rapid-acting insulin for that meal would be 90/15 or 6 units. This amount would be in addition to a correction dose if the pre-meal glucose level was high or above your goal range (discussed below). Someone with type 2 diabetes may have a ratio of 10:1 and would take 9 units for the same meal. By pre- and postmeal testing, you can determine your appropriate ratio.

It is important to note that many people with type 1 and especially type 2 diabetes do pretty well guesstimating their dose based on past experience and trial and error. For many of us, we are creatures of habit and eat the same amounts and types of food most of the time. I suggest using an insulin algorithm based on personal experience, trying different doses with certain types and amounts of food. In a short time, with the help of premeal and postmeal home glucose monitoring, most of us will have a fairly well-defined mental "insulin menu." An insulin menu is basically how much insulin you need for a certain type of food. For example, when I eat my usual three slices of pizza, I always add an extra 8 to 10 units of my rapid-acting insulin to my usual dose in order to avoid excessively high postmeal glucose values (**Table 8**-4). In summary, it is important to figure out your dose of insulin at mealtime for the amount of food you are going to eat and correct for a high blood glucose level if you have one.

Table 8-4

Example of an "Insulin Menu" Using Steve Edelman's Eating Habits

Usual Meals	Usual Rapid-Acting Insulin Dose[a]
Breakfast	
Just coffee with milk (no food)	3 units
Bagel with cream cheese	10 units
Bowl of cold cereal with milk *(I love Trix!)*	12 units
Bowl of hot cereal (no milk)	7 units
Pancakes or French toast	15 units
Scrambled eggs (2) with buttered toast (1 slice)	6 units
English muffin with peanut butter	3.5 units
Lunch	
Tuna, turkey, or veggie sandwich	10 units
Veggie burger	12 units
Soup and salad	8 units
Dinner	
Typical pasta dinner	14 units
Large salad with fresh bread	10 units
Chicken, fish, or meat dinner	12 units
3 Large slices of pizza	18 units

Unusual Meals

Restaurants

Usually add 5 to 10 units to my normal dose because I always find myself eating more in a restaurant than I do at home

Desserts (Yes, I do eat desserts once in awhile!)

Small scoop of ice cream	3 units
Large bowl of ice cream	8 units
Cookies (2 or 3)	5 to 7 units
Small piece of chocolate cake *(when no one is watching me)*	6 to 8 units
Pudding (I love butterscotch)	4 to 5 units

[a] These doses are my usual normal premeal dose of Apidra, Humalog, or Novolog.

How to "Catch Up": Insulin Algorithms, Sliding Scales, and Correction Factors

In addition to determining how much insulin you need for a meal, it is important to figure out if you need to "correct" for a high blood sugar. It doesn't make any sense to give the same amount of Regular or fast-acting insulin every day before every meal, no matter if the blood glucose is 80 or 350 mg/dL. It always boggles my mind to hear my patients tell me that their blood glucose was high before a meal and that they did not take any extra rapid-acting insulin to help compensate for it. Insulin algorithms, sliding scales, and correction factors are phrases to describe different methods to correct for a high glucose level between meals and at mealtimes. They are an important part of achieving glucose control on a day-to-day basis, in addition to helping make decisions about long-term adjustments. It turns out that all three terms are variations on the same theme. The problem is that many caregivers and patients may not know how to design or utilize a proper algorithm, sliding scale, or correction factor. As a result, these valuable tools are not widely used, and their use is sometimes inappropriately discouraged.

An example of an insulin algorithm or sliding scale is shown in **Figure 8**-**4**. As you can see, once the glucose value goes above 150 mg/dL, the dose of insulin increases one unit for every 50 mg/dL. This would also be called a correction factor of 1:50—one unit of rapid-acting insulin should be added to the total dose of rapid-acting insulin to be given for every 50 mg/dL above 150 mg/dL measured. Everyone needs to figure out what his or her correction factor is by lots of pre- and posttesting. For example, if you had breakfast at 7 AM, and at 10

Figure 8-4
Sample Algorithm of Case Presentation for "Sandy"

Name: Sandy

Date: December 15, 2012

Provider: Dr. Edelman

Phone: 858-552-8585

Time between injection and meal (minutes) Apidra, Humalog, or Novolog	Blood glucose value (mg/dL)	Breakfast	Lunch	Dinner	Bedtime	Bedtime snack size
0	< 80	5	3	7	Ø	large
5	81 to 150	6	4	8	Ø	medium
5 to 15	151 to 200	7	5	9	Ø	small
15 to 30	201 to 250	8	6	10	3	none
30	251 to 300	9	7	11	4	none
30+	301 to 350	10	8	12	5	none
30+	351 to 400	11	9	13	6	none
30+	401 to 450	12	11	15	7	none
30+	451+	13	13	17	5	none

AM long-acting insulin dose _____

PM long-acting insulin dose _20 units Lantus or Levemir_ ☐ Take before dinner ☒ Take at bedtime

AM your glucose value is 276 mg/dL (damn pancakes will do it to you every time), and you would like to be close to 150 mg/dL at lunchtime in a few hours. If your correction factor is 1:50, you would take 2 to 3 units of rapid-acting insulin at 10 AM (276 [current blood glucose] minus goal of 150 divided by 50 equals 2 to 3 units). You need to decide on what your goal blood glucose is and how many mg/dL your blood glucose will drop after 1 unit of rapid-acting insulin. If you are a type 1 diabetic, your correction factor will most likely be around 1:50; if you are a type 2 diabetic, your correction factor may be closer to about 1:25. It is important to test before and after taking insulin to find the correct factor for you, as it is different for everyone. The dose of insulin does not matter. What does matter is your glucose level.

The 1800 rule is used if you are taking rapid-acting insulin to estimate what your correction factor may be. You take the total amount of insulin you use per day (both long- and short-acting insulin) and divide the total into 1800. For example, if you use 40 units of insulin per day (20 units of Levemir and 20 units of Novolog), an estimate of your correction factor would be 1800 divided by 40, which equals 45 or 1:45. You would then use this correction factor at meal times and between meals to correct for an elevated glucose value over what your goal is, which will be between 100 and 150 mg/dL, depending on what you and your doctor mutually decide. The 1500 rule works in the same manner if you are using the older Regular insulin instead of a rapid-acting insulin.

Insulin Pens

Insulin pens not only allow for an easier and more convenient way to take insulin, but they also help protect the insulin from light, agitation, and heat (all of which can lead to reduced activity of the insulin). Insulin pens are used by 90% to 95% of insulin-treated patients in Europe, Asia, and Scandinavia with excellent results. Insulin pens are severely underutilized in the United States (used by only about 12% of insulin users), mainly because of ignorance by caregivers and PWD. They just do not know about them and have never seen one. In addition, many health care systems do not offer them because they are slightly more expensive than using a vial and syringe.

Insulin pens are small, pen-size devices that contain a reservoir and needle for the accurate and convenient delivery of the various types of insulin (**Figure 8-5**). They are either totally disposable or reusable, replacing only the cartridge of insulin. Normally insulin pens are used for

Figure 8-5

Examples of Insulin Pens

Disposable Pens	Insulin Delivered	How Supplied
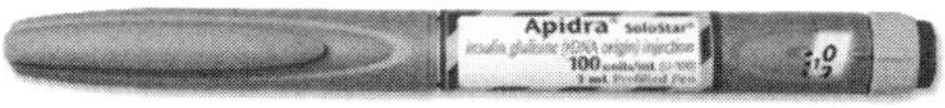 Apidra SoloStar (Sanofi US)	Glulisine (rDNA origin)	3-mL SoloStar pen
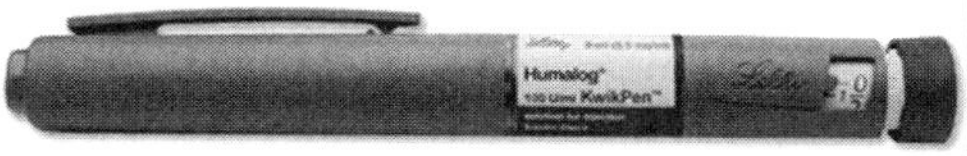 Humalog KwikPen (Eli Lilly & Co)	Lispro (rDNA origin)	3-mL KwikPen
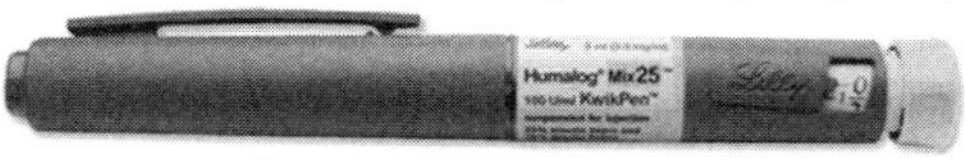 Humalog Mix 75/25 KwikPen (Eli Lilly & Co)	Lispro (rDNA origin)	3-mL KwikPen
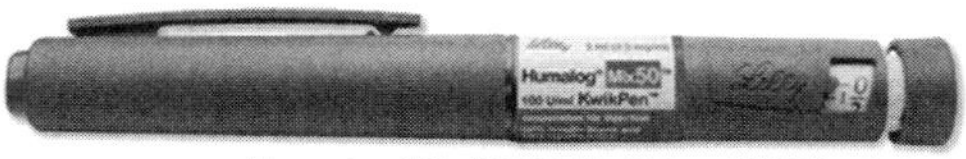 Humalog Mix 50/50 KwikPen (Eli Lilly & Co)	Lispro (NPH-like insulin)	3-mL KwikPen
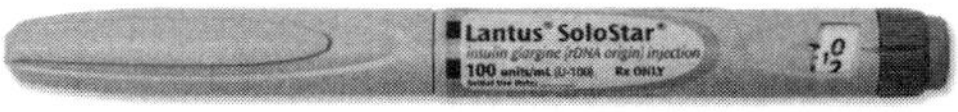 Lantus SoloStar (Sanofi US)	Glargine (rDNA origin)	3-mL SoloStar pen
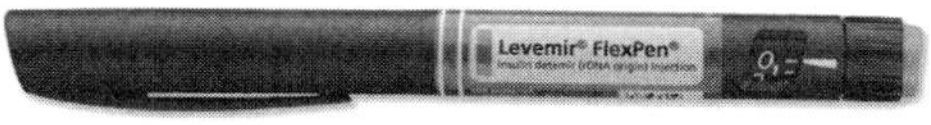 Levemir FlexPen (Novo Nordisk, Inc)	Detemir (rDNA origin)	3-mL FlexPen
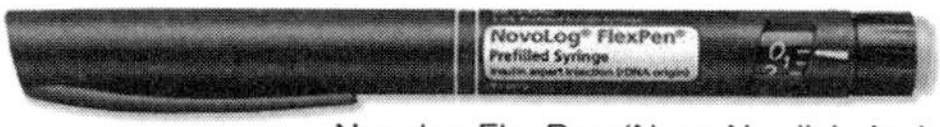 Novolog FlexPen (Novo Nordisk, Inc)	Aspart (rDNA origin)	3-mL FlexPen
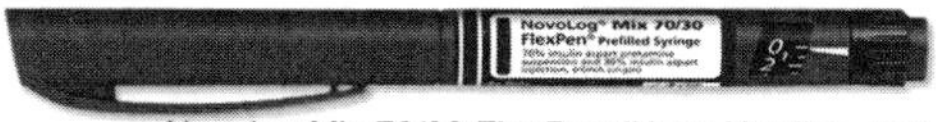 Novolog Mix 70/30 FlexPen (Novo Nordisk, Inc)	Aspart (rDNA origin)	3-mL FlexPen
Refillable Pen		
NovoPen 3 (Novo Nordisk, Inc)	Aspart (rDNA origin)	3-mL PenFill cartridge
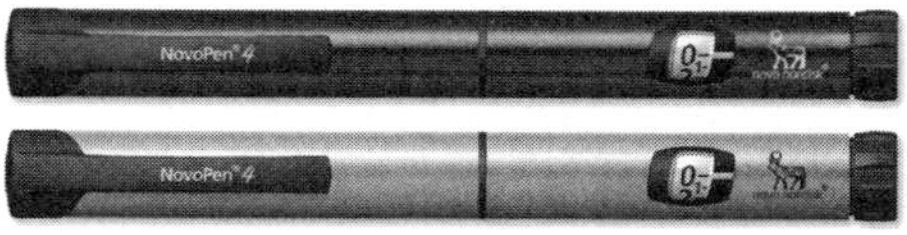 NovoPen 4 (Blue, Silver) (Novo Nordisk, Inc)	• Aspart • Detemir and degludec • NovologMix 70/30	3-mL PenFill cartridge (color coded for different insulins)

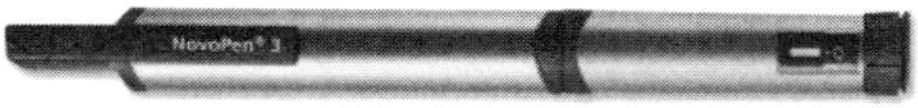

All images provided as a courtesy from Eli Lilly & Company, Novo Nordisk Inc, and Sanofi US.

the premeal injections of rapid-acting insulin; however, insulin pens can also deliver the long-acting and premixed insulins. Don't forget that the needle of an insulin pen does not get dull because it is not shoved through the thick rubber stopper of an insulin vial. One can unofficially use insulin needles multiple times before discarding them if you are somewhere without a new needle tip, but in reality, they should be changed each time. I find that the injection from an insulin pen is much less painful than even pricking my finger to test my blood glucose level.

The Role of Home or Continuous Glucose Monitoring

It is important to emphasize that there is no way to achieve glycemic control without the proper use of home or continuous glucose monitoring, especially if you are on a multiple daily injection regimen or insulin pump. In fact, giving yourself insulin without knowing what your blood sugar is, from where it has come, and what direction it is going can be dangerous. Home glucose monitoring or continuous glucose monitoring is essential to determine how much rapid-acting insulin to give yourself before each meal and how long to wait between the injection of insulin and consumption of the meal. Glucose monitoring after meals will also help to figure out if you gave yourself too much or too little insulin. Home glucose monitoring or continuous glucose monitoring will also help with avoiding hypoglycemia, planning exercise, and making long-term adjustments in your insulin regimen (**Table 8-5**). Please, see *Chapters 10, 11,* and *12* to help analyze your own glucose results.

Adjusting for Exercise

If you are lucky, you can fit exercise into your daily schedule on a regular basis at the time most desirable for you. If you are like me and most other people, it is a constant battle to find any time to exercise, let alone a desirable time. I love to exercise because I like the way it makes me feel and it's good for me. Unfortunately, it can be really upsetting when you have to stop exercising because of low blood sugars. There is nothing more frustrating for me than starting exercising and having to stop in 5 minutes to eat and drink. I didn't start exercising to help me eat MORE!

It is important to know how exercise affects your glucose control. Much of the information will come from pre- and postexercise home glucose monitoring or continuous glucose monitoring and a mental diary of how certain types of exercise (including the length and degree of intensity) bring down your blood glucose level and by how much. There are no shortcuts or fancy formulas to predict how you will respond to certain types of exercise. You must test a lot and learn from experience. The best prediction of what will happen to your blood glucose is what has happened in the past during similar types of exercise. See *Chapter 6* for much more on exercise.

Table 8-5

Importance of Home and Continuous Glucose Monitoring in Achieving Glycemic Control

- *Determining the premeal dose of Regular or rapid-acting insulin:* It is important to adjust the premeal dose of insulin, depending on the premeal glucose value as well as the size of the meal and anticipated exercise.

- *Timing of the insulin injection in relation to consuming the meal:* You should wait at least 30 minutes after you inject before eating if you are using the older Regular insulin and only 5 minutes if you are using the new rapid-acting analogues (Apidra, Humalog, and Novolog). This time period is appropriate only if your premeal blood glucose value is within the normal range. However, if your premeal glucose value is higher than normal, you should wait longer to give the insulin a chance to bring down your abnormally high value before you consume more calories. The timing of your insulin dose in relation to your meals is of utmost importance and is usually ignored by most patients and physicians.

- *Determining if you gave yourself too much or too little premeal insulin:* Testing your blood glucose value 1 to 2 hours after eating is important to determine whether you gave yourself too little or too much rapid-acting insulin. This postmeal testing is especially important if your premeal glucose was high or if you ate an unusual amount or type of food. If your blood glucose is too high after eating, a small extra dose of rapid-acting insulin is usually warranted. If your postmeal glucose is too low, consumption of extra calories may be appropriate to avoid a severe low blood glucose, especially if you are planning on exercising

- *Avoidance of hypoglycemia:* Home glucose monitoring and especially continuous glucose monitoring are important tools to help you avoid serious hypoglycemia. By knowing when your insulin will be peaking, you can use home and continuous glucose monitoring to detect a low blood glucose before a severe low blood glucose reaction occurs..

- *Exercise planning:* Home and continuous glucose monitoring before, after, and sometimes during prolonged exercise can give you important information for a safe and effective workout. Glucose testing before exercise is important, not only to avoid hypoglycemia but also to detect and treat severe hyperglycemia, which will definitely affect your workout. In addition, sometimes prolonged and strenuous exercise can cause delayed and severe hypoglycemia that needs to be monitored.

- *Make long-term adjustments in your insulin regimen:* Using home glucose monitoring or continuous glucose monitoring is not only important for making short-term daily adjustments in your insulin dose, it is crucial that appropriate long-term changes be made as well. For example, if the prebreakfast glucose value is consistently high, requiring the need for extra Regular or rapid-acting insulin every morning, then more evening or bedtime long-acting insulin is needed in order to avoid the morning high glucose value in the first place.

In general, if you know you are going to exercise within 2 to 4 hours of your last dose of a rapid-acting insulin, you should reduce that premeal dose by 20% to 50%, depending on the intensity and duration of the exercise (**Table 8-6**). My usual exercise is either 45 to 60 minutes on an exercise bike, a 2- to 3-hour ride on my bike or a 3- to 4-mile run. I reduce my premeal rapid-acting insulin dose by approximately 25% if I exercise fairly soon after eating. You may not need to reduce your dose as much if you are using a rapid-acting insulin such as Apidra, Humalog, or Novolog, since they leave your system much more quickly than the older Regular. In order to avoid problems, it is best to exercise when your Regular or rapid-acting insulin is not peaking. If you are one of those exercise freaks who run marathons in your spare time, you need to reduce your long-acting basal insulin as well by 20% to 50%.

Always test your blood glucose value before and after exercising, and every 1 to 2 hours during prolonged strenuous routines. If your blood glucose is over 250 mg/dL, you should consider giving yourself a

Table 8-6
General Recommendations for Exercise and Insulin Regimens

- For anticipated mild-to-moderate exercise 1 to 3 hours after eating, reduce your premeal dose of Regular or rapid-acting insulin by approximately 20% to 50%
- For anticipated strenuous exercise over an extended period of time, not only reduce your premeal dose of Regular or rapid-acting insulin by 30% to 50%, but also reduce your long-acting insulin or basal rate by 20% to 50%
- Always test your blood glucose before exercising. Consider testing your blood glucose after exercising, especially if you are developing your mental diary on how exercise affects your diabetes. Testing every 1 to 2 hours during prolonged exercise, and better yet wearing a CGM, may be extremely helpful in avoiding severe hypoglycemia and hyperglycemia, improving your workout
- Always carry something with you to treat a low blood glucose reaction. The day you forget will be the day you get low… Murphy's law!
- If you are a hard-core athlete, definitely joint Team Type 1 (*www.team type1.org*), Insulin Dependence (*www.insulindependence.org*), or other sports-minded diabetes groups for mentorship, advice, and support. These organizations are for the novice athelete as well.
- None of these recommendations is written in stone. You have to do whatever works for you, and sometimes it is trial and error that gives you the most information.

small amount of rapid-acting insulin, depending on the time of your last dose and how sensitive you are to insulin. If your last dose was within 1 or 2 hours, it might be safer to not take any extra insulin. If your blood glucose level is in the low or normal range (less than 120 mg/dL), you should consider taking in some carbohydrates before exercising. Once again, if your last injection was within 1 or 2 hours, it is more likely that your blood glucose level will become low during exercise than if your last injection was given over 5 hours prior to the activity.

Case Presentations of Commonly Used Insulin Regimens

We have discussed a lot of different types of insulin, insulin mixtures, and Symlin. You may begin feeling like there is just too much information! Well, I find when you give some real-world examples, it helps to make everything more clear. For people with type 1 diabetes, there are two main effective regimens, which include the basal/bolus or basal/prandial or multiple daily injection regimen (all names used to describe the same thing) and insulin pump therapy, discussed in detail in *Chapter 9*.

The regimens most commonly used in people with type 2 diabetes are combination therapy (oral agents during the day plus a basal insulin), the split-mixed and premixed regimens, and the basal/prandial approach. I will describe an example of each one to give you an idea of what they entail. Let's start with some type 2 diabetic examples. I'll start by giving the case example and then giving my take on the regimen. Please, note for all you type 2s reading this chapter that the issue of combination therapy is discussed again with a different example in *Chapter 7*.

Combination Therapy: Oral Medications During the Day and a Basal Insulin

Combining medication(s) taken during the day with a single injection of a long-acting insulin at bedtime can be an effective way to achieve 24-hour glucose control. Combination therapy is important because the use of insulin plus daytime medications is a natural extension of daytime medications alone. This regimen was especially attractive when the sulphonylureas (SFUs) were the only oral medications available in the United States and incretin hormones were not yet developed; however, this type of combination should work with any of the oral agents on the market today as well as with Byetta.

This combination therapy is effective in many individuals because the evening insulin works mainly during the night and early morning to improve the fasting or prebreakfast glucose level to normal. When you start off the day with a good blood glucose value, the daytime medications work much better to control the blood glucose value during waking hours.

There are a number of practical reasons why combination therapy can be beneficial. You do not need to learn how to mix different types of insulin, and it is more desirable to be on a single injection of insulin rather than a multiple-injection regimen. In addition, you do not have to carry the insulin with you during the day since you take it only at bedtime. You can also estimate the initial dose and safely start 5 to 10 units of Lantus, Levemir, or NPH insulin if you are not overweight (10 to 15 units if you are overweight) at bedtime (about 10 PM ± 1 to 2 hours). Obviously, you will need to discuss the details of your regimen with your caregiver.

In either case, the dose is increased in 2- to 5-unit increments every 3 to 4 days until the fasting or prebreakfast blood glucose levels are consistently within the 80 to 130 mg/dL range. It is recommended that you remain on your current dose of oral medication(s); however, if the daytime blood glucose level starts to become excessively low, the dose(s) of the daytime medications must be adjusted downward. If this occurs, it is a good indication that combination therapy is successful. Your physician may also instruct you to make your own insulin adjustments using home glucose monitoring (**Table 8-7**). An even simpler method is to increase the dose of insulin by 2 units if the average of the previous three morning values was not under 120 mg/dL.

Daytime Oral Agents and Predinner Premixed Insulin

Another great clinical tool is to take a premixed insulin before

Table 8-7

Instructions for Adding Bedtime Insulin to Daytime Oral Medication(s)[a]

- Start with a dose of __10__ units of NPH/Lantus/Levemir insulin given just before bedtime
- If your morning blood glucose level is higher than 130 mg/dL for more than 3 days in a row, increase the dose of bedtime NPH insulin by __3__ units
- If your morning blood glucose level is less than 80 mg/dL for 2 days in a row, decrease your bedtime NPH dose by __3__ units
- It is extremely important that you not increase your dose of insulin more frequently than every 3 days
- If you have any questions, call your caregiver who prescribed this regimen.

[a] This type of regimen must be prescribed by your caregiver. Do not change or start therapy on your own.

dinner instead of bedtime insulin. A premixed insulin such as Humalog mix 75/25 or Novolog Mix 70/30 has 70% to 75% intermediate-acting insulin, similar to NPH, and 25% to 30% rapid-acting insulin (Humalog or Novolog). Humalog Mix 50/50 is now available as well. In this manner, the premixed insulin will help to control blood glucose immediately after dinner as well as with overnight control. I usually try this regimen when the postdinner and morning blood glucose levels are both consistently too high (**Table 8-8**).

When the fasting blood glucose in the morning is brought under control, the success of combination therapy is dependent upon the ability of the daytime medication(s) to maintain glucose control throughout the day. If this cannot be achieved, some or all of the pills should be stopped and an insulin regimen started.

Case #1: Type 2 Diabetes

John is a 65-year-old Hispanic male with type 2 diabetes for 12 years. When he was first diagnosed, he was on diet and exercise alone but soon after, both glyburide and Glucophage (metformin) were added to get his glucose level under control. This worked for a few years. Later, Actos was added to his regimen, which helped, but his A1C was still above goal at 7.4%. John's home glucose monitoring data showed that his fasting glucose level in the morning was in the mid 200-mg/dL range. His caregiver prescribed 10 units of long-acting basal insulin Levemir at bedtime and slowly increased the dose to 55 units over the next few weeks to get his

Table 8-8

Instructions for Adding Predinner Premixed Insulin to Daytime Oral Medication(s)[a]

- Start with a dose of _1Ø_ units of Humalog Mix 75/25, Humalog Mix 50/50, or Novolog Mix 70/30 given just before dinner

- If your morning blood glucose level is higher than 130 mg/dL for more than 3 days in a row, increase the dose of predinner Humalog Mix 75/25, Humalog Mix 50/50, or Novolog Mix 70/30 by _3_ units

- If your morning blood glucose level is less than 80 mg/dL for 2 days in a row, decrease your predinner Humalog Mix 75/25, Humalog Mix 50/50, or Novolog Mix 70/30 dose by _3_ units

- It is extremely important that you not increase your dose of insulin more frequently than every 3 days

- If you have any questions, call your caregiver who prescribed this regimen

[a] This type of regimen must be prescribed by your caregiver. Do not change or start therapy on your own.

morning blood glucose level in the 80- to 130-mg/dL range. His dose of oral medications was not changed and his A1C eventually came down to 6.5% with no episodes of hypoglycemia and a weight gain of only 3 pounds.

Our Take...

This is a very common scenario in patients with type 2 diabetes. As I mentioned above, most patients with type 2 diabetes will progress to the point that they require insulin therapy. Typically, patients will be on several oral medications but not reaching A1C goals. The initiation of a once-daily insulin injection, typically at night, is an easy transition to get familiar with insulin injections and dosing. One piece of good news is that when you start insulin therapy, it may be possible to come off some of the oral medications you are taking in time. While John and his caregiver chose Levemir for his basal insulin, the other available long-acting insulin is Lantus. There are differences between these insulins so it wise to discuss them with your caregiver. If combination therapy does not get the A1C to goal, it may be necessary to advance the insulin regimen to a split-mixed or basal/bolus strategy, which will be discussed next.

The Split-Mixed/Premixed Regimen

Case #2: Type 2 Diabetes

Brenda is a 47-year-old overweight woman who has had type 2 diabetes since the age of 39. She did not respond well to oral agents and is currently treated with 25 units of NPH and 15 units of Regular before breakfast and 20 units of NPH and 12 units of Regular units before dinner. Her overall glycemic control is poor with an A1C of 8.2%. Her home glucose monitoring records show that her blood glucose is bouncing all over the place from high (over 200 mg/dL) to low (below 60 mg/dL); however, there are two consistent trends: The trends show that her postbreakfast and postdinner blood glucose levels are too high, commonly in the 300 mg/dL range.

Our Take...

She is currently being treated with a split-mixed insulin regimen. This regimen consists of an injection of a combination of NPH and Regular insulin prior to breakfast and dinner. Although this regimen is used quite frequently in type 2 diabetes and rarely in type 1 diabetes, it has some pros and cons when compared to a basal/bolus regimen including:

PROs:
■ Patients with type 2 can occasionally generally get 24 hours of insulin coverage with only two injections.
■ Pre-mixed formulations are available to simplify dosing.
No lunchtime dose is required; however, with a large lunch, the afternoon glucose values may be higher than desired *(see below)*.

CONs:
■ As there is no Regular or rapid-acting insulin given for lunch, hyperglycemia is not uncommon in the early afternoon.
■ The morning NPH peaks 6 to 8 hours after injection, leading to hypoglycemia in the late afternoon, especially if the midday meal is light or is missed.
■ The NPH given before dinner usually peaks in the early morning, leading to hypoglycemia during the night (1 am to 3 am).
■ Since the evening NPH is given before dinner (around 6 pm to 7 pm), it loses effectiveness by the next morning, and it is not uncommon to have persistent prebreakfast hyperglycemia or high blood glucose.

Brenda's main problem was high postmeal glucose values. She was switched to the mixture that contained the rapid-acting analogue Novolog (Novolog Mix 70/30) to help improve her postbreakfast and postdinner blood glucose level. She also reduced the calorie content of her midday meal so that her postlunch blood glucose value was improved. After the changes, she noticed:

1. Her postmeal glucose level improved tremendously.
2. She enjoyed a little more flexibility in the timing of her insulin dose since the rapid-acting insulin analogue given before or soon after the meal have the same results in glucose control.

Brenda's A1C value came down to 7.1% about 5 months after making the changes. She loved the convenience of the Novolog Mix 70/30 FlexPen. Her A1C drifted below 7.0% over the next 6 months with no changes in her weight.

The Basal/Bolus or Basal/Prandial Regimen

Case #3: Type 2 Diabetes
Sandy is a 50-year-old, obese woman who has had type 2 diabetes for the past 5 years. She originally was treated with a split-mixed regi-

men but was changed to a basal/bolus regimen several years ago when she started to work the graveyard shift (11 PM to 7 AM) as a surgical nurse. Her daily schedule consists of going home after work and going straight to bed until 1 PM or 2 PM without eating anything. She then has a regular type of lunch consisting of a sandwich or salad. Her dinner is normally at 8 PM every night with her husband. She has breakfast at the hospital during one of her breaks between 4 AM and 6 AM, although this eating time is variable since emergency surgeries are not predictable.

Sandy's regimen has changed through the years but currently consists of 25 units of the basal insulin Levemir given at around 8 AM before she goes to sleep, with a few units of Novolog only if her glucose level is high (above 180 mg/dL). She also takes 15 units of Levemir at dinner (8 PM) along with her Novolog dose, according to her premeal blood glucose value (insulin algorithm). She gives herself small boluses (about 8 to 15 units) of Novolog before breakfast, lunch, dinner, and other small snacks. She does pretty well adjusting her dose and does not use carbohydrate counting. She loves the Novolog and Levemir Flex pens, which make her daily life with diabetes easier. One year ago, Sandy started Symlin as her postmeal value was difficult to get below 200 mg/dL and she was well over her ideal body weight. She eventually got her A1C below 7% and lost a significant amount of weight (13 to 15 lb) at the same time.

Our Take...

Sandy's regimen is a great example of a custom-fit insulin regimen. Her basal/bolus regimen is designed to fit her schedule. She has a good baseline insulin dose with long-acting Levemir given about 12 hours apart and the rapid-acting insulin analogue Novolog given before each meal. She has the freedom to eat her meals at any time that is convenient for her. She also has the freedom to skip meals, provided she checks her blood glucose value to make sure it is not too low or too high. A good baseline insulin dose should not allow your value to get too low or too high, even if you do not eat. If your blood glucose level gets too low in the fasting state, your long-acting insulin dose is too high and must be adjusted. On the other hand, if your glucose value goes too high in the fasting state, your long-acting insulin dose needs to be increased. This case also shows how the addition of Symlin to your insulin regimen can help you get that extra little help you need to get your A1C to goal while potentially helping you lose weight.

The Basal/Bolus or Basal/Prandial Regimen in Type 1 Diabetes

Case #4: Type 1 Diabetes

Kirk is a 45-year old man who has had type 1 diabetes for 22 years. He is a construction worker and sometimes has a problem with consistent meal times and doing regular exercise. Many years ago, he was switched from NPH twice a day to Lantus 25 units at bedtime and he is also on the rapid-acting analogue Apidra, given before meals. He learned to count his carbohydrates and his ratio is 15:1 (for every 15 grams of carbohydrates consumed he takes 1 unit of Apidra) and his correction factor is 1:50 (for every 50 mg/dL he is above his goal of 120 mg/dL, he will take an extra 1 unit of Apidra). He adjusts his Lantus dose based on his morning glucose value and his Apidra dose is based on his postmeal glucose value. He is also on Symlin 60 mcg with each major meal. His A1C has been in the low 7% range with 1 to 2 hypoglycemic reactions a week. He recently got a Dexcom continuous glucose monitor (see *Chapter 12*), which has allowed him to fine-tune his regimen and reduce his A1C to 6.7%, in addition to almost eliminating completely his low blood glucose reactions.

Our Take...

The basal/prandial regimen is the most physiologic regimen, in addition to insulin pump therapy. The basic concept is to try and mimic the normal insulin secretory pattern of a nondiabetic. The pancreas of a normal nondiabetic secretes a little bit of insulin all the time (basal rate), even in the fasting state, and puts out little squirts or boluses for every meal. Lantus and Levemir are basal insulins that have been chemically altered to be longer acting, similar to any sustained-release medication.

Finally, most insurance companies are approving CGM devices for people with type 1 diabetes. There is sometimes resistance but it is a battle worth fighting! The information these devices provide can make it easier to determine your basal and bolus doses. This technology is also available for type 2 diabetics, but currently it is much more difficult to get insurance to cover it (see the *Chapter 12*).

Insulin Pump Therapy

Case #5: Type 1 Diabetes

Mary is a 22-year-old female with type 1 diabetes since the age of 5. She has been on insulin pump therapy using Humalog for the past several years and loves the freedom it gives her in terms of the ease of boluses and controlling her blood glucose values overnight. Her basal rate is set at 0.7 units an hour except between the hours of 3 AM to 8 AM, when it automatically goes up to 1.0 units per hour.

Our Take...

This increase in her basal rate of insulin is to counteract the dawn phenomenon (see *Chapter 9* and *Chapter 12* on pump therapy and CGM for more details of pump therapy and the dawn phenomenon). One real benefit of pump therapy is the ability to change your basal rate during the day. Once-daily Lantus is nice, but the dose is constant during the day. With a pump, you can increase the basal rate during the morning when most of us require a little more insulin. Her carbohydrate-to-insulin ratio is 20:1, and her correction factor is 1:60. She is obviously more sensitive to insulin than Kirk. She also uses CGM, which helps her prevent her blood glucose level from going too low at night, especially important since she lives alone.

Summary

Designing an insulin regimen that fits your lifestyle is important for achieving and maintaining glycemic control (**Table 8-9**). To do this successfully, you must have a basic understanding of the time course of action of the different insulins, as well as know the benefits of Symlin. You must also not only perform home glucose monitoring at the appropriate times and strongly consider CGM, but you must also be well informed on how to respond to your glucose values. The use of an insulin algorithm or correction factor is vital to make the day-to-day decisions in your treatment plan as well as making long-term adjustments. Every dose of premeal insulin must be guesstimated, keeping several facts in mind, including the premeal glucose value, amounts and types of food (carbohydrates) to be ingested, and anticipated exercise. With experience and time, you will develop mental diaries and insulin menus of how certain types of meals and exercise routines affect your diabetes. You will be able to use this information in addition to carbohydrate counting to come up with the best guesstimate of what insulin dose should be given at any particular time or in any situation. Eventually, adjusting your daily insulin regimen will be as easy and routine as brushing your teeth. You have the ability to have a flexible lifestyle while achieving excellent glycemic control on insulin. Being educated and motivated to work with your caregiver to design the perfect insulin regimen for you is the key. We now have many new insulins and Symlin to choose from, and with the advent of continuous glucose monitoring, excellent control with minimal hypoglycemia is easily possible.

Table 8-9

Insulin Regimens Commonly Utilized

Type 1 Diabetes
- Basal/bolus regimen (also called basal/prandial)
- Insulin pump therapy

Type 2 Diabetes
- Combination therapy (oral agents during the day in addition to a basal insulin)
- Premixed or free-mixed regimen (intermediate-acting and rapid-acting insulin given 2 or 3 times a day)
- Basal/bolus regimen
- Insulin pump therapy

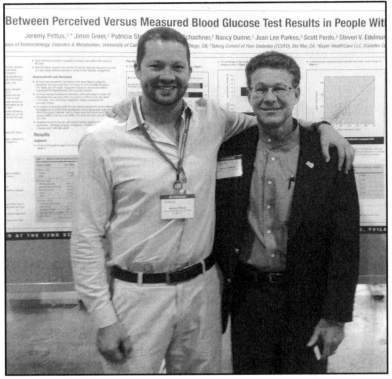

Dr. Jeremy Pettus with Steve Edelman presenting our data at a diabetes conference

9

Today's New and Improving Insulin Pumps

by John Walsh, PA and Ruth Roberts, MA

Introduction

The use of insulin pumps has risen dramatically over the last 30 years to nearly a million people worldwide. These numbers grow as pump, continuous glucose monitor (CGM), and closed-loop technologies, along with their benefits for control, continue to evolve.

Enthusiastic pump wearers of all ages propel this growth when they share their experiences with others. A pump is often seen as a turning point in diabetes care. People say "For the first time in years, I can eat when I want to," or "I can really control my blood sugar now and I feel better, too."

Benefits include fewer injections, the ability to easily give insulin for spontaneous events, and quicker insulin adjustments when your eating or activity changes. A pump uses only a rapid-acting insulin and eliminates the large depot of long-acting insulin that may absorb differently from day to day as temperature or activity changes.

A pump offers convenience, more consistent insulin action from day to day, easier problem solving, easier tracking of insulin use, less hypoglycemia, less risk of hypoglycemia unawareness, and fewer morning and postmeal highs. A built-in bolus calculator (BC) uses personalized settings to make bolus doses more accurate and less likely to cause insulin stacking from prior boluses. The pump keeps a history of insulin doses and glucose readings for a handy record that helps the wearer and their physician assess control issues.

Pump features include:
- A BC with settings for a carb factor, correction factor, target glucose, and duration of insulin action
- An integrated glucose meter, as well as a CGM display in some pumps
- Carb-counting aids
- Tracking of bolus on board (BOB) to reduce insulin stacking

- An accurate history of actual insulin usage (basal/carb bolus balance, correction bolus percentage, etc) and glucose values
- Helpful reminders and alerts.

With training and support, an insulin pump helps a person feel better, live more freely, and have fewer diabetes-related health problems. This is especially true when a pump's precise insulin delivery is paired with feedback from a CGM. A CGM helps prevent highs and lows, and lets the wearer see where problems arise. The results of undercounting carbs, late boluses, overtreatment of lows, and being on too little or too much insulin can be quickly seen in CGM trend lines (**Figure 9-1**).

As the reliability and accuracy of CGMs continue to improve, glucose readings will eventually be directly entered into the pump for basal and bolus adjustments, resulting eventually in an artificial pancreas. Although full integration of pumps and CGMs will take time, early features, such as stopping basal insulin delivery for a period of time when the glucose is going low and combining the delivery of insulin plus glucagon in a dual-chamber pump to automate glucose control, are starting to appear.

Figure 9-1
Line Pump

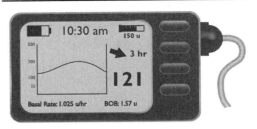

This demo insulin pump shows CGM reading, glucose trend line, battery life, time, units of insulin left in the reservoir, current basal rate, and how many units of bolus on board (BOB) are still lowering the glucose.

Diabetes devices are evolving with improved control procedures, better CGM integration, smaller sizes, color screens, more infusion set choices, faster insulin analogues, trend analysis, and pattern recognition. The Medtronic pump displays CGM results on the pump screen. A new and more accurate Dexcom CGM will soon be integrated into Animas, Accu-Chek, OmniPod, and Tandem pumps to allow them to display CGM readings in a single device.

Today's insulin pumps help wearers manage the complex interactions between insulin levels, glucose, and carbs with less effort (**Table 9-1**).

Benefits of a Pump
Better Control and More Stable Readings

Research studies show that people on pumps have lower A1C values, less hypoglycemia, and more stable glucose readings compared with people using multiple daily injections.[1-7] In one study of 225 pumpers, severe hypoglycemia dropped from 138 events for every 100 years in the previous year on MDI to 22 per 100 years in the first year of pump use and throughout this 4-year study.[8]

A pump's precise insulin dosing usually gives the wearer fewer lows overall and less rapid declines in glucose. Consequently, the wearer has more time to recognize symptoms and consume carbs.[9] By avoiding frequent lows, stress hormone levels can be rebuilt and enable stronger and earlier hypoglycemia symptoms the next time the glucose goes low.

Hypoglycemia unawareness occurs when someone is no longer aware that they are going low. Symptoms become so reduced by frequent low readings that thinking is already severely impaired before symptoms begin. This is more common in those who have had diabetes for many years, especially when excessive insulin doses and frequent lows have depleted typical stress responses. It becomes especially dangerous if no one else is around to help.

Nighttime is especially problematic since many undetected lows and most episodes of hypoglycemia unawareness occur during sleep. A pump helps, because it can be programmed to deliver nighttime basal rates that better match a person's real need. A CGM used day and night with a pump stops many low blood sugar levels by tracking glucose trends and alarming when the glucose crosses a low or high glucose threshold, or if the glucose is falling or rising faster than desired. Prevention of nighttime lows usually allows a pump wearer to again sense their daytime lows.[10]

Table 9-1
Insulin Delivery with an Insulin Pump

Basal—a continuous 24-hour delivery that matches background insulin need. The basal is given as units per hour, ranges between 0.3 and 2.0 units per hour for most pumpers. Basal rates usually make up about half of the total daily dose (TDD) of insulin.

Carb Bolus—a spurt of insulin delivered quickly to match the carbohydrates in a meal or snack. Most pumpers use 1 unit per 4 to 20 grams of carb.

Correction Bolus—a spurt of insulin designed to bring a high glucose back to target. For most pumpers, 1 unit lowers the blood glucose between 15 and 120 mg/dL (1 to 6.7 mmol/L)

Convenient Dosing

Daily work or school hours can vary, events pop up, and meals be delayed or missed from day to day. On weekends, you may want to rise early or sleep late and be more or less active at different times of the day. Larger family or holiday meals and late dining are easier to manage. Insulin doses from a pump can be more easily adapted to life's variety. Plus, you no longer need to carry an insulin vial and syringe or an insulin pen to give insulin at a restaurant, or go to a public rest room to give an injection.

More Precise Bolus Doses

Precision is important for most insulin users, but benefiting the most are adults and children who use so little insulin per day that one unit lowers their glucose by 100 mg/dL (5.6 mmol/L) or more. Even a small dose miscalculation can spell disaster. A pump's precise delivery often gives those who use less than 35 to 40 units a day more stable glucose levels.

Easier Problem Solving

If a glucose goes high or low on injections, it is difficult to determine whether the long-acting insulin is peaking erratically, or a rapid-acting insulin dose was the wrong amount or given at the wrong time. On a pump, you simply test and adjust basal delivery until it keeps your glucose steady when you are not eating. Once the basal rate has been tuned, any high or low reading after meals suggests that the carb amount and carb bolus was the cause. The carb factor or carb count is then adjusted to keep the glucose controlled after meals with a minimum of lows and highs.

A pump's history helps you and your doctor know exactly how much insulin you use each day and helps identify where control problems may arise. Basal/carb bolus imbalances are easy to identify. All these make troubleshooting easier. Once you know your average insulin total daily dose (TDD), you and your doctor can select more accurate pump settings for better readings. The 5th edition of *Pumping Insulin* (2012, Torrey Pines Press) shows how to use your TDD to select accurate pump settings.

Pump Choices

Pump wearers can choose between standard infusion set (line) pumps or patch pumps (**Figure 9-2**).

Infusion Set (Line) Pumps

Powered by a rechargeable battery, or by AA or AAA batteries, a line pump is a pager-sized device that delivers insulin via tubing to an infusion set on the skin. Some current line pump manufacturers include Animas, Accu-Chek, Medtronic, Sooil, Tandem, and soon Asante (**Figure 9-3**).

New line pumps include Tandem's small 300-unit t:slim pump that has an eye-popping iPhonelike touch screen, a precise pressure motor, and an easy-to-program interface (**Figure 9-3**). The t:slim allows all pump programming to be done from a single screen.

Another California company, Asante, will release its Pearl pump in 2013 (**Figure 9-3**). The Pearl uses prefilled 300-unit insulin pen cartridges to eliminate the preparation and filling of reservoirs, rewinding the pump motor, and tap-

Figure 9-2
Insulin Pump Choices: Infusion Set or Patch

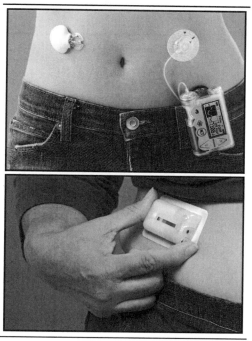

Medtronic MiniMed Paradigm Real-Time Revel is an example of an infusion set (line) insulin pump *(top)*. The V-Go by Valeritas is a disposable, spring-driven patch pump *(bottom)*.

ping for air bubbles. Priming of the infusion line is done automatically. Small, sleek, and lightweight, the Pearl uses a novel method to detect occlusions and has an easy-to-read screen.

A third line pump made by Cellnovo will be available first in Europe (**Figure 9-3**). Designed with a unique wax motor, this very small 200-unit pump weighs only 1.2 ounces when filled with insulin. This allows it to be attached to the skin near an infusion site. Its communication system operates over a secure, dedicated phone line that allows users to transfer glucose data to a central database where it can be rapidly accessed by health care professionals or others with whom the wearer wants to share their data.

Figure 9-3
Today's Insulin Pumps Offer Variety

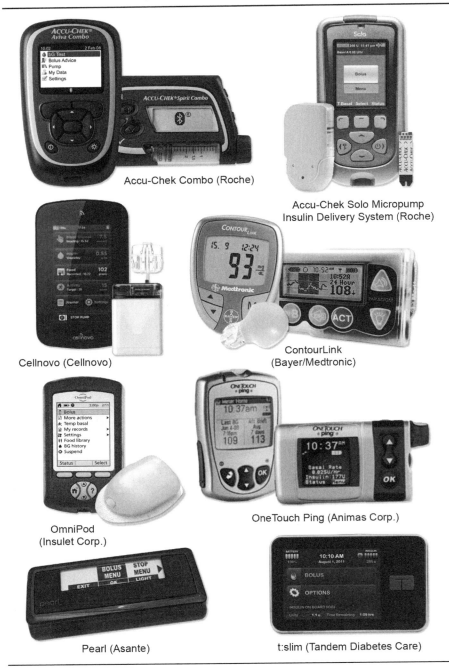

Accu-Chek Combo (Roche)

Accu-Chek Solo Micropump
Insulin Delivery System (Roche)

Cellnovo (Cellnovo)

ContourLink
(Bayer/Medtronic)

OmniPod
(Insulet Corp.)

OneTouch Ping (Animas Corp.)

Pearl (Asante)

t:slim (Tandem Diabetes Care)

Photos provided as a courtesy by Animas, Asante, Bayer, Cellnovo, Insulet,
Medtronic, Roche, and Tandem; manufacturers of insulin pumps.

Infusion Sets

At least 15 varieties of infusion sets are available with numerous connections and catheter and line lengths. With a smaller size compared with patch pumps, infusion sets can be placed on more body areas. Both Teflon and metal needles are available. Metal needles are comfortable, have the lowest profile on the skin, and tend to have the highest reliability. A super short 1.5-mm microneedle is currently in development by Becton Dickinson that is expected to speed up insulin action. Both Teflon and metal needles tend to be more reliable and last longer when the wearer routinely anchors the infusion line with tape. Anchoring the line near the infusion set stops most leaking and dislodgement that can cause unexplained highs and even ketoacidosis.

Patch Pumps

Patch pumps have a pod with an insulin reservoir and motor that attach directly to the skin, and usually have a separate controller. Patch pumps require more skin area and this reduces site options. They do not have an infusion line, which is the most vulnerable part of a standard pump. Even so, insulin leaks and detachment can occur with patch pumps, as well as kinking of the Teflon catheter during insertion, similar to what can happen when an autoinserter is used to place a standard infusion set.

The OmniPod was the first patch pump that provided automatic insertion and priming of a small cannula for insulin delivery (**Figure 9-3**). The pod, batteries, motor, and electronics are replaced every 48 to 72 hours. The current OmniPod requires a separate controller to give boluses. The wearer needs to keep the controller or an insulin pen with them at all times to give boluses.

Other patch pumps, like the Accu-Chek Solo and another by Medtronic, available sometime in 2013, will have bolus buttons on the pod itself so manual boluses can be given if the controller is left behind (**Figure 9-3**). Newer patch pumps will have a reusable modular design where the motor and electronics are used for 3 to 6 months rather than being discarded every 3 days. If a modular patch pump is dislodged, only the base cradle needs to be replaced resulting in additional savings in electronics and insulin.

Two simpler patch pumps have also been developed that use buttons on the device to deliver bolus doses and do not require a separate controller. One from Valeritas, called the V-Go (**Figure 9-2**), is a simple, disposable, spring-driven patch pump for adults with type 2 diabetes. The V-Go is replaced daily and offers basal delivery choices of

20, 30, or 40 units a day (0.83 U/hr, 1.25 U/hr or 1.67 U/hr, respectively), with a 2-unit manual bolus increment that can deliver up to 36 units of bolus insulin a day to cover meals and high glucose readings.

A second inexpensive patch pen not yet available, called Finesse, was developed by a California company called Calibra and later purchased by Lifescan (Animas). This bolus-only manual pump can switch between 1 or 2 unit bolus increments per button push. It holds 200 units and provides a convenient bolusing option for people with type 1 or type 2 diabetes who use a long-acting insulin.

Pump Features

Training before and after a pump is started is necessary to understand and benefit from all the pump features that are listed below. Read your pump manual carefully, work with your health care professionals, and talk with other pumpers for the best results.

Bolus Calculator

The pump BC allows bolus recommendations to match the carbs you eat, bring down high readings, and minimize insulin stacking.

For optimal glucose results, these BC settings are adjusted:
- Basal rates
- Carb factor (CarbF)
- Correction factor (CorrF)
- Correction target or target range
- Duration of insulin action (DIA).

The pump BC uses these settings and its internal logic, plus a carb count and glucose reading from the wearer, to recommend accurate bolus doses. There are, however, some differences in how pumps calculate bolus doses. All BCs count carb boluses and correction boluses as *bolus on board* (BOB, *discussed below*), except the 2012 and earlier Omnipods that do not include carb boluses in BOB.

However, most current BCs do not subtract excess BOB from carb boluses. This can cause excessive bolus recommendations in some situations, such as when someone wants to eat carbs at bedtime, but they have BOB with a relatively normal glucose reading. It is important to know how your pump handles active insulin or BOB when boluses are given. This is detailed in the 5th edition of *Pumping Insulin*.

Dr. Irl Hirsch at the University of Washington suggests that the BC bolus recommendation may need to be overridden as often as 25% of the time to give a more appropriate bolus in light of circumstances the wearer knows, but the pump does not. Recommended bolus doses can usually be more accurately adjusted by a pumper when they wear a CGM that shows their glucose trend.

Basal Insulin and Basal Rates

Basal rates from a pump provide an around-the-clock delivery of rapid-acting insulin that replaces the long-acting insulin doses taken by those on injections. The major role for basal rates is to stop the liver from making and releasing excess glucose into the bloodstream. Different pumps can change basal delivery every 1 to 30 minutes in increments as small as 0.01 to 0.025 unit per hour.

Accurate basal rates keep glucose readings level overnight or when meals are skipped during the day. When someone has their basal rates set correctly, their glucose will rise or fall no more than 30 mg/dL (1.7 mmol) during 8 hours of sleep or during any 5-hour period of fasting while they are awake.

Basal rates usually make up about 50% of the TDD of insulin.[11,12] Effective basal rates rarely fall below 40% and occasionally rise above 60% of the TDD. Carb boluses make up most of the remainder, with a small percentage of the TDD, usually less than 9%, used for correction boluses.

Many teens and adults require a higher basal rate in the predawn hours to counteract a natural increase in growth hormone production that starts about 3 AM each day. This normal rise in glucose production is called the dawn phenomenon. If no extra insulin is provided, the glucose will rise and be high when the person wakes up. As a person approaches middle age, the dawn phenomenon often declines or disappears entirely.

To accommodate changes in basal need, pumps provide *temporary basal rates* that can be increased or decreased in 1% to 10% increments for 1 to 72 hours as needed for illness, exercise, or other situations. Temporary rates can be increased to handle occasional illnesses or decreased during and after long periods of exercise or activity.

Most pumps also allow for *alternate basal profiles* to be entered into a pump. Someone wearing a pump can also switch between alternate basal profiles if their insulin needs differ on weekends vs weekdays, or on several days a month during menses for women. Alternate basal profiles can be especially helpful for people whose activities vary from day to day.

Alternate basal profiles currently adjust only basal rates, not the CarbF and CorrF that accompanies the basal profile. Future pumps may allow carb and correction factors to be adjusted in tandem with the basal profile.

Boluses

Boluses are short spurts of insulin given to cover the carbs in meals and snacks and to lower any high readings that may occur. Unlike basal rates, boluses are not programmed ahead of time but are given in the appropriate amount when they are needed. Once a pump BC is programmed with a carb factor and a correction factor by the user and health care provider, the user simply enters how many carbs they plan to eat and their current glucose. The bolus recommendation from the BC can always be adjusted by the wearer as needed for exercise, illness, or stress.

Carb Boluses

The more carbs in a meal or snack, the larger a carb bolus needs to be. Accurate carb counting or a very consistent diet is critical to obtain accurate bolus doses. Although carbs are the primary reason that the glucose rises after a meal, meals with large amounts of protein or fat may require larger bolus doses or a combo bolus.

A personal CarbF programmed into the pump makes carb coverage easier and more accurate. The CarbF determines the size of the bolus that will be recommended for the grams of carb in a meal. Calculated with the help of your health care provider, *a CarbF is how many grams of carb 1 unit of insulin will cover.* Like basal rates, the CarbF can be adjusted as needed to improve control, and different CarbFs can be entered for different times of the day. The pump divides the total carbs in a meal or snack by the CarbF to determine the carb bolus it recommends for the food. Some pumps offer a built-in carb database to simplify carb counting.

Carb Bolus Types

With a standard carb bolus, all of the bolus is given over a short period of time. A pump is also flexible and can also delay some or all of its bolus delivery to accommodate low glycemic index or high-fat meals. Combo or extended boluses can be used with medications like Symlin (pramlintide) or GLP-1 inhibitors like Byetta (exenatide) that delay food. They are also helpful when digestion has been slowed by gastroparesis.

A combination or dual-wave bolus gives some of the bolus now and the rest over time, while an extended or square-wave bolus is like a temp basal increase where all of the bolus is given over a period of time.

For example, a combo bolus may best match the digestion of specific foods with part of the bolus given immediately and the rest over the next 90 or 120 minutes.

Carb Bolus Timing

Even on an insulin pump, insulin action is still relatively slow. Carb boluses are not delivered directly into the blood like the insulin delivery from a pancreas. Instead, the pump infuses insulin into fat below the skin from where it is gradually absorbed into the bloodstream.

This delay in uptake means that carb boluses have to be given well before a meal begins to have their best effect. *Boluses are ideally given 15 to 20 minutes before eating for better postmeal glucose levels unless the glucose is low.* When carbs are accurately counted and matched with a premeal bolus using an accurate CarbF, the postmeal glucose will ideally rise no more than 40 to 80 mg/dL (2.2 to 4.4 mmol) and return to the target glucose within 4 to 5 hours.

If a meal bolus is given right before eating for convenience, the glucose often spikes after the meal and raises A1C levels. This spiking can easily be seen on a CGM. Faster insulins are under development that may eventually better match the digestion times typically seen with carbs. This would allow boluses to be given closer to meal time with less risk of delayed hypoglycemia.

Correction Boluses

Someone with a normal pancreas and counterregulatory system never sees a high or low glucose reading. With diabetes, a high glucose level will occur whenever there is a deficit in a basal rate or a carb bolus dose. Other things like menses, stress, pain, or infection can also cause high readings. Even those with excellent glucose levels average about two correction boluses a day.[12]

The higher the glucose, the larger the correction bolus that will be needed to bring it down. *A CorrF, called an insulin sensitivity factor (or ISF in some pumps) is how many points the glucose will fall per unit of insulin.* It is used to determine how much bolus insulin to take to bring a high reading down to target without going low. Once the CorrF is programmed into a pump BC, correction boluses will be automatically calculated, with reductions made as needed for any active BOB (**Table 9-2**).

The infusion set and pump should be thoroughly checked for leaks anytime there is an unusual or unexplained high glucose. If an infusion site failure or mechanical problem causes a high glucose level, a correction dose should be given by syringe or insulin pen to ensure delivery. Always take action to lower your glucose before getting involved in troubleshooting the pump.

Glucose Target

A glucose correction target or target range is the target to which you want your glucose brought down. It can be entered into the pump BC as a single target for the entire day or as a different target for each meal and at bedtime.

Your correction target differs from the wider glucose goal range in which you would like your glucose to stay. Your correction target is used by your pump BC to calculate the bolus dose you need to reach this glucose 4 to 5 hours later. For example, if a reading of 140 mg/dL (7.8 mmol) is desired

Table 9-2

Today's Pumps Excel at Stable, In-Target Glucose Levels

- Precise insulin delivery allows most pumpers to achieve glucoses within an acceptable target range most of the time. If you use a smart pump and your glucose often goes too high or too low, your TDD, basal rates, carb factor, correction factor, or duration of insulin action can be changed to better fit your needs

- Never accept a high A1C or erratic glucoses on a pump. A pump should deliver excellent overall results. If it does not, modify your lifestyle or work with your health care professional to tweak your pump settings until it does

near bedtime at 10 PM, this target would be set in the pump by 5 PM to allow time for the pump to achieve this goal. If you select a wide range for your correction target, your pump BC's aim becomes less precise. A single correction target like 110 mg/dL (6.1 mmol/L) or a narrow range is preferred.

Duration of Insulin Action

The DIA or duration of insulin action is how long a bolus lowers the glucose. An accurate DIA must be entered in the pump to prevent insulin stacking when boluses are given close together. Stacking can occur any time a previous carb and correction bolus is still lowering your glucose when a new bolus is given. An accurate DIA time allows the BC to properly calculate subsequent carb and correction boluses once the first bolus of the day has been given.

It takes a minimum of 4 to 6 hours for all of the glucose-lowering activity of a recent bolus of rapid-acting insulin to stop lowering the glucose. Insulin has little effect on the glucose for the first 15 to 20 minutes, reaches a halfway point in activity at just over 2 hours, and has the other half of activity tail off over about 5 to 6 hours after the bolus is given.

Today's pumps allow the user to select a wide range of times for the DIA with possible settings between 1.5 and 8 hours in most pumps. This wide range is designed to handle faster, genetically engineered insulins that may appear in the future, as well as older Regular insulin. However, this range is far wider than the action time for the rapid-acting insulins currently in use. Every pump comes with a default setting for DIA. This default setting can often be changed to a more effective and sometimes safer setting.

An appropriate DIA setting for today's insulins (Novolog [aspart], Apidra [glulisine], and Humalog [lispro]) is between 5 and 6 hours.[13-18] A DIA time shorter than this will hide bolus insulin activity and hide insulin stacking. *Pumping Insulin* has a full discussion of how to avoid hidden insulin stacking.

Bolus on Board

Frequent boluses are easy to give on a pump, but this can also lead to insulin stacking of BOB. *BOB is the insulin that remains active from one or more recent boluses.* When a carb bolus is given for dinner, another for an unplanned dessert, and then a correction bolus is needed for the high reading that follows, the resulting insulin pileup or stacking can make it difficult to determine the amount of bolus insulin remaining in the body at bedtime. This is critical when deciding whether you need more insulin to cover a high reading, or whether you need to eat carbs to prevent your glucose from going low.

When a high glucose reading is entered into the pump before giving a correction bolus, pump BCs take into account the current BOB (insulin on board or active insulin) to prevent insulin stacking. This is especially helpful for those who live alone, those who have hypoglycemia unawareness, and those with a history of frequent lows.

Unfortunately, the pump user still has to know whether and how their pump subtracts BOB from carb boluses when the pump BC makes its bolus recommendations. In some situations, this will prevent getting too large a bolus. For instance, a high bedtime reading may require no correction bolus if enough BOB remains to bring the glucose down, while a glucose near your target at bedtime may be dangerous if you do not account for any BOB that is still active.

When the current glucose reading is entered into the pump or, even better, sent automatically from a glucose meter, the pump BC can reduce the bolus recommendation to avoid insulin stacking from bolus insulin on board. Today's insulins lower the glucose for 4.5 to 6 hours after a bolus. To accurately measure BOB, the DIA time must be correctly set in the pump.

Reminders and Alerts for Safety

Reminders and alerts on pumps can be customized for safety and to improve control. For instance, a postmeal reminder can be set to recheck your blood glucose 1.5 or 2 hours after a bolus has been given. Postmeal testing lets you evaluate the meal bolus. You may need extra carbs to prevent a low or a correction bolus, because the meal bolus was too small. Postmeal testing helps prevent lows and speeds correction of highs.

Reminders can also be set to ensure that boluses are given at specific times of the day. Some pumps can be set to sound an alarm if no bolus is given at the usual time, such as between 11:45 AM and 12:30 PM for lunch. If a bolus dose was started but never completed due to a distraction, a helpful pump would alert the wearer that they never completed the bolus. Another reminder can sometimes be set to remind the user to retest their glucose 15 to 30 minutes after a low glucose level to ensure that the treatment corrected the low reading or 90 minutes to 2 hours after a high reading to ensure a correction bolus is working. Helpful reminders like these minimize human error and improve control.

An auto-off feature can be a lifesaver for those who travel or live alone. When auto-off is activated, the pump turns itself off if one of the pump buttons has not been pressed within a determined amount of time, such as 8 or 9 hours overnight. This protects against the continuation of basal insulin delivery if the wearer becomes incapacitated due to hypoglycemia. Read your pump manual to learn about the options it offers.

Basal/Bolus Balance and Correction-Bolus Tracking

Basal and bolus doses have to be balanced for optimum control. The pump wearer's basal/bolus balance can be calculated manually from the average insulin doses given over several days or may be calculated by the pump itself and shown in a history screen. This lets you see how your insulin is used and can help spot causes for any problems that may arise. For adults with type 1 diabetes, glucose control is usually best when basal insulin delivery makes up 40% to 65% of the TDD. If control problems occur, the pump's memory can be quickly checked to determine the percentage of the TDD currently used for basal rates, carb boluses, and correction boluses. Many diabetes clinicians check basal/bolus balance at each clinic visit because it gives helpful insight for improving control.

Some pumps track correction bolus doses to determine how much correction bolus insulin has been used over the last 2 to 30 days to bring down high readings. Correction boluses usually make up less than 9% of the TDD. If more than 9% of the TDD is used to bring down high readings, the basal rates or carb bolus doses need to be increased.

Pump-Meter Combos

Many pumps have an associated meter that sends glucose readings directly into the pump for convenience and helps the pump calculate an accurate correction bolus to prevent insulin stacking. Direct entry ensures accurate data entry, reduces human error, speeds bolus calculations, and guarantees that every glucose reading is used by the BC to suggest appropriate boluses after accounting for BOB. If your meter does not automatically enter readings into your pump or you use more than one meter, be sure to enter a test each time it is taken. Only when you enter your glucose into your pump will it account for BOB in its bolus recommendations.

Choosing a Pump and Infusion Set

When choosing a pump, take the time you need to make a good choice. You will depend on this pump for 4 to 5 years, so discuss different pumps and pump options with your doctor and health care team to select the features that will be most helpful.

Ask local pump representatives to demonstrate their pumps. Ask lots of questions and discuss the advantages of each pump and assess the support provided. Look for a pump support group or go to a diabetes conference where pumpers are discussing their pumps and pump vendors are showing their products. This may take some time, but you will be better informed and able to make a better decision.

The pump company will prepare the paperwork to submit to your insurance carrier or Medicare to cover their share of the pump and supplies and can help you deal with any insurance questions.

Things to Consider for Insulin Pumps

Insulin pumps differ in their features and ease of use. Your needs may make one pump a better choice than another. When selecting a pump, consider the following:

1. What appeals to you about the pump? Look, feel, and color, features, accessories?

2. How easy is the pump to program and use? Is the screen easy to see?
3. How easy are the buttons to push? A bolus should be easy to deliver, but giving a bolus accidentally while gesturing, reaching into a pocket, or displaying the pump to inquisitive friends should not.
4. What reminders and alarms does the pump have?
5. How finely can basal rates be programmed for children and insulin-sensitive adults who require low basal rates? How often does basal delivery occur?
6. How easy is it to stop a bolus?
7. Can you hear or feel the alarms? Will you know if your insulin delivery has stopped?
8. How much information is stored in the pump's memory? How easy is it to access? This is important if you get distracted and forget to give a bolus, if you want to check on your current BOB or active insulin, or if a parent wants to verify bolus delivery by a child.
9. If required, can the pump survive rough use? Is the pump waterproof? Is it easy to disconnect before showering or swimming?
10. How many infusion sets can the pump connect with?
11. With patch pumps, will the adhesive keep it from being knocked off? Can you bolus if you forget your controller?
12. What level of customer service is provided by the manufacturer? 24-hour telephone support? Assistance with insurance coverage? Warranty? Ease of upgrading to a newer pump? Trial period? Shipment of temporary supplies to different addresses? How soon will a replacement arrive if needed?

Things to Consider for Infusion Sets and Patch Pumps

Using an infusion set that works well is one of the more important steps in making your pump experience successful. Having a secure attachment of the infusion set or pod is the most important link for successful pumping. If a particular set causes skin irritation, falls off when swimming or sweating, or is easily dislodged, problems with your control will occur. For infants and young children with diabetes, and during pregnancy, metal infusion sets are preferred for their reliability and ease of use.

For success with a pump, the attachment of infusion sets or pods must be secure and comfortable. When selecting an infusion set, consider:
1. How much body fat do you have?

2. Which sites on your body are best to use?
3. Does your belt or clothing choices limit wearing a set near the waist?
4. Does your activity level limit you to certain sites?
5. Which type and size infusion set will work best for the body locations you prefer?
6. Is disconnection easy? Does it disconnect right at the infusion site or have a connector that is located a few inches away?
7. Will you need an insertion device for this infusion set?
8. Straight-in metal sets have the smallest guages and are easiest to insert, even using only one hand. Slanted Teflon sets may be more reliable for some users than straight-in Teflon sets. Auto-inserters can introduce some problems of their own, but they tend to work best with straight-in Teflon sets.
9. Unless you experience leaking or control problems, the shortest metal needle or Teflon catheter lengths usually work best. If infusion set problems arise, make sure to anchor the infusion line with tape. If you are doing this already, try a different type of insulin set. Discuss your options with your health care professional.

Most infusion sets are reliable and work well. However, problems with a particular set, like a tendency to detach, crimping of the Teflon when an automatic inserter is used, or a series of unexplained high glucose readings caused by set failure, will not be apparent until a set is worn for some time. A particular infusion set may cause a skin rash or irritation while another one will not. A trial run with various sets often helps the wearer select a set that works well for them. If there is an infusion set problem, finding an infusion set that works reliably can dramatically improve satisfaction. Fortunately, there are many good choices.

Good technique when applying an infusion set is important and can avoid many control headaches. See *Pumping Insulin* for the latest information on how to succeed with infusion sets and pods.

Drawbacks

An insulin pump can have drawbacks. For example, if the site-preparation technique is poor, an infection or abscess may occur at the infusion site. If an infusion set or patch pump comes loose or detaches entirely, this can lead to ketoacidosis, especially if testing is infrequent. Attachment to a pump can be perceived as a drawback or be a real one that needs to be dealt with by those who swim or play contact sports. A pump can never be more successful than the ability and effort of the person responsible for its use.

Summary

When a pump is used well, the wearer feels better, lives more freely, and is far less likely to have diabetes-related health problems. Confidence about good diabetes management enables the wearer to be more in charge of their life. The improved sense of well-being and better quality of life that come from improved glucose stability motivates many pumpers to do even better as time goes on.

On a pump, it requires less effort to improve glucose readings and there is less impact on daily life. Pumpers appreciate the sense of security and improved quality of life, along with the added benefit of knowing they are preventing future health problems through improved glucose levels. When the pros and cons are carefully weighed, a pump clearly offers significant advantages for people who want a healthy and enjoyable life.

More pump information and hundreds of pumping tips are available in the totally-revised 5th edition of *Pumping Insulin*, available at *www.diabetesnet.com*.

References

1. Willi SM, Planton J, Egede L, Schwarz S. Benefits of continuous subcutaneous insulin infusion in children with type 1 diabetes. *J Pediatr*. 2003;143(6):796-801.

2. Linkeschova R, Raoul M, Bott U, Berger M, Spraul M. Less severe hypoglycaemia, better metabolic control, and improved quality of life in type 1 diabetes mellitus with continuous subcutaneous insulin infusion (CSII) therapy; an observational study of 100 consecutive patients followed for a mean of 2 years. *Diabet Med*. 2002;19(9):746-751.

3. Hanaire-Broutin H, Melki V, Bessières-Lacombe S, Tauber JP. Comparison of continuous subcutaneous insulin infusion and multiple daily injection regimens using insulin lispro in type 1 diabetic patients on intensified treatment: a randomized study. The Study Group for the Development of Pump Therapy in Diabetes. *Diabetes Care*. 2000;23(9):1232-1235.

4. Sulli N, Shashaj B. Continuous subcutaneous insulin infusion in children and adolescents with diabetes mellitus: decreased HbA1c with low risk of hypoglycemia. *J Pediatr Endocrinol Metab*. 2003;16(3):393-399.

5. Weintrob N, Schechter A, Benzaquen H, et al. Glycemic patterns detected by continuous subcutaneous glucose sensing in children and adolescents with type 1 diabetes mellitus treated by multiple daily injections vs continuous subcutaneous insulin infusion. *Arch Pediatr Adolesc Med*. 2004;158(7):677-684.

6. Pickup J, Mattock M, Kerry S. Glycaemic control with continuous subcutaneous insulin infusion compared with intensive insulin injections in patients with type 1 diabetes: meta-analysis of randomised controlled trials. *BMJ*. 2002;324(7339):705.

7. Colquitt JL, Green C, Sidhu MK, Hartwell D, Waugh N. Clinical and cost-effectiveness of continuous subcutaneous insulin infusion for diabetes. *Health Technol Assess*. 2004;8(43):iii, 1-171.

8. Bode BW, Steed RD, Davidson PC. Reduction in severe hypoglycemia with long-term continuous subcutaneous insulin infusion in type I diabetes. *Diabetes Care*. 1996;19(4):324-327.

9. Hirsch IB, Farkas-Hirsch R. Cryer PE: Continuous subcutaneous insulin infusion for the treatment of diabetic patients with hypoglycemia unawareness. *Diabetes Nutr Metab*. 1991;4:41-43.

10. Fanelli CG, Epifano L, Rambotti AM, et al. Meticulous prevention of hypoglycemia normalizes the glycemic thresholds and magnitude of most of neuroendocrine responses to, symptoms of, and cognitive function during hypoglycemia in intensively treated patients with short-term IDDM. *Diabetes*. 1993;42(11):1683-1689.

11. Walsh J, Roberts R, Bailey T. Guidelines for insulin dosing in continuous subcutaneous insulin infusion using new formulas from a retrospective study of individuals with optimal glucose levels. *J Diabetes Sci Technol*. 2010;4(5):1174-1181.

12. Walsh J, Roberts R, Bailey T. Guidelines for optimal bolus calculator settings in adults. *J Diabetes Sci Technol*. 2011;5(1):129-135.

13. Heinemann L. Time-Action Profiles of Insulin Preparations. Mainz, Germany: Verlag Kirchheim & Co. GmbH; 2004.

14. Heinemann L, Weyer C, Rauhaus M, Heinrichs S, Heise T. Variability of the metabolic effect of soluble insulin and the rapid-acting insulin analog insulin aspart. *Diabetes Care*. 1998;21(11):1910-1914.

15. Vaughn DE, Yocum RC, Muchmore DB, et al. Accelerated pharmacokinetics and glucodynamics of prandial insulins injected with recombinant human hyaluronidase. *Diabetes Technol Ther*. 2009;11(6):345-352.

16. Steiner S, Hompesch M, Pohl R, et al. A novel insulin formulation with a more rapid onset of action. *Diabetologia*. 2008;51(9):1602-1606.

17. Rave KM, Nosek L, de la Peña A, et al. Dose response of inhaled dry-powder insulin and dose equivalence to subcutaneous insulin lispro. *Diabetes Care*. 2005;28(10):2400-2405.

18. Rave K, Bott S, Heinemann L, et al. Time-action profile of inhaled insulin in comparison with subcutaneously injected insulin lispro and regular human insulin. *Diabetes Care*. 2005;28(5):1077-1082.

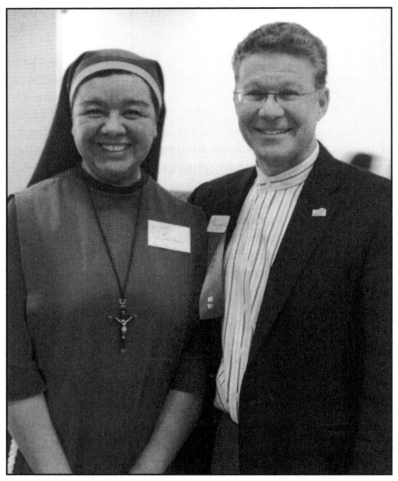

Got to make sure you get everyone you can to be on your side.

10

Using Technology to Take Control of Your Diabetes

Your Glucose Meter Is Your Own Personal Lab in the Palm of Your Hand

by Timothy S. Bailey, MD, FACP, FACE, CPI

Introduction

We know that blood glucose control predicts risks for eye, nerve, and kidney damage and now even heart attack. To better manage your blood glucose levels and fine tune insulin or medication doses, your doctor and nurse educator have probably suggested that you keep a record of your readings. They have probably even handed you countless varieties of logbooks that over the years have kept local paper recyclers in business.

Logbooks are a time-honored way for people with diabetes to communicate what is going on in their life with their diabetes caregiver. The recording/logbook theory goes as follows:
- You keep a record of everything that affects your blood glucose since the last visit
- You understand your diabetes better after recording these events
- Your doctor, after finding the time to look at your record book, understands exactly what is going on and may prescribe a change in therapy that will improve your diabetes control
- The blood glucose levels are better controlled due to more appropriate treatment.

Have you considered using a computer or your favorite mobile device to track and manage your blood glucose levels? Technology can help you:
- Collect data from blood glucose meters, certain insulin pumps, and other new devices such as continuous glucose monitors (CGMs)
- Create charts and graphs that reveal trends and patterns in your blood glucose values for better treatment
- Provide an accurate record that both you and your caregiver can use to improve your readings.

A variety of computer programs have been available since the 1980s to assist with diabetes management. Similar to the way a computer organizes your financial data, it can also organize your blood glucose data. More recently, software apps for smartphones have been introduced that allow you to have similar functionality in your favorite mobile device. Don't miss out on these great tools that can help you to better understand your diabetes. Today's meters, pumps, and CGMs can automatically upload blood glucose values and other data right into your computer or device.

Get Ahead With Today's Meters

Most blood glucose meters today store information about the tests you perform and also let you recall the date and time that you checked it. More advanced meters even store data such as low blood glucose reactions, insulin doses, activity levels, the amount of carbohydrates consumed, and even your A1C levels. CGMs typically generate 288 readings a day, so software is a must.

Until recently, tapping into the information in your meter required a cable to connect it to a PC and software to analyze the data. Typically, each meter has a proprietary cable, meaning you will need a different cable for each brand of meter you wish to upload. Cables may be obtained from each meter manufacturer and usually come with software. The cable connects the meter's data port to your computer's USB port or a small box that communicates over the phone or Internet independent of a computer. For those of you with Macintosh computers, there are fewer options, as most software is designed to work under Windows. You need to check your meter's downloading capability.

If you are in the market for a new meter, consider the following features in making your selection:

- How easily does this meter store the data I need?
- How well does it display the data I collect and can I use this to improve my control?
- What information can I store (blood glucose values, medication dose, food intake, activity, etc)?
- How much information will the meter hold?
- What do I need to connect the meter to my computer (and what will it cost)?
- What software is available that will "talk" with it?

Newer meters have higher-resolution screens which allow them to display more information in bright colors. Also some meters can spot patterns and provide general suggestions for you to consider. There are now several products that can connect from the meter to a smartphone for better data display, either by plugging in directly or wirelessly.

A comparison of available blood glucose meters can be found at *http://forecast.diabetes.org/magazine/features/blood-glucose-meters.*

Uploading Other Devices

Continuous glucose monitors that measure blood glucose as frequently as every 5 minutes are now available. For short-term control decisions, the trend line, trend arrows, and alerts from one of these devices work well. For a bigger picture to see patterns in your readings, however, a computer download really helps you to organize all the data.

Today's smart insulin pumps are loaded with the data you need to manage your diabetes, such as basal and bolus insulin doses, grams of carbohydrate eaten, and often the blood glucose data from a meter or continuous monitor. They have a data port and, therefore, uploading capabilities. They can provide printouts of the doses of insulin you take and general pump settings.

Other "smart" diabetes devices, such as insulin pens that record time, insulin doses, and carbohydrate intake, and smart phones that also test and transmit your blood glucose values and contain a large food database are now available. Smart devices will turn your treatments and carbohydrate intake into a complete record. This will let you record more easily, as well as let you analyze your information will less effort. These devices along with a health care provider, can assist you in achieving much better control of your diabetes.

Uploading your data is not the end but the beginning of your quest for control. Keep your thinking cap on, along with an open mind and your best analytic tools handy when you review your data.

Put the Internet and Your Computer to Work

Once your meter is connected to your computer, you need software to make the magic of uploading occur. Until recently, you had to purchase software. Each device company (eg, Roche, Bayer, LifeScan, and Abbott) developed software systems that only work with their meters. These were designed primarily with the physician in mind and so far have still not gained a dominant following with either physicians or patients. The proprietary nature of these programs precludes their effective use in situations where different brands of meters are being used, such as occurs in many diabetes clinics or homes. In response to this need, several independent companies have developed programs that upload multiple meter types. A comprehensive list of available software can be located at *www.mendosa.com/software*.

The newest development in uploading is brought to you courtesy of the Internet. Web-based tools for diabetes record keeping are now available. Most of these are free and only require a web browser and Internet connection. These systems allow you to access your information from anywhere—with some, you can even use your cellular phone. Recently the first meter with a built-in cell phone chip was introduced to the market. With this, or with a meter connected to your smartphone you can send your data easily to the "Cloud." In this way, downloading happens in the background so there is nothing to remember to do. Your provider can access the information with your permission, making communication easier. If you choose a meter that can send data to the Cloud without requiring a computer, your records can be kept up to date automatically after checking your blood sugar.

However, as with online banking and shopping, you need to ensure the security of your data. To evaluate the trustworthiness of a website, start with the privacy policy. It must be clear that your data will only be shared with your caregiver and only with your explicit permission. Then read more about the company to see if its purpose is something you agree with. Next, register anonymously—the best sites will allow this, further increasing your confidentiality. Finally, enter your data and take advantage of the tools available with the suggestions below.

How Software Helps Reveal Glucose Patterns and Variability

There are many graphs that you can use to better understand your blood glucose readings. Here are a few that are becoming standard in the diabetes information field:

Standard ("Modal") Day

This graph arranges blood glucose readings from the meter so it looks like a whole week or even months of values happen in 1 day. This chart is important because it shows at what time of the day blood glucose levels are in or out of control. This helps you and your health care professionals pinpoint what may be causing the problem. This chart also has a goal area (the shaded area) so it is easy to tell at a glance if a blood glucose value is too high, too low, or within the goal range.

Before-Meal and After-Meal Glucose

These are pie charts that show the percentages of time that blood glucose levels are high, low, or within the blood glucose goal range. These charts are great motivational tools because they immediately show how well you're doing and help keep you on track. They also help health care professionals see how meals are affecting your blood glucose.

Combination Line Graph

This type of chart shows the different factors that affect your blood glucose, including medication dosage (including basal rates for pumps), food (carbohydrates consumed), events, and exercise.

Glucose Line Chart

All of your blood glucose levels are graphed in chronological order in a glucose line chart. It lets you see long-term trends in your blood glucose and whether you're in or out of your goal range.

Glucose Statistics

The latest concern in diabetes monitoring is glucose variability. Until recently, the focus of all efforts was to improve A1C (which reflects the average glucose). It might appear obvious to you that the ups and downs of blood glucose matter. However, the notion that this is important to developing long-term complications is relatively new.

So how can we get a handle on this? One approach is to look at the glucose line chart. You can get an overall impression that the more jagged the lines appear, the more variability there is. A better approach is to use something from statistics called a standard deviation (SD).

Standard deviation reflects the spread around the average with a single number. You can calculate this based on values from entire days or just specific times of day (eg, before-breakfast readings). Dr. Irl Hirsch of the University of Washington created a useful and easy benchmark—the SD multiplied by 2 should not exceed the mean. For super control, the SD multiplied by 3 should be less than the mean. If your SD is high, this means that better coordination of meals, activity, and treatment might be needed.

We will now examine some of these graphs in action in a person with diabetes.

Case Presentation

Dan is a 39-year-old man who developed type 1 diabetes at age 11. He has been followed annually by his family physician since he was a child and was told of the development of background retinopathy 6 years ago by his eye doctor. He recently read an article in a magazine about the chronic complications of diabetes and is concerned that the blurring of his vision over the past few weeks could be due to his diabetes. Both feet have been burning and tingling at night for several months. Additionally, he has occasional nightmares and has been given juice at night several times by his wife because he appeared confused. He has been faithfully taking two daily mixed injections of NPH and Regular insulin (25 N and 20 R every morning and 20 N and 15 R every evening). A1C values have been between 9% and 10% (normal range <6%) on most occasions, and he has made every attempt to follow a healthy diet. He monitors his blood glucose level every morning and states that it is usually 100 to 200 mg/dL. He exercised daily in the past, but attributes his current sedentary lifestyle to the demands of his present employment.

Dan's wife bought him a new blood glucose meter last month that stores his blood glucose information, insulin doses, and carbohydrate intake. He hooked up his meter to his personal computer, using a data cable and a new software package that he had heard about from his diabetes educator. He then entered his blood glucose goals that he had decided on in consultation with his physician and diabetes educator. The information contained in his meter is uploaded to the computer.

With the click of a button, you can display a choice of pie graphs. This one (**Figure 10-1**) shows how Dan is doing overall—in this case, 28.4% of his readings were within his goal range, 61% were higher, and 10.6% were lower. He wants to increase the slice of the pie representing his goals.

Using his computer, Dan decides to analyze his blood glucose patterns by creating a chart showing a standard (modal) day. Here it appears as if the whole weeks or months of values all happened in 1 day. This chart shows that he is checking his blood glucose levels at breakfast and dinner and makes it clear that they are running high. You can also see that he has never checked his blood glucose during the night or at lunch (**Figure 10-2**).

Dan now decides how he will fix those high morning blood glucose levels. His diabetes educator says that he will need to have a good sampling of blood glucose levels before his medication doses can be adjusted with confidence. He decides to test his blood glucose at least 4 times a day to learn more about his diabetes patterns. He checks his blood glucose several times halfway between bedtime and breakfast (often about 3 AM) as well as several times 1 to 2 hours after meals. He

Figure 10-1
Pie Graphs

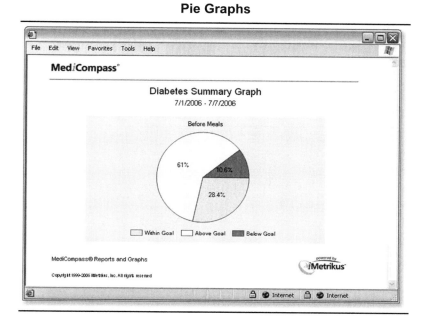

Figure 10-2
Blood Glucose Patterns Analysis

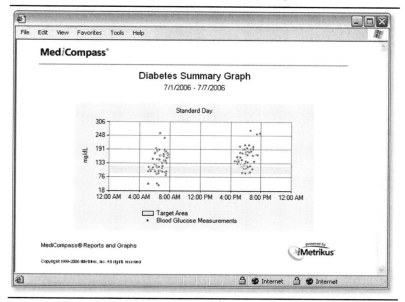

fires up his computer, plugs in the meter, and uploads it to display this new information.

Figure 10-3 shows the logbook automatically generated by the computer program from information in Dan's meter. Such a logbook can be printed out easily and quickly to bring to your next appointment.

Figure 10-3

Logbook Generated by Computer From Meter

MediCompass®

Patient Name: _____   Patient ID: _____

Glucose Logbook
7/6/2006 - 7/12/2006

Date	Before breakfast	After breakfast	Before lunch	After lunch	Before dinner	After dinner	Bedtime	Night
7/12/2006	150 6:18AM		52 10:56AM		142 6:00PM			
7/11/2006	105 5:22AM	167 9:07AM	85 10:31AM		123 6:04PM		179 8:43PM	52 2:59AM
7/10/2006	126 5:58AM	176 7:27AM	46 11:26AM		134 5:55PM			
7/9/2006	152 5:43AM		208 11:30AM		192 5:39PM	272 6:36PM	196 10:23PM	70 3:41AM
7/8/2006	146 6:33AM		74 11:59AM	196 12:13PM	180 6:27PM			
7/7/2006	172 7:10AM	163 7:10AM			198 6:06PM			
7/6/2006	169 6:52AM				204 5:13PM			

MediCompass® Reports and Graphs

Copyright 1999-2006 Metrikus, Inc. All right reserved

powered by iMetrikus

Another way to examine the patterns is to click on the button for the computer to do a blood glucose frequency analysis (**Figure 10-4**). This shows Dan where the blood glucose readings cluster according to time of day. You can see that 50% of the blood glucose levels during the night were below 70 mg/dL. Also 5% of the before breakfast and 30% of the before lunch glucose levels were also below 70 mg/dL. After breakfast, 85% of the values were between 160 and 200 mg/dL. Compared with simple averages, this better illustrates the distribution of blood glucose levels over multiple ranges.

Dan brought these with him to his next appointment with his physician and diabetes educator. They recommended that he move his dinner NPH insulin from dinner to bedtime so that the NPH would peak later to avoid low blood glucose levels in the middle of the night. They also

200

Figure 10-4

Glucose Frequency Analysis

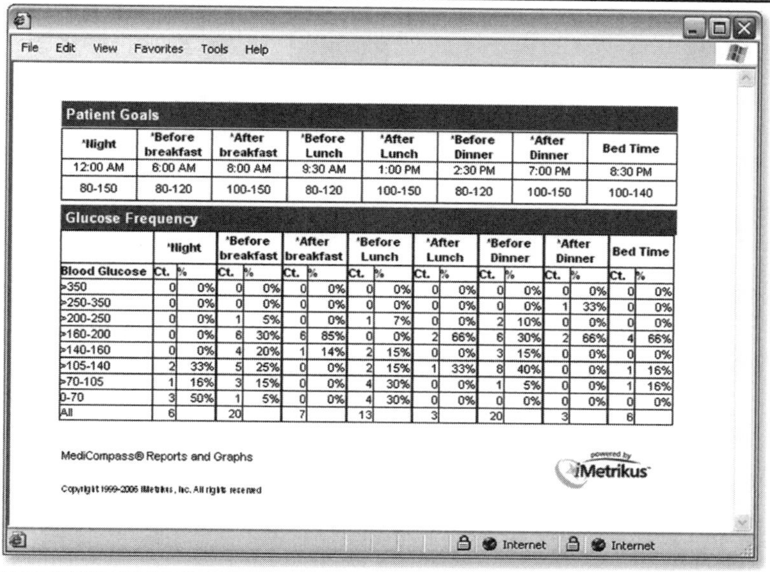

Patient Goals

	Night	Before breakfast	After breakfast	Before Lunch	After Lunch	Before Dinner	After Dinner	Bed Time
	12:00 AM	6:00 AM	8:00 AM	9:30 AM	1:00 PM	2:30 PM	7:00 PM	8:30 PM
	80-150	80-120	100-150	80-120	100-150	80-120	100-150	100-140

Glucose Frequency

Blood Glucose	Night Ct.	%	Before breakfast Ct.	%	After breakfast Ct.	%	Before Lunch Ct.	%	After Lunch Ct.	%	Before Dinner Ct.	%	After Dinner Ct.	%	Bed Time Ct.	%
>350	0	0%	0	0%	0	0%	0	0%	0	0%	0	0%	0	0%	0	0%
>250-350	0	0%	0	0%	0	0%	0	0%	0	0%	0	0%	1	33%	0	0%
>200-250	0	0%	1	5%	0	0%	1	7%	0	0%	2	10%	0	0%	0	0%
>160-200	0	0%	6	30%	6	85%	0	0%	2	66%	6	30%	2	66%	4	66%
>140-160	0	0%	4	20%	1	14%	2	15%	0	0%	3	15%	0	0%	0	0%
>105-140	2	33%	5	25%	0	0%	2	15%	1	33%	8	40%	0	0%	1	16%
>70-105	1	16%	3	15%	0	0%	4	30%	0	0%	1	5%	0	0%	1	16%
0-70	3	50%	1	5%	0	0%	4	30%	0	0%	0	0%	0	0%	0	0%
All	6		20		7		13		3		20		3		6	

MediCompass® Reports and Graphs

Copyright 1999-2006 iMetrikus, Inc. All rights reserved

powered by
iMetrikus

suggested changing Regular insulin to a new rapid-acting insulin and decreasing his morning and dinner shorter-acting insulin doses by 2 units and that he try to decrease his food intake at lunch. The diabetes team suggested that he track his food intake by counting carbohydrates. Dan let them know that he had also decided to try exercising daily in the afternoon.

Dan uploaded his meter a week later and viewed the glucose line graph shown in **Figure 10-5** on his computer. The difference that these changes made over time is clearly seen. Dan is so pleased with his improvements that he sends these graphs every 2 to 3 weeks to his physician directly from his computer. His physician is also pleased with this information and sends Dan encouragement and suggestions for further refinement of his blood glucose control.

Online Resources for Patients and Health Care Providers

In the past, it was traditional to list resources for patients separately from those aimed toward health care professionals. With the explosion of online information available, this distinction is less clear. The best sites will have links to other relevant or related sites. Be sure to discuss what you find with your health care professional before changing your treatment.

Figure 10-5

Glucose Trend Over Time

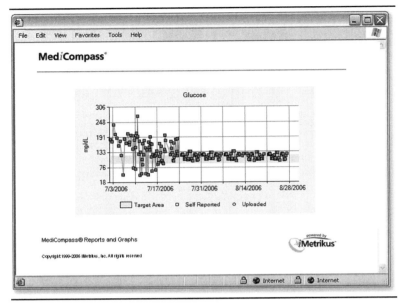

Summary

With a little initial effort, you can use current technology to provide a more complete and accurate record than by using a conventional logbook or diary. This can help you learn to recognize important trends in your diabetes. It may also empower you to better communicate with your health care professional and receive better advice. This is one more useful option to help you take the next step toward controlling diabetes.

11

Know Your Numbers

Test for Yourself Primarily and for Your Caregiver Secondarily

Checking Basal Dose of Insulin While on Pump

Todd is a 36-year-old man taking 23 units of Lantus (long-acting basal insulin) at night and 5 to 10 units of Apidra (fast-acting insulin) before each meal. He was having problems with high blood sugar in the afternoon and before dinner, and thought it was because he was not on enough Lantus. His morning numbers were very good, however, and I was concerned that increasing his Lantus may cause low blood sugar in the early morning.

	B	P B	L	P L	D	P D	HS	Notes
Monday								
Tuesday	112		123	190	186		178	
Wednesday	97		151	179	162		155	
Thursday	124		132	128	121		173	FASTING UNTIL DINNER
Friday	107		162	185	202		141	

When he came to see me, I suggested that he test his basal dose of insulin by fasting from the morning until dinnertime, and testing periodically throughout the day, especially in the afternoon. This is the best way to examine whether or not the basal dose is accurate.

When he did this, his blood glucose levels were stable all day until dinner. This indicates that his dose of Lantus is perfect. If his basal dose of Lantus was insufficient, then his blood sugar levels would have started to creep up in the afternoon. In order to lower those afternoon and predinner blood sugar levels, he needed more fast-acting insulin with lunch and not an increase in his Lantus. Fasting and checking frequently is the best way to determine if your basal dose of insulin or basal rate on your pump is adequate.

High Bedtime Values

The logbook is from Betty, a 67-year-old woman with type 2 diabetes, currently on two oral medications for her diabetes (glucophage and rosiglitazone), as well as 45 units of Lantus at bedtime. Her A1C is 7.5% (goal is less that 7%). As you can see, the glucose values in the morning and during the day are really pretty good. It is mainly the bedtime values that are consistently high. She does not snack after dinner and has cut back on the carbohydrates with that meal.

	Usual Target Before Meals: 70-130	**BLOOD GLUCOSE**		Usual Target 1-2 Hours After Meals: 70-180				
DATE	INSULIN TYPE / AM / PM	BREAKFAST BEFORE / AFTER	LUNCH BEFORE / AFTER	DINNER BEFORE / AFTER	BED TIME	OVER NIGHT	COMMENTS	
S		96	89	—	231			
S		104	—	108	267			
M		85	—	122	244			
T		117	125	106	219			
W		92	113	—	199			
Th		88	—	124	258			
F		126	110	—	221			

Her basal insulin, Lantus, is perfectly adjusted because her morning values are excellent and she is on the maximum dose of her other medications. This woman clearly needs some fast-acting insulin to address the rise in blood sugar following dinner (Apidra, Humalog, or Novolog). The typical starting dose is 5 or 10 units, but one thing must be remembered with this effective and focused strategy. If you normalize the bedtime glucose values by giving fast-acting insulin at dinner, you must also proactively lower the amount of basal insulin at bedtime to avoid overnight hypoglycemia. At the current time, her 45 units of Lantus work well to bring down her bedtime values (which are well over 200 mg/dL) into a very good range but if the bedtime values were suddenly improved and the dose of Lantus not adjusted downward, hypoglycemia would surely occur.

Lifestyle Changes to Help Consistency

What is clear from Kevin's logbook is that on a daily basis, the numbers jump from as low as 35 mg/dL to as high as 478 mg/dL. What must be so frustrating for this fellow is that there are no consistent trends, which makes it almost impossible as a provider to make any adjustments in the dose of insulin or oral medications. For example, if the morning pre-breakfast values were always high, then increasing the nighttime dose of medication would be appropriate; however, if one third of the numbers are low, one third are high, and the last one third are just right, then any adjustment would not be appropriate and could possibly be dangerous. What is amazing is that the A1C was 7.1%, indicating great control, but it is important to remember that the A1C is just an average and does not reflect the day-to-day ups and downs. Usually, in cases like this one, the person will need to improve the consistency of his/her daily eating and exercise schedule in order to reduce the day-to-day fluctuations.

Day	Breakfast		Lunch		Dinner		Bedtime	Other/Snack
	Pre Post	Carbs Insulin	Pre Post	Carbs Insulin	Pre Post	Carbs Insulin	Carbs Insulin	Carbs Insulin
M	72		234		111		263	
T	144				94		179	
W	356	65	166				105	
T	42	115					39	
F	121	35			279		38	
S	225	478	315				119	
S	127				60		156	
Avg.								

Continuous Glucose Monitor

Megan is a 30-year-old female with type 1 diabetes and has been living with this condition for many years. She is frustrated trying to control her diabetes. She has an insulin pump and recently began using a continuous glucose monitor (CGM). Her A1C is not that bad, however, she seems to yo-yo up and down on a daily basis. She tries to be as consistent as possible but travels a lot, which makes things difficult.

Her carbohydrate-to-insulin ratio is 10:1, and her correction factor is 1:35 with a goal of 100 mg/dL. See the download of a typical day. What could be the cause(s) of her erratic control?

Although easier said than done, trying to keep her glucose levels in a good "zone" while avoiding the extreme highs and lows is the key to success. First of all, when she is high, she must make sure that she is using the appropriate correction dose (if you are giving yourself more than you need, it will drive you down into the low range). Also, she should be careful not to "stack" her dose by taking several correction doses too closely together in time (typically you should wait at least an hour before giving a second correction dose).

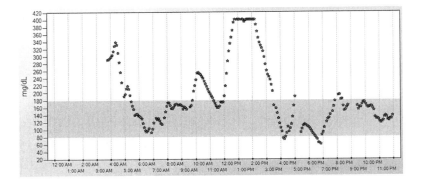

On the other end of the spectrum, she doesn't want to overtreat her lows, which will drive her back up too high, as then she will definitely be on the roller coaster. Also, she should test to make sure her carbohydrate-to-insulin ratio is appropriate (pre- and postmeal testing), because if she is not giving herself enough insulin with meals, she will commonly be too high after eating, creating the up and down cycle. Upper and lower alert levels should be set appropriately (ie, 80 mg/dL for the low and 180 mg/dL for the high). It will defeat the purpose of having a CGM device if the limits are too high and too low. Megan must remember to pay attention to the alerts and do something when she crosses the line in order to avoid the extremes.

It will take several months to learn how to correctly interpret CGM readings and make the appropriate micro-adjustments throughout the day.

Multiple Daily Injection Regimen

Wilson is a 54-year-old male with type 2 diabetes who has recently started using insulin. His current regimen includes 90 units of Lantus at night and about 15 units of Novolog before meals. Wilson eats a pretty consistent breakfast, lunch, and dinner at 7 am, 12 noon, and 6 pm, respectively. As you can see from his logbook, he is frequently getting low over night and in between meals, just before lunch, and in the afternoon. He is on too much insulin, but which one? Lantus or Novolog?

	Breakfast			Lunch			Dinner			Bedtime		Night	Comments
	Blood Sugar Before	Insulin Units/Type	Blood Sugar After	Blood Sugar Before	Insulin Units/Type	Blood Sugar After	Blood Sugar Before	Insulin Units/Type	Blood Sugar After	Blood Sugar Before	Insulin Units/Type	Blood Sugar	
Mon	79		67	156	81					121			
Tues	54	65 glucose tabs	89	—		111				142			Low 3am
Wed	101		—		171	92				166			
Thurs	63			102		55				151			Low 2AM
Fri	59 shakey		84		64					—			
Sat	96		—		—					179			Low 5am
Sun	44 (Low)		71		59					184			

When an individual on a multiple daily injection regimen, consisting of a basal and bolus insulin, the ratio should be close to 50% of each. This is not a hard and fast rule but in this case, it appears that he is on too much basal insulin since he gets low in between widely spaced meals and in the early morning. His current ratio of basal-to-bolus insulin is 90:45 or 67% basal and 33% fast-acting. This lopsided ratio may indicate too much basal or not enough bolus insulin, and in Wilson's case, it is the former.

Prediabetes in a 56-Year-Old Man

Peter is a 56-year-old man with a history of being overweight, along with high blood pressure and abnormal cholesterol levels. His mother, brother, sister, and two paternal uncles have type 2 diabetes. He came to my office to ask what he can do to prevent diabetes.

	Usual Target Before Meals: 70-130			BLOOD GLUCOSE					Usual Target 1-2 Hours After Meals: 70-180	
DATE	INSULIN			BREAKFAST	LUNCH		DINNER		BED TIME	OVER NIGHT	COMMENTS
	TYPE	AM	PM	BEFORE				AFTER			
				102				—			
	TYPE	AM	PM	86				—			
	TYPE	AM	PM	98				187			
	TYPE	AM	PM	—				145			
	TYPE	AM	PM	123				198			
	TYPE	AM	PM	—				—			
	TYPE	AM	PM	117				141			

I gave him a loaner glucose meter and he came back with the results shown in his logbook. As you can see, his before-breakfast numbers range from 86 to 123 mg/dL and his after-meal values go as high as 198 mg/dL. The official ranges before food in the morning (fasting) is less than 100 mg/dL for normal individuals and over 126 mg/dL in people with diabetes (in between is called prediabetes). The postmeal glucose value for people who are normal is less than 140 mg/dL and over 200 mg/dL in people with diabetes (again, in between is called prediabetes).

Peter's values are not normal, but nor are they within the diabetes range. He clearly has prediabetes. I recommended a good dietitian and exercise physiologist to slowly begin practical lifestyle changes that will help him to avoid developing full-blown diabetes.

After we see how his blood glucose does with lifestyle modifications, I will make sure Peter is aware of medication options to see if he wants to be aggressive about attempting to prevent diabetes.

High Glucose Levels in the Morning

This logbook is from Katie, a 27-year-old female with type 2 diabetes for 3 years, who is currently on two oral agents during the day (Glucophage and Januvia), as well as an injection of a long-acting basal insulin (insulin detemir or Levemir) at night. As you can see from her logbook, the bedtime blood sugar values are consistently high (well over 200 mg/dL). The numbers are also not at goal first thing in the morning before breakfast, however, they are not as high as the bedtime values. She was asked to gradually increase her bedtime Levemir dose of insulin by 2 units every night until her morning numbers were consistently below 140 mg/dL. After several weeks, she has gone from her starting dose of 10 units at night up to her current 62 units. Will she ever get her mornings down to her goal? Well, one of the most important trends I see is that the bedtime numbers are extremely high, and one of the first goals is to bring those down to less than 180 mg/dL at bedtime in order for the overnight basal insulin to work more effectively. She will need to reduce her calories at dinner, exercise after dinner, or take a dose of fast-acting insulin with her dinner in order to improve her nighttime numbers, since increasing her basal insulin at night is not addressing the main problem.

🍎 = Pre-meal   ⚕ = Post-meal

Day	Breakfast 🍎	Breakfast Medication/Insulin	Breakfast ⚕	Lunch 🍎	Lunch Medication/Insulin	Lunch ⚕	Dinner 🍎	Dinner Medication/Insulin	Dinner ⚕	Other	Comments bedtime
M	237			193			133			243	
T											
W	244			161			151			224	
Th	218			182			146			217	
F	205			221			178			298	
S											
S											

Diabetes and Steroids

Dan is a 65-year-old man, currently on Glucophage, glyburide, Lantus, and Byetta for his diabetes. His blood sugars have gone haywire and he cannot figure it out. He is not taking any new medications and is eating the same things. He isn't exercising as much due to back pain.

As you can see, on October 25th, his blood sugar levels started to rise extremely high. We spent at least 30 minutes together on the phone trying to figure out the cause. We discussed several issues:

1. Were any of his diabetes medications (including his insulin) expired?
2. Was his insulin exposed to excessive heat or frozen by accident?
3. Did he start taking any new medications?
4. Was he eating new types of food or consuming excessive calories?
5. Was he experiencing any emotional stressors?

As mentioned above, the only change to his daily routine was the back pain that lead to reduced exercise. At the end of our conversation, Dan told me that the orthopedic surgeon had injected something into his back, but he did not know what it was. I replied with, "Do you mean to tell me that a doctor injected something into the space around your spinal cord (epidural) and you did not know what the heck it was?" It turned out that he was given a huge dose of Kenalog, a very strong steroid, into his spinal canal to relieve pain, and neither the doctor nor nurse warned him about what it would do to his diabetes. Well, this situation could have been avoided entirely if the doctor or Dan had a clue about the effect of steroids on blood sugar. Dan could have been given a proactive plan for adjusting his insulin to account for the presence of the steroid.

	Before Meals			Between Meals		
Date	Fast	B	L	D	3:00	Bed Time
Need						
10/22		139	157	284	196	131
10/23		121	90	144	284	208
10/24		150	170	148	213	229
10/25		148	194	218	198	237
10/26		215	245	311	298	332
10/27	442					

Strong Family History of Diabetes

This logbook is from a 58-year-old male named John who has a strong family history of diabetes, obesity, and heart disease. Both of his parents and several uncles and aunts have type 2 diabetes and are well above their ideal body weights. John's father died of a heart attack at the age of 55, and his sister just had a stroke at the age of 59. John's two kids are heavy and look just like their dad. His doctor recommended occasionally testing his blood sugar levels at home. Testing with a home glucose meter is more practical and realistic than using a formal oral glucose tolerance test (OGTT). OGTT consists of fasting overnight and then swallowing 75 grams of glucose. Blood glucose levels are taken just before and 2 hours after the ingestion of the sweet syrup.

As you can see from John's logbook, his morning (or fasting) values are between 100 and 126 mg/dL and his post-dinner values are typically above 140 mg/dL but not above 200 mg/dL. John eventually got an A1C value, and it was 5.8%. His diagnosis is "prediabetes."

Day	Breakfast ●	Medication/Insulin	☓	Lunch ●	Medication/Insulin	☓	Dinner ●	Medication/Insulin	☓	Other	Comments
M	111								—		
T	—								153		
W	109								—		
Th	—								175		
F	124								151		
S	99								139		
S	112								142		

Type 2 Diabetes and Alcohol Consumption

This logbook is from Christi, a very active 38-year-old female who has had type 2 diabetes for 5 years and is on a multiple daily injection regimen (40 units of Lantus at night and 10 to 15 units of Novolog with each meal). She is single and goes out with her girlfriends to a local bar one to two times a week. As you can see from her logbook, she tested very frequently on Friday night and gave herself several extra doses of Novolog. She likes to drink wine and typically has three to four glasses, along with the free nuts and pretzels that are in bowls all over the bar. A 4-ounce glass of wine is about 90 calories, pretzels are very rapidly absorbed carbs, and nuts have tons of calories. She does a pretty good job of correcting her elevated glucose levels, but testing frequently while drinking is the key. Her friends know she has diabetes, and there is always a designated driver in this group of fun-loving women (they take turns).

		BREAKFAST		LUNCH		DINNER		NOTES						
		Pre	Post	Pre	Post	Pre	Post							
Friday	Time					6:50pm	8:30pm	9:30pm	10:30pm	11:30pm	12:30am	1:30am		
	BS					121	225	189	145	265	219	188		
	NL					15 NL	5 NL	0 NL	0 NL	8 NL	0 NL	0 NL		
Saturday	Time	10:00am		2:00pm		7:00pm								
	BS	157		171		109								
	NL	14 NL		10 NL										

Type 1 Diabetes and Alcohol Consumption

Andrea is a 21-year-old college student living with type 1 diabetes since the age of 11. Her diabetes is well controlled and she is on an insulin pump. Andrea is an avid runner, putting in between 4 to 6 miles almost every day immediately after her classes in the late afternoon, As you can see from her logbook, Andrea has been having problems with low blood sugar reactions at bedtime and in the early hours of the morning.

I stared and stared at her numbers but could not discover any trends or clues that could explain why she was having these sporadic lows. Her blood sugar readings are pretty good before and after dinner, as she really tries to be consistent with the amounts and types of food she eats from the school cafeteria.

After multiple conversations with Andrea, it turns out that she goes out drinking with her buddies a few nights a week... the same nights she has problems with the lows. She drinks rum and diet coke, tests her blood sugar levels frequently while drinking, and has not had any problems while out bar hopping. Alcohol can inhibit the body's ability to produce glucose mainly by the liver (hepatic glucose production). Because Andrea exercises regularly and intensely, her body's glucose stores in her liver are low. When she drinks alcohol, this inhibits her natural glucose stores from being replenished, and this puts her at risk for delayed hypoglycemia. If her glucose control was not so good, she may not have experienced the problem; however, her basal rate was perfectly adjusted for the nights she did not "party" with her friends.

I am a sucker for a glass of Baileys on cracked ice here and there but because of all the calories (carbs and fat), my problem is hyperglycemia! People with diabetes can have alcohol in moderation, but they need to be knowledgeable about how it can affect their bodies and their diabetes. Drink diabesponsibly!

					BREAKFAST		LUNCH		DINNER		BED TIME	OVER NIGHT	COMMENTS
DATE	INSULIN	TYPE	AM	PM	BEFORE	AFTER	BEFORE	AFTER	BEFORE	AFTER			
S					98		151	127			133	55	2 a.m. low
S					76	122	140		169				
M							139	86			142		
T					102		137	92	106	148			
W							133	119			132		
Th					88		141	129	153	168		47	3 a.m. low
F					65		118	146		122			

Usual Target Before Meals: 70-130 — BLOOD GLUCOSE (2:30 pm pre-run) — Usual Target 1-2 Hours After Meals: 70-180

12

Continuous Glucose Monitoring

Technology That Can Take Some of the Unpredictability Out of Diabetes Management

by Jeremy Pettus, MD, with
Timothy S. Bailey, MD, and
Steven V. Edelman, MD

Introduction

Back in the time of the dinosaurs when Dr. Edelman was diagnosed with type 1 diabetes, the only way to know your glucose level was to check your urine. The problem with urine testing is that it represents what your blood glucose was *hours* ago, and even then, it doesn't give you a precise value for your blood glucose. Controlling your diabetes was like swinging at a piñata with a blindfold on. Thankfully, home glucose monitoring (HGM) became available, and patients could rapidly and accurately know their blood glucose level. With this new accuracy, insulin regimens could be tightened and overall diabetes control could be improved. Now everybody has perfect blood glucose control and we all live happily ever after, right?

We wish that was the case—even though HGM has helped diabetes care tremendously, it still has limitations. Even if you are fanatical about checking your blood sugar and check 15 times per day, that means that you know what your blood sugar is for 15 minutes of the day. Well, there are 1440 minutes in a day, so you can see that HGM gives you only a snap shot of what is happening. Continuous glucose monitoring (CGM) can now fill those wide and potentially dangerous gaps.

For the past almost 20 years, I (Jeremy Pettus) have struggled to control my blood glucose level the best I could. Even with all of the knowledge that I have and tools at my disposal, it was difficult to achieve the control goals that I wanted. I would have unexpected high glucose readings, frequent nocturnal hypoglycemia (low blood sugar), and so on. When I finally got my first CGM, it was like somebody removed my blindfold and now I was free to swing away at that piñata.

The challenge now is to get this technology into the hands of the people who could benefit the most. This will take a concerted effort to educate the people living with diabetes, the professional community, and the insurers. This chapter is designed to get you up to speed on what the technology is, what the benefits are, who should use it, and how it should be used. Since this is such a new technology, a lot of these points are changing rapidly.

What Is a Continuous Glucose Monitor and Who Should Use It?

A CGM system is a device that measures glucose levels 24 hours a day. The devices provide measurements every 5 minutes or up to 288 values every 24 hours. The device works by having a sensor inserted under the skin (which you can do easily at home in about 1 minute). The sensor takes glucose measurements at frequent intervals. It then transmits these values wirelessly to a handheld, cell phone-sized device, which enables you to see glucose values and trends. Depending on the device, these sensors can stay in place for 3 to 7 days before they must be changed, and companies are working on extending the interval for continual usage. CGM is primarily for people with type 1 diabetes, insulin-requiring type 2 diabetes, gestational diabetes, and anyone with hypoglycemia unawareness.

At the current time, CGMs are not meant to replace traditional blood glucose meters—they work together with fingerstick readings to give you a more complete understanding of what is happening to your glucose level. You should always confirm your CGM readings with a fingerstick before you take any action such as taking an insulin dose.

Figure 12-1 shows CGMs that are currently available.

Benefits of Continuous Glucose Monitoring

The continuous readings that are provided every 5 minutes create a trend line, which you can use to help understand how insulin, food, exercise, and other variables affect your glucose values. Traditional fingersticks provide a point-in-time glucose value, but do not tell you whether your glucose levels are rising or falling, or how fast these changes are happening.

Continuous monitoring allows you to see these trends in glucose and, after confirming with a fingerstick, to make adjustments to your insulin or take other appropriate action. Trend arrows, which tell you what direction your glucose levels are going, can really help you predict future highs and lows. Trend arrows must be looked at when calculating an insulin dose, planning exercise, during exercise, and many other situations that may affect your glucose control (**Figure 12-2**). Alert levels can be individually set for both high and low glucose levels, helping

Figure 12-1

CGM Systems Currently Available

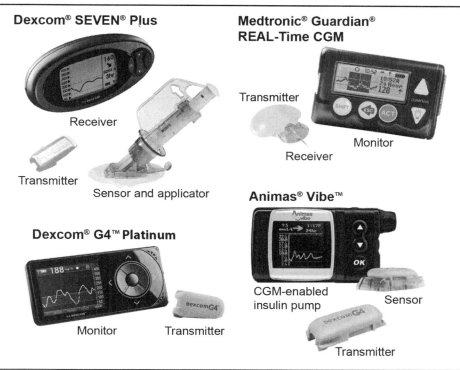

Dexcom® SEVEN® Plus

Receiver

Transmitter

Sensor and applicator

Dexcom® G4™ Platinum

Monitor   Transmitter

Medtronic® Guardian® REAL-Time CGM

Transmitter

Monitor

Receiver

Animas® Vibe™

CGM-enabled insulin pump

Sensor

Transmitter

The value of a CGM system over point-in-time finger sticks is that glucose values are determined on a minute-to-minute basis (gives a new reading every 5 minutes based on the average) while the system is attached to the body. An insulin pump delivers insulin via an infusion set inserted into the abdominal region. The glucose values are then sent by a transmitter, via radio frequency wireless technology, to the pump where the numbers and graphs are displayed to the user. The transmitter is linked to a sensor attached to the abdomen by a tiny wire through the skin that measures glucose levels in the cellular fluid. The Dexcom® SEVEN® Plus, Dexcom® G4™ Platinum (*www.dexcom.com*), and Guardian® REAL-Time Continuous Glucose Monitoring System (*www.minimed.com*) are currently available in the United States. In Europe you can get an Animas® Vibe™ (pump-Dexcom combination) that displays the CGM results on the screen as does the Medtronic Gardian CGM system.

Photos courtesy of Dexcom and Medtronic Diabetes.

you better detect and manage hyper- and hypoglycemia. CGM can help you respond more quickly to changing glucose levels and take control of your diabetes management by using the information provided from continuous monitoring (**Figure 12-3**).

Lower Your A1C

Multiple trials have now shown that using a CGM can help improve your diabetes control. The evidence at this point is most convincing in type 1 diabetes, but more studies are underway in type 2 diabetics.

Figure 12-2
CGM Trend Arrows Defined

➡	**Constant**: your glucose is steady (not increasing/decreasing more than 1 mg/dL each minute)
↗	**Slowly rising**: Your glucose is rising 1-2 mg/dL each minute
↑	**Rising**: Your glucose is rising 2-3 mg/dL each minute
↑↑	**Rapidly rising**: Your glucose is rising more than 3 mg/dL each minute
↘	**Slowly falling**: your glucose is falling 1-2 mg/dL each minute
↓	**Falling**: your glucose is falling 2-3 mg/dL each minute
↓↓	**Rapidly falling**: your glucose is falling more than 3 mg/dL each minute
no arrow	**No rate of change information**: the receiver cannot always calculate how fast your glucose is rising or falling

Trend arrows tell you the rate of change of your glucose values and should be used to adjust your insulin calculations either up or down, depending on the direction and steepness of the arrow and other lifestyle factors.

One important point is that CGMs only lower A1C levels in patients that use the device on a consistent basis. In other words, if you only wear it 1 or 2 days a week, it isn't going to help you. This is something you need to wear consistently in order to get good at using the extra information it provides.

No More Unexpected Highs

One of the most frustrating things that would happen to me when I was using home glucose monitoring is when I would check my blood glucose and it would be sky high. I would say to myself, "How long has my blood glucose been that high?!" This would really bother me when it was my morning reading because that probably meant that it was high all night. Also, starting your day with a really high reading usually meant the rest of my day was going to be a mess blood glucose-wise.

Fortunately now that I have a CGM, I can set it to alarm when by blood glucose is high (I have mine set at 180). That way I know exactly when I need to take action to bring it back down. I find this is particularly useful at night. I wake up with a buzz that my blood glucose is

Figure 12-3

Examples of Four Fingersticks Taken and Values From CGM During 24 Hours

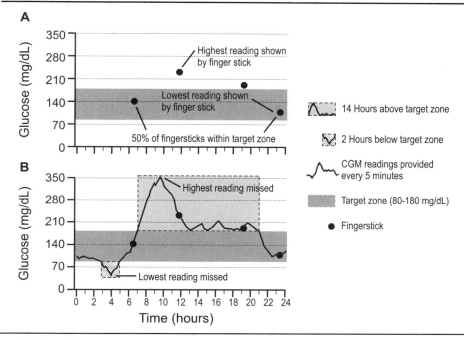

A) These fingerstick point-in-time readings show that half of the values throughout the day were within the target zone (80-180 mg/dL) and half were outside. None of the four readings fell below the target zone (potentially dangerous glucose levels). The highest reading shown was 230 mg/dL. *B)* CGM readings of the same patient in the same day reveal substantially more information. Higher glucose readings (over 330 mg/dL) on this same day as well as lower glucose readings (under 60 mg/dL) are recorded, both of which were missed by fingerstick readings alone. About 16 hours were spent outside of the target zone. A portion of this time outside the target zone was unknown to the person, because fingerstick readings did not show glucose values or trends between these points.

180, I take a couple units of insulin, go back to sleep and wake up with a perfect blood glucose. That sure beats waking up with another 300 reading and pulling out my hair.

Beyond how it works for just me, clinical research shows that using CGMs can help you spend less time hypoglycemic, less time hyperglycemic, and more time in your target zone. CGMs allow you to set a range of target control, including the high and low levels that are recommended by your caregiver or diabetes management team. You can customize these levels at your doctor's office or at home. CGM uses three zones: target, high, and low (**Figure 12-4**).

Less Hypoglycemia

Another frustrating (and dangerous) situation for me before I started using a CGM was hypoglycemia; specifically hypoglycemia at night. I would wake up only when my body felt that I was low, but when I would wake up has changed over time. I used to wake up when my blood sugar was 70 or so, but as time has gone on, I find that I only wake up now when my blood sugar is closer to 40. This is a common phenomenon in diabetes called hypoglycemic unawareness. I would wake up confused, stumble into the kitchen, and eat absolutely everything in sight. No matter how many times I told myself to just drink a little juice, it didn't matter. I would

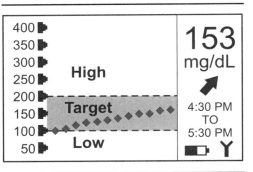

Figure 12-4

**Three Zones of CGM:
High, Target, and Low**

The dashed lines in this graph show a sample target glucose zone of 100 mg/dL (low) to 200 mg/dL (high). When glucose goes above the high target level or below the low target level, the CGM will alert you to let you know that you are outside of your target zone. Once you are alerted, you have the option to take action early in order to avoid wide swings in glucose values. The trend arrow gives an idea in which direction your glucose values are going. In this example, the trend arrow is indicating a slow rise of 1-2 mg/dL per minute.

absolutely demolish the pantry. Then, of course, I would wake up with a blood glucose over 300 and have to take a ton of insulin.

Now that I sleep with my CGM next to me, it alarms when my blood sugar is 80. I wake up in a much more reasonable state of mind, drink just a little juice, and get back to sleep. Not only does this save me from taking in an extra thousand calories that I don't need, it also is a much safer situation. People often ask me, "Does the alarm always wake you up?" It's a great question. It almost always wakes me up, but one time it didn't. My blood sugar was crashing and I wasn't waking up. Thankfully, it did wake up my wife next to me. She jumped into action and got me the sugar I needed. I honestly think the device may have saved my life that night. It at least prevented a trip to the emergency room.

In clinical trials, CGMs have been shown to allow patients to tighten their blood glucose control and lower their A1C, without any increase in hypoglycemia. This is actually fairly significant. In all previous clinical trials, tightened glucose control with intensive insulin therapy always came at the cost of more hypoglycemia. Fortunately, CGM devices are giving patients the ability to tighten their control while still avoiding hypoglycemia.

If you want to see how CGM has changed my life at night, go to YouTube and type in "hypoglycemic blues." You can see my life before and after I got a CGM!

Fine-Tune Your Basal Rate/Dose

An important component of insulin therapy is finding the right basal dose for you. Whether you use a long-acting insulin like Lantus/Levemir or you are on an insulin pump, you need to know what your basal insulin requirements are. The role of a basal insulin is to keep your blood sugar constant during the day when you aren't eating. A CGM can really help you accomplish this. When I first got my CGM, I noticed that my blood sugar would creep up during the day, even when I wasn't eating. I was able to increase my Lantus dose and take care of this problem.

Another important consideration is the dawn phenomenon. We have talked about this several times in this book, but it is when your blood sugar increases in the early morning hours. With a CGM, you can determine exactly at what time of the early morning your blood sugar starts increasing. People using insulin pumps can take this information and adjust their basal rate appropriately to counteract the dawn phenomenon.

Download Glucose Data

I look at my CGM multiple times during the day and take different actions all the time. However, sometimes it is hard to see the big picture when you are making all these little changes. Fortunately, all CGM devices allow you to download all your data onto the computer. The software included with the devices shows you your glucose ranges over a long period of time. It can tell you how much time you are in range, and importantly can show you trends about times of day. For example, you might see that you are constantly high after breakfast. Downloading this information can give you information about patterns you are developing overtime. You can also download this information with your healthcare provider, and the two of you can review the data together (**Figure 12.5**).

Figure 12-5
CGM Downloads

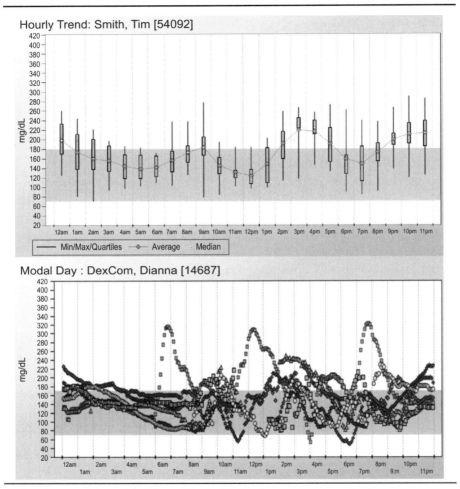

Hourly trend download from Tim's CGM. As you can see he bounces up too high after lunch and dinner. The Modal Day download is from Dianna and shows that she is really in range most of the time but had only one bad day over the time frame.

Glucose Trends

Without a CGM, I would test my blood sugar and if it were high, I would have to give myself a correction bolus. Say my blood glucose reading was 200. I would need to give myself a correction bolus of about 2 units to bring that glucose reading down. However, sometimes I found that the 2 units wouldn't do anything at all, and sometimes it would make my blood glucose crash. What was going on? This situation usually has a lot to do with not just what your glucose is, but where it is going. For example, if my glucose was 200 and rising quickly, that 2 units may just keep my glucose where it is. However, if my glucose was 200 and crashing, that 2 units may send me into hypoglycemia. The direction of your glucose can be just as important as the reading itself.

I like to use the metaphor of a plane in flight. If I told you that the plane was at an altitude of 10,000 feet, you might think nothing of it. However, that altitude doesn't tell you anything about what the plane is doing. It could have just taken off and be rising toward its cruising altitude, or it could be in a free fall heading to crash. The direction the plane is going in will dictate what action the pilots need to take. Similarly, the direction of your blood glucose can drastically change how you decide to act. Let me show you some examples.

Rising Trend

In **Figure 12-6**, the glucose value is above the target zone and is continuing to rise. After confirming the reading of 220 mg/dL with a fingerstick, a rising trend may prompt you to take additional insulin or begin exercising.

Falling Trend

In **Figure 12-7**, the glucose value is falling and headed back into the target zone. After confirming the reading of 220 mg/dL with a fingerstick, a falling trend may prompt you to watch and wait. If the trend continues to fall rapidly, even if the glucose reading is still within the target zone, it may prompt you to eat some fast-acting carbohydrates.

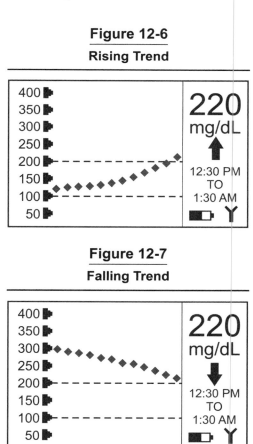

Figure 12-6

Rising Trend

Figure 12-7

Falling Trend

Constant Trend

In **Figure** 12-8, the glucose value is above the target zone and is constant. After confirming the reading of 220 mg/dL with a fingerstick, a constant trend may prompt you to take additional insulin or begin exercising.

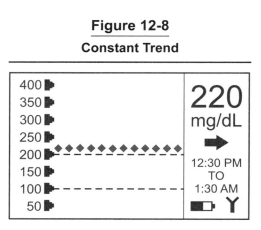

Figure 12-8
Constant Trend

Don't Overreact—Understand "Turnaround Time"

Turnaround time is the time it takes to reverse a trend. There is a delay that it takes for insulin to take effect once it is administered, even with rapid-acting insulin such as Novolog or Humalog. When your glucose trend is going up, it may still rise for a while before it comes down if you take insulin. When your glucose trend is going down, you may still go down for a while before it comes up if you take glucose or other carbohydrates. In some cases, it is best to watch and wait before you react to a slowly rising or slowly falling glucose level.

Three Views of the Same Trend at 3 PM

These charts in **Figure** 12-9 are the same trend line shown over different periods of time: 1 hour, 3 hour, and 9 hour. This person ate a meal and took insulin at noon, and soon after you can see the glucose trend starting to rise. Although glucose initially went up, the 3-hour trend graph shows that it began to level off and then went back into the target range (as insulin began to take effect and brought the glucose level back down). The 1-hour and 3-hour glucose-trend graphs are the best graphs to show that the rise in glucose is leveling off, indicating that a watch-and-wait approach may be appropriate. This turnaround time needed to reverse the trend is shown in the shaded area of each of the three graphs. The 3-hour and 12-hour glucose-trend graphs show that the total turnaround time in this example was about 2 hours.

CGM Considerations

When evaluating CGM devices, it's important to recognize that CGM is a relatively new technology that may not work consistently all the time. This is definitely *not* a "set it and forget it" type of device. In order to get the most out of your CGM, you need to wear it constantly, interact with it frequently, and continue to check your blood sugar on your home glucose meter. Also, CGM technology continues to improve; if you tried CGM a few years ago and were disappointed, it makes sense to re-evaluate it, as what is available now is much better. Issues to consider when using a CGM are discussed in the following sections.

Sensor Inaccuracy and Errors: Control Your Expectations

The sensors that these products use are getting better and better but still do have some issues with inaccuracy, especially in the lower glucose ranges. With that in mind, you can use your CGM to guide your day-to-day decisions but you should always check your blood sugar with your HGM if you feel the CGM is reading inaccurately. Also, the sensors can experience errors in which they stop functioning and will need to be replaced. These issues can be extremely frustrating if you are not expecting them when you start using CGM. CGM technology is improving at a rapid pace so, in the

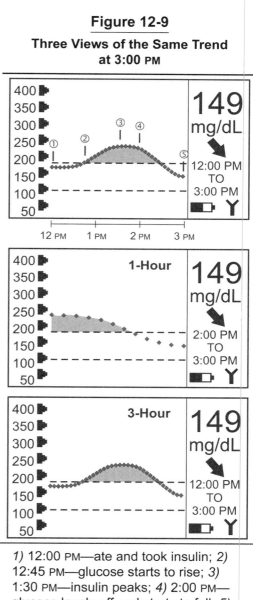

Figure 12-9
Three Views of the Same Trend at 3:00 PM

1) 12:00 PM—ate and took insulin; 2) 12:45 PM—glucose starts to rise; 3) 1:30 PM—insulin peaks; 4) 2:00 PM—glucose levels off and starts to fall; 5) 3:00 PM—current glucose reading is 149 mg/dL; no action required at this time as glucose is within target zone, but watch for continued lowering.

mean time, don't freak out if your CGM value does not perfectly match your HGM number. Be grateful that this technology is here!

Wearing the Sensor

Sensors are currently approved to be worn on the abdomen. That being said, many patients place them on their thigh, their buttocks, or on their triceps area. Although these areas are not officially approved for wear, most patients report good results when using the devices in these areas. Like anything attached to your body (such as an insulin pump), it can take some getting used to. Thankfully, the sensors are small and generally out of the way. If you have issues with them falling off, you can check the company support lines about use of other adhesive materials that would prove to be more durable. The sensors are waterproof and can be taken into pools, etc, but the receivers are not. Finally, as these are a new technology of which most people are not aware, expect to be pulled out of an airport security line from time to time to explain what you have attached to you! It might expedit getting through security if you were to give the screening personnel advance notice to expect the device attached to your body. A doctor's note confirming that you have diabetes would also help in this effort. This can also potentially save you the embarrassment of being pulled out of the line.

Start-Up Period and Calibrations

Each time you insert a new sensor, there is a start-up period that typically lasts about 2 hours. After the 2 hours is up, the machine will ask you to calibrate with a blood sugar from your HGM. The device will start recording your continuous glucose readings from that point forward. Once you are up and running, most CGM devices require two to four fingersticks each day to keep the system calibrated. This is extremely important to keep in mind as it highlights that the CGM devices are not currently able to *replace* your HGM and you will still be required to do fingersticks. Although you won't be able to stop doing fingersticks completely, most patients end up doing fingersticks much less frequently than they were before starting CGM. As CGM devices improve, the calibration requirements may not be needed in the future.

Margins of Difference and Lag Time

Even with calibration, the CGM device will generally not provide the exact same glucose value as your blood glucose meter. On average, most CGM device readings are about 5% to 20% different from those of your blood glucose meter. As the technology improves, the CGM devices will achieve better accuracy. Furthermore, as the sensor is lying in your subcutaneous tissue, it is not actually measuring your "blood" sugar. The glucose readings in your subcutaneous tissue lag behind what is happening in your blood by less than 10 minutes. You need to keep this in mind when your blood sugar is changing rapidly. For instance, if your CGM shows you are at 200 and crashing but your HGM reading is 135, this might not be an issue of your CGM being wrong. Rather, your CGM is reflecting your blood sugar about 10 minutes ago. In another 10 minutes, your CGM will likely catch up and read at 135. Generally, you should avoid calibrating your CGM during times of rapid glucose change.

Reimbursement

Health insurances have begun to cover the cost of CGM. Generally speaking, most type 1 diabetic patients can get the technology covered, and companies are beginning to cover type 2 diabetics as well. Patients with hypoglycemic unawareness can often get coverage more readily. Additionally, the device can be used in pregnancy. Finally, insurance may cover the device for a temporary period of time in which you wear it for several weeks to a month and then get feedback with your doctor on how you have been doing. With more and more data coming in confirming the benefit of CGMs, insurance coverage will likely expand to cover more patients. In the meantime, ask your health care provider about your options. You may be able to use one temporarily or enroll in a clinical trial to get the device paid for. You can always pay out of pocket, but the devices will cost you around $1000 to get started with an additional $200-$400 dollars a month for the sensors. This is a price tag that not many people can afford, but the CGM companies may work with you to lower your payments if you are paying out of pocket. The lack of insurance coverage can be frustrating and although it is much better than it was, there still is a long way to go.

How to Get the Most Out of This Chapter

Following are three clinical situations that you may encounter while using a CGM. Each example will begin with a real-life situation and the corresponding 1-hour glucose-trend graph and, in many cases, the 3-hour glucose-trend graph as well. In cases that involve overnight glucose control problems, the 12-hour glucose-trend graph will also be shown. After you read the case history, you will be asked questions. You should try to answer each question as best you can, then read the explanation that follows each question. If you select an incorrect answer, please read the explanation very carefully before you go on to the next question.

This chapter is meant to illustrate how to interpret the information provided by your CGM device. Our hope is that by the time you review the case scenarios, you will be able to make more effective and safe decisions regarding your diabetes care.

Section I: Blood Glucose Levels on the Rise
Scenario #1

John is a 32-year-old male who has had type 1 diabetes for 20 years. He is currently on 25 units of Lantus at bedtime as his basal insulin and a rapid-acting insulin (Apidra [glulisine]), which he takes before meals and for correction boluses. His correction factor is 1:50, which means that 1 unit of a rapid-acting insulin like Apidra, Novolog (aspart), or Humalog (lispro) will lower his glucose level about 50 mg/dL. His carbohydrate-to-insulin ratio is 15 to 1, which means that for every 15 grams of carbohydrates consumed, he will take 1 unit of Apidra. John's blood glucose upon awaking was 72 mg/dL, and he ate breakfast at 8 AM (60 grams of carbohydrates). He took 4 units of Apidra, calculated this way:

60 grams carbohydrates in meal ÷ 15 grams/unit (insulin ratio)
= 4 units for meal dosage

At 9:20 AM, the high alert (set at 180 mg/dL and shown by the upper dashed lines in the graphs below) went off. John did a fingerstick to confirm his glucose level, reviewing the 1-hour (**Figure 12-10**) and 3-hour (**Figure 12-11**) glucose-trend graphs.

Question 1a. Options for Treating High Glucose Levels

Which of the option(s) below is the best suggestion for John to follow at 9:20 AM when his high alert went off? (There may be more than one correct answer.)

A. Watch and wait (give no additional insulin)
B. Walk for an hour at a brisk pace
C. Give a correction dose of 2 to 3 units
D. Adjust the carbohydrate-to-insulin ratio to 12:1 at breakfast if this scenario repeats itself every morning

Explanation

The correct answers are B, C, and D, depending on the situation. Watching and waiting when the glucose level is rising fairly steeply after a meal usually means that not enough rapid-acting insulin was given with that meal. Blood glucose levels are not always the same after meals, even if we have had that same meal numerous times before. There are so many variables that affect the glucose readings, including stress, exercise, medications, etc. This is why it is important to be able to use a correction dose to account for unexpected elevations in your glucose values. Normally, if you just tested your blood glucose with your blood glucose meter 2 hours after a meal and got a 182-mg/dL reading, you might have been perfectly satisfied. However, the CGM data clearly show that if nothing is done, the blood glucose level may continue to rise and stay elevated for hours.

One question you might ask is: Given that the correction factor is 1:50 and that 2 to 3 units of Apidra (answer C) would drop the blood glucose level 100 to 150 points, if John is only at 182 mg/dL, shouldn't this amount of insulin cause hypoglycemia? The big difference in this situation is that you have important trend information that tells you not only that the blood glucose level is 182 mg/dL, but also that it is rising steeply. This really helps you give a more appropriate correction dose and limit the amount of time spent in the hyperglycemic range.

Aerobic exercise for an hour (answer B), especially within 1 to 2 hours after your last injection of a rapid-acting insulin such as Apidra, will help to lower your glucose level. If you have an opportunity to exercise, you would not give any insulin and would watch to see what happens to your number while you exercise. If it does not come down, you can give a correction dose later (with an amount determined by your blood glucose level and trend over time as well).

Answer D is also correct—if you find that your blood glucose level is above 180 mg/dL morning after morning, you need to make the long-term adjustment by changing your breakfast carbohydrate-to-in-

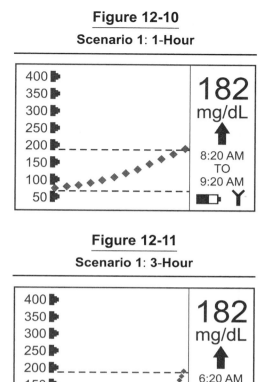

Figure 12-10

Scenario 1: 1-Hour

400
350
300
250
200
150
100
50

182
mg/dL
↑
8:20 AM
TO
9:20 AM

Figure 12-11

Scenario 1: 3-Hour

400
350
300
250
200
150
100
50

182
mg/dL
↑
6:20 AM
TO
9:20 AM

sulin ratio. It is usually recommended to make small changes slowly and wait several days to see how your adjustment affects your glucose levels.

Question 1b. Avoiding Postmeal Highs

John gave himself a correction dose of 3 units of Apidra at 9:20 am. Over the next 90 minutes, his glucose level peaked at 232 mg/dL, but started to trend downward. By noon, it was 122 mg/dL with a flat or level trend (**Figures 12-12** and **12-13**).

What could John do differently in the future in order to avoid the same situation of high postmeal glucose values in scenario 1? (More than one answer may be correct.)

A. Take 2 to 3 extra units on top of his usual 4 units when he eats the same type of breakfast that he ate that day (eg, only when he eats 60 grams carbohydrates such as Cheerios with milk)

B. Change the carbohydrate-to-insulin ratio from 15:1 to 12:1 for the breakfast meal

C. Eat only two thirds of his normal breakfast

D. Change the composition of the breakfast to include fewer refined carbohydrates and more protein and fat

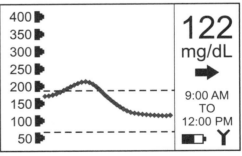

Figure 12-12

Scenario 1/Question 1b: 1-Hour

Figure 12-13

Scenario 1/Question 1b: 3-Hour

Explanation

Answers A, B, C and D could all be correct, depending on the situation. Taking 2 to 3 extra units of a rapid-acting insulin (answer A) is a viable option. The correction dose of 2 to 3 units that John gave himself at 9:20 AM worked well. Thus the same correction dose could be given at the beginning of the meal, in addition to his calculated initial dose, in order to avoid the high postbreakfast blood glucose level in the first place. If this scenario happens most of the time, answer B would be appropriate. Changing the carbohydrate-to-insulin ratio is an excellent option if John is going to eat the same type of breakfast on most days. This would work since his postmeal values are typically high when he uses the 15 grams of carbohydrates to 1 unit of rapid-acting insulin ratio. Reducing the carbohydrate-to-insulin ratio allows for a higher dose of rapid-acting insulin per serving and in this scenario would indicate that John should take 5 units for breakfast instead of 4 units:

$$60 \text{ grams carbohydrates in meal} \div 12 \text{ grams/unit (insulin ratio)}$$
$$= 5 \text{ units for meal dosage}$$

If this change does not solve the problem, he could try a 10:1 ratio for breakfast. It is important to look for trends and patterns and not make long-term changes based on one blood glucose result. Last, John's carbohydrate-to-insulin ratio of 15:1 may be perfectly adequate at lunch and dinner.

Eating two thirds of his normal breakfast (answer C) would help his postmeal glucose values. However, if that leaves John hungry after breakfast and leads to snacking and overeating at lunch, this would not be the best option. This option would improve or solve the problem, but John would have to make that decision himself. All changes really are up to the individual living with diabetes and his or her diabetes care team.

Changing the composition of the breakfast from a refined carbohydrate meal, such as cold cereal and milk, to one that has more fat and protein (answer D) would reduce postmeal glucose values. One must be aware of his or her limitations for fat if high cholesterol is a problem or of limitations for protein if kidney problems are present. Normally, a balanced breakfast of carbohydrate, fat, and protein is the best choice; however, personal preferences, living situation, budget, etc., may limit the ideal choices. Now that we have rapid-acting insulin, Symlin, and CGM, we can control postmeal glucose values regardless of the amount or type of foods eaten.

Section II: Blood Glucose Levels on the Way Down
Scenario #2

Ruth is a 76-year-old woman with insulin-requiring type 2 diabetes. She has many relatives with diabetes, and when she retired from her job as a banker at age 65, she was diagnosed with diabetes. After taking oral medications for 5 years, her average blood glucose level rose to more than 200 mg/dL, and she started taking insulin. She now takes 60 units of Lantus (long-acting basal insulin) at bedtime, 20 units of Apidra (rapid-acting insulin) with breakfast, 10 units of Apidra with lunch, and 25 units of Apidra with dinner. She also takes 1000 mg of oral metformin (Glucophage) twice daily. She weighs 169 pounds and is 5'4" tall.

She is meticulous with her diabetes treatment. Last month, she purchased a CGM and has been using it every day. She set her low blood glucose alert to 60 mg/dL and high glucose alert to 200 mg/dL. Her last A1C value was 6.2%, and she has been able to avoid many complications of diabetes. However, she has macular degeneration (damage to the macula or the eye), and her vision is not as good as it once was.

Ruth went to Napa, California, to spend a week tasting wine with her husband. She went to bed at 11:15 PM with a glucose level of 128 mg/dL and took her usual 60 units of Lantus. Within 45 minutes of injection, she was awakened by a low-glucose alarm. Her monitor read 53 and showed a sharp decline in blood glucose (**Figures 12-14** and **12-15**).

Figure 12-14
Scenario 2: 1-Hour

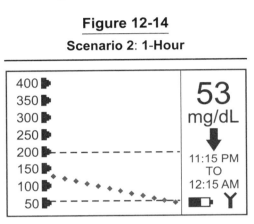

___

Question 2a. Using Different Insulins

What answer do you think is most likely to have caused Ruth's blood glucose level to drop? (Only one answer is correct.)

Figure 12-15
Scenario 2: 3-Hour

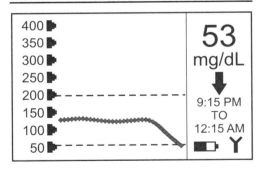

A. Ruth forgot to have her bedtime snack

B. Ruth mistakenly took 60 units of Apidra at bedtime (instead of Lantus)

C. The batteries were low in the receiver, which led to a falsely low reading

D. The insulin went bad and was working too quickly

Explanation

The correct answer is B. While this may seem improbable for a woman as careful as Ruth, it happens not infrequently. It may be due in part to all of the newer insulins being clear or colorless and, therefore, difficult to distinguish from one another.

Prior to the introduction of Lantus and Levemir, all clear insulins were faster-acting products. NPH is cloudy and easy to distinguish from clear, short-acting insulin. Currently, there is no consistent way to distinguish commonly used insulins other than by reading the labels, which is difficult for people with limited vision. To minimize the potential for confusion, some doctors suggest using insulin pens for meal therapy and a vial and syringe for long-acting insulin therapy.

Missing a bedtime snack (answer A) can cause problems for people who are taking excessive basal insulin. However, it usually results in a much slower decrease than that seen here, so answer A is incorrect. However, if Ruth drank a great deal of alcohol during her wine tours, it could have made her more vulnerable to hypoglycemia, as drinking alcohol can lower glucose levels.

Answer C is also incorrect. When the monitor's batteries are low, there is a low-battery indicator. The low-battery state does not lead to false readings. The monitor is designed to shut off the display of readings in case of suspected inaccuracy of the device.

When insulin is exposed to extreme temperatures or used beyond its expiration date, there is generally a reduced potency. An increased insulin effect has not been seen, so answer D is incorrect.

Question 2b. Options for Treating Low-Glucose Levels

Ruth took four glucose tablets and woke her husband. What should she do next? (Only one answer is correct.)

A. Call her doctor and ask for further advice
B. Call room service to order some desserts
C. Confirm that her glucose level is really low by a fingerstick test and continue to take glucose tablets and any other available carbohydrates until the CGM shows a glucose level greater than 100 mg/dL and a rising trend
D. Inject herself with 1 mg of Glucagon and call the paramedics immediately

Explanation

The correct answer is C. Treatment of her accidental mistake is urgent, and quick action is required to avoid severe hypoglycemia. The insulin she took will keep her at risk for hypoglycemia for at least 4 hours, so she should not go back to sleep. Having a CGM will allow her to closely watch her blood glucose level.

Answer D would be correct if she was unable to take anything by mouth. If she had type 1 diabetes and took this amount of rapid-acting insulin and was not very close to a hospital, taking Glucagon and calling the paramedics would not be an unreasonable choice.

Calling the doctor (answer A) would be a good idea if Ruth didn't know what to do or if she didn't realize her mistake. However, patients using CGMs tend to be among those most informed about diabetes.

Answer B is unwise for short-term treatment, due to the unpredictable time it may take to get the food. In addition, answer B has the potential for overtreatment (depending on the type and amount of desserts eaten) and could lead to high blood glucose levels. However, ordering a small snack from room service may make all of those glucose tablets more palatable.

Ruth has had a rough night so far. Her initial glucose level when she confirmed it by fingerstick with her blood glucose meter was 68 mg/dL. It has been 2 hours since her low glucose alarm went off. She has not only exhausted her supply of glucose tablets, but she also ate a bagel leftover from lunch and drank the only 2 bottles of regular soda that were in her minibar. Her husband has finally come back with dessert. Look at her 1-hour and 3-hour glucose-trend graphs in **Figures 12-16** and **12-17** and decide what she should do next.

Figure 12-16

Scenario 2/Question 2b: 1-Hour

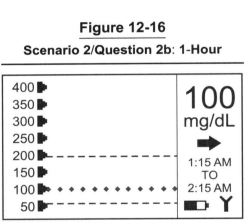

Question 2c. Treatment Following a Low Glucose Value

What should Ruth do now? (Choose the one best answer.)
  A. Decide not to eat the desserts and go to sleep, as she was confident her glucose was not going to drop further
  B. Have a decaf cappuccino and watch the monitor closely for another hour before doing anything else
  C. Continue eating, but more slowly
  D. Give 10 units of Apidra to prevent rebound hyperglycemia

Explanation

Answer B is the best option, since she has reversed the falling glucose trend and has a glucose level high enough to be reasonably safe.

Remember, she has type 2 diabetes, and because of the associated insulin resistance, overdoses of insulin are less catastrophic (as compared with such a high dose of Apidra in a thin person with type 1 diabetes).

Figure 12-17

Scenario 2/Question 2b: 3-Hour

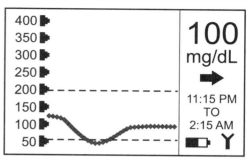

Answer A is incorrect. Although Apidra is a rapid-acting insulin, it remains active for 4 to 5 hours, and she is not out of the woods yet with regard to hypoglycemia risk.

Answer C might be an option if glucose levels begin to trend downward again.

Answer D would be unwise as the time frame during which she is at risk for hypoglycemia has not passed. Most likely, Ruth's glucose level will not be in the normal range in the morning due to overtreatment of her lows with food. However, this is preferable to hypoglycemia. With the use of CGMs, both overtreatment of hypoglycemia and risk of hypoglycemia can be safely reduced.

Question 2d. Adjusting Your Target Range

Which setting change on her CGM receiver should Ruth consider? (Choose the one best answer.)
   A. Raise the high-glucose alert to 250 mg/dL
   B. Raise the low-glucose alert to 100 mg/dL
   C. Call the manufacturer of the company to change the fixed low warning of 55 mg/dL
   D. Turn off the audible alarms

Explanation

Answer B is the correct answer. Raising the threshold for a low alarm can improve safety, as it gives you more time to anticipate a potential low. Although the alarm on the device may annoy you, the increase in safety from hypoglycemia can be worth it (particularly if you have hypoglycemia unawareness).

Raising the high-glucose alert in Ruth would offer no benefit (it is already somewhat high at 200 mg/dL), so answer A is incorrect.

Answer C is incorrect because the low-glucose alarm warning (set at 55 mg/dL) cannot be altered. This option would also be unwise because of safety concerns.

Answer D would be unwise as the audible alerts might be very helpful to Ruth, particularly during the night.

Section III: Blood Glucose Levels During the Night
Scenario #3
Mary is a 19-year-old college student who has been living with diabetes for less than a year. She uses an insulin pump with the basal rate set at 0.6 units per hour for 24 hours (a basal rate is a constant amount of insulin delivered throughout the day and night by an insulin pump in very small increments). The basal rate maintains blood glucose values in the normal range between meals, overnight, and during periods of fasting. Mary's correction factor is 1:50 and her carbohydrate-to-rapid-acting insulin ratio is 15:1. She commonly goes to bed with a good blood glucose level, but it is high upon awakening in the morning. She has dinner at 6 PM on most nights and does not snack after dinner. She usually goes to bed around 11:00 PM. Please see her 12-hour glucose-trend graphs in **Figures 12-18**, **12-19**, and **12-20** from the previous 3 nights.

Question 3a. Nocturnal Hyperglycemia—Second Culprit
Which option below best explains what is happening with Mary overnight? *(Only one answer is correct.)*
  A. Mary is experiencing the Somogyi reaction (rebound hyperglycemia as a result of a hypoglycemic reaction)
  B. Mary's insulin pump is malfunctioning
  C. Mary is experiencing the dawn phenomenon, which is early morning resistance to insulin
  D. Mary has gastroparesis

Explanation
Option C is the correct answer. The dawn phenomenon is a well-characterized problem that is common in people with diabetes. People without diabetes commonly need more insulin in the early hours of the morning to keep the blood glucose levels from rising. This need for more insulin is thought to be due to natural circadian (natural biologic cycle of the body) elevations in anti-insulin hormones such as the growth hormone. If you do not have diabetes, the pancreas merely secretes a little more insulin during this time period, which is normally between the hours of 3 AM and 7 AM. However, if your pancreas does not secrete enough insulin because you have diabetes, your glucose level will go up during this time unless you compensate for it.

Answer A is not correct. The Somogyi reaction is a situation where there is rebound hyperglycemia after one has a hypoglycemic reaction.

When one has a hypoglycemic reaction, there is sometimes a natural physiologic response to protect one from extremely low glucose values by secreting hormones such as epinephrine (also called adrenalin) and glucagon that raise the glucose levels. As you can see from the 12-hour displays, Mary is not getting into the hypoglycemic range, so this option is not correct.

There is no reason why the pump would malfunction at such a specific time period, so answer B is not correct.

Gastroparesis, delayed absorption of food after it enters the stomach, which is further described in *Chapter 19*, would not take 12 hours to cause hyperglycemia, so answer D is not correct. Mary eats dinner at 6 PM and the glucose values do not go up until around 3 AM. Gastroparesis usually causes a delay in postmeal glucose elevations of about 2 to 4 hours.

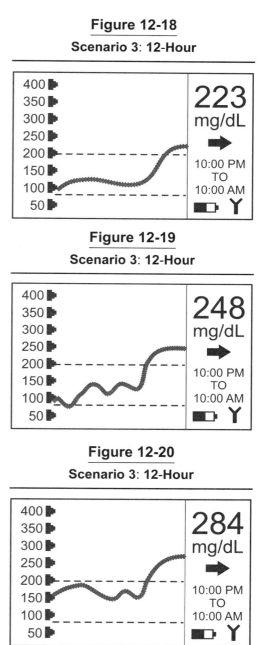

Figure 12-18
Scenario 3: 12-Hour

Figure 12-19
Scenario 3: 12-Hour

Figure 12-20
Scenario 3: 12-Hour

Question 3b. Preventing This Phenomenon

Which of the options below might help to prevent this situation causing elevated glucose level in the early morning? (There is one best answer.)

A. Have Mary take an injection of NPH insulin at bedtime
B. Program a second basal rate into Mary's pump where the rate is increased by 30% to 0.8 units/hour, starting at 3 AM until 7 AM
C. Have Mary do 30 to 45 minutes of aerobic exercise starting at 3 AM

D. Have Mary change her normal sleep hours, so that she goes to bed much later than 11 PM

Explanation

Option B is the best answer. One advantage of insulin pump therapy is that you can have more than one basal rate throughout the day and night. You can adjust your basal rate according to your activities, including exercise and whether you experience the dawn phenomenon. Having an increased basal rate during the time of the dawn phenomenon is normally very effective at preventing the rise in glucose in the early morning hours. CGM is really ideal for making the diagnosis quickly and accurately. It can also help you make the correct insulin adjustment.

Giving NPH at bedtime (answer A) would also help the situation; however, the timing of NPH insulin is not as precise as increasing the basal rate on an insulin pump. In addition, adding intermediate-acting insulin such as NPH at night to a patient on a pump adds unnecessary complexity to the insulin regimen. Changing Mary's sleep habits (answer D) and exercising in the middle of the night (answer C) are unreasonable options.

CGM Products Available

Now that we have reviewed how to use a CGM appropriately, you may be curious about what devices are available. Currently, there are only three CGM devices available on the market in the United States (**Figure 12-1**). This is good news in that you can be familiar with all the options, but bad news in that the options are limited. The devices are made by Dexcom and Medtronic. Each has some pluses and minuses that I will discuss briefly.

Dexcom SEVEN Plus

Pluses:

- The Dexcom device benefits from its longer sensor wear. Sensors are approved to be worn for up to 7 days at a time (while Medtronic device is only 3 days currently)
- Easy and relatively pain-free insertion
- Strong adhesive that generally holds the sensor in place without extra tape
- Simple and user-friendly display
- Loud high/low alerts
- Calibrations can be entered at any time regardless of glucose changing

Minuses:
- Taking Tylenol (acetaminophen) or any acetaminophen-containing products will cause very inaccurate readings. Therefore you *cannot* take Tylenol (acetaminophen) while using this device
- No current integration with insulin pumps
- Sensor does not store any information when out of range from the receiver

Dexcom G4 Platinum

The Dexcom G4 Platinum is the 4th generation CGM from Dexcom and, in a similar manner to the 3rd generation SEVEN Plus, consists of three parts: a sensor, transmitter, and monitor. The sensor, about the diameter of a human hair, is inserted by the user under the skin, and a small transmitter sends data wirelessly to an ergonomic monitor and provides data every 5 minutes for up to 7 consecutive days.

The Dexcom G4 Platinum CGM compared with the G3 SEVEN Plus:
- The monitor does not need to be charged as frequently
- It can pick up the readings at a much greater distance from the sensor (~20 feet)
- It is more consistently accurate.

Any CGM device, including the G4, needs to be prescribed by a health care provider covered by most insurance plans for people taking insulin and is indicated for use as an adjunctive device to complement, not replace, information obtained from standard home glucose monitoring devices.

Medtronic Guardian REAL-Time
Pluses:
- The main advantage of the Medtronic Guardian is that it can be incorporated with an insulin pump so both the CGM data and insulin pump control is all on one device
- Customize alerts by time of day so you can be more aggressive with glucose control depending on the time
- Statistics are displayed on screen and do not require downloading to a computer to view
- Predictive alarms that will alarm if your current glucose rate of change will put you into the hyperglycemic or hypoglycemic range
- Sensor stores up to 40 minutes of data if you are out of range from the receiver
- Can take Tylenol (acetaminophen) without problems

Minuses:

- Sensors only last 3 days
- Insertion process is slightly more complicated and can be painful
- Calibrations should only be done with relatively stable glucose readings
- Sensors often require more adhesive or tape to keep in place
- Patients complain that the high/low alerts are sometimes not loud enough

So there you have it. People always ask me, which device is the best. You need to look at each product carefully, and pick the one that is best for your needs. The CGM environment is changing rapidly and this information will quickly become out of date. Both Medtronic and Dexcom are developing next-generation products that promise longer durability and better accuracy. Furthermore, more combinations with CGM and pumps are in the works. Ask your health care provider about what is currently available. With that in mind, let me talk briefly about some cool new products and what is coming in the future.

Medtronic mySentry

Medtronic has recently released this new product called mySentry. The CGM products on the market currently require that the receiver be very close to the sensor to transmit information. In other words, you need to carry the receiver on you for it to work (the new Dexcom G4 Platinum has a range of 20 to 25 feet). This is fine if you are only using the information for yourself, but what if you want to transmit the information farther away? This is particularly an issue for parents of children with type 1 diabetes who want to monitor their child's blood sugar overnight. This new product greatly amplifies the signal from the sensor so the information can be transmitted to another room. I liken this product to a diabetes baby monitor. It is a step toward giving parents peace of mind when their child is sleeping.

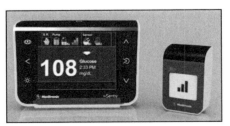

Medtronic's mySentry remote glucose monitor is designed for enhanced nighttime protection with sensor alerts and alarms that can awaken you to important information.

Photo courtesy of Medtronic, Inc.

Medtronic Veo

As I mentioned above, the Medtronic CGM device has the advantage of being incorporated with an insulin pump. Your blood sugar is displayed right on the pump screen. However, regardless of what your blood sugar is, the insulin pump does not change what it is doing unless you tell it to. In other words, although the devices share a screen, they don't "talk" to one another. Medtronic has taken the first step toward making this happen. They have a device called the Veo that will suspend insulin delivery when your blood sugar is low. This is an important safety feature. Currently, if you were sleeping at night and didn't wake up to your CGM low alarm, your insulin pump would continue to deliver insulin and make the situation worse. With the Veo, the insulin delivery would shut off automatically to help your body recover. This device is not yet available in the United States but is available in other countries.

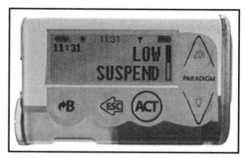

The Veo Paradigm pump/cgm system.

Medtronic Enlite Sensor

Medtronic has launched the Enlite Sensor, their most advanced CGM sensor in more than 35 countries outside of the United States (not currently approved for use in the United States).

When the Enlite Sensor is used with the predictive alerts feature on Medtronic systems, diabetes patients have access to hypo detection and helps give early warning to prevent dangerous hypoglycemia. The Veo medtronic pump *(see above)* in Europe combined with the Enlite sensor (Veo Paradigm insulin pump/cgm system) will turn off the delivery of insulin for two hours if the user does not respond to the low blood glucose alarm, which is actually the first step in developing an artificial pancreas.

Artificial Pancreas

The Veo is the first step in the process toward what we call "closing the loop." What that means is that we are all working toward a device that will be fully integrated between the CGM and an insulin pump. Ideally the device would adjust your insulin levels depending on your CGM results. If this was the case, you wouldn't need to take boluses, adjust insulin, or really do any work at all. This would be an artificial pancreas. As CGM devices are getting more accurate and insulin pumps are more sophisticated, many believe that the artificial pancreas is a real and achievable goal in the next 10 to 15 years!

Summary

For people on insulin and with hypoglycemia unawareness, CGM is one of the more important advances in the past several decades. In our opinion, the vast majority of folks with type 1 diabetes could benefit greatly from CGM. In addition, people with type 2 diabetes on multiple daily injections or an insulin pump may also benefit from CGM technology. Home glucose monitoring only captures a snapshot of what is happening throughout the day and night, while CGM provides much more information on trends and patterns. CGM allows many people with diabetes (including me) to achieve a better A1C in a safe manner with less hypoglycemia. Please go to the TCOYD web site (*www.tcoyd.org*) to watch the TCOYD-TV episode on continuous glucose monitoring.

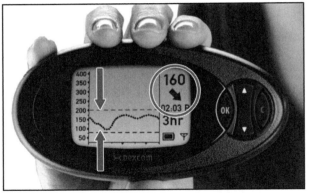

CGM monitor showing patient and physician choosen upper and lower alarm levels, real time blood glucose level, and trend arrow.

13

Hypoglycemia

Origins, Prevention, and Proper Management

by Patrick J. Boyle, MD

Introduction

Hypoglycemia (low blood glucose) is undoubtedly the limiting factor preventing many motivated patients with diabetes from achieving their goal of near-normal blood glucose concentrations. So, quite correctly, hypoglycemia prevents us from preventing long-term complications. If it were easier to achieve better glucose control without substantial hypoglycemia risk, then diabetes would, in part, be much less of a national health care dilemma.

Common Themes With Type 1 and Type 2 Diabetes

First, you need a bit of general background information on hypoglycemia. The body has a series of redundant hormonal responses for limiting how low of a blood glucose one can have. These systems also allow recovery from hypoglycemia. The first line of defense should be a reduction in insulin production as the blood glucose falls just below the normal range.

Insulin's primary function is to tell your liver not to make glucose. Without insulin, your body can make extraordinary amounts of glucose (even running into concentrations in the thousands of milligrams per deciliter [mg/dL]). Insulin can entirely shut off liver glucose production. In fact, we try to take advantage of this fact by having patients take their insulin before meals in order to give the liver the signal that making glucose will not be necessary while food is being absorbed. The absence of insulin-producing beta cells results in the loss of this important buffer against low blood glucose in patients with type 1 diabetes. When a person with type 1 diabetes gets a low glucose concentration from injection of relatively excessive amounts of insulin, there is no capacity to regulate the body's total insulin concentration – once it is injected beneath the skin, there is no taking it back!

Patients with type 2 diabetes are not sensitive to the insulin that they do make. Therefore, if hypoglycemia begins to occur, their insulin-producing beta cells simply shut down the production of insulin and the body runs off of what was put under the skin. So hypoglycemia in patients with type 2 diabetes is much less common compared with that in type 1 diabetes patients. However, it must be underscored that patients with type 2 diabetes can experience a substantial increase in risk if the A1C target is selected to be as low as 6%. At A1C values of 7%, using conventional intensified therapy including higher dose insulin treatment, patients with type 2 diabetes can be at increased risk of cardiovascular mortality.

The next line of defense is release of glucagon, a hormone produced in cells adjacent to the insulin-producing beta cells in the pancreas. Glucagon goes to the liver and tells it to release stored glucose and to make new glucose. But there's a problem here, too. The alpha cells that make glucagon become dysfunctional and fail to respond to hypoglycemia the longer one lives with either type 1 or type 2 diabetes. The exact reason for this failure is not known, although it is generally believed that the alpha and beta cells communicate back and forth with one another through chemical and nerve signaling in order to cause release of glucagon when you need it. Unfortunately, when the beta cells are destroyed, the communication becomes one-sided, and appropriate glucagon release is lost in the face of low glucose concentrations. Abnormally low, but not absent, glucagon responses are also known to be part of the type 2 diabetes picture.

When glucagon is not available to correct low glucose concentrations, there is another backup plan. The adrenal glands, which sit on top of the kidneys, release the hormone adrenalin (or epinephrine), which tells the liver to break down stored glucose and make new glucose. Adrenalin is like glucagon in this sense, but it induces its effect from completely independent biochemical steps.

During hypoglycemia, rising adrenalin concentrations also tell muscles to stop using glucose and redirect the fuel to the brain. Humans can develop deficiencies in either glucagon or adrenalin and they can still have perfectly normal glucose concentrations. Coupled with diabetes and the need to inject insulin, the defect in glucagon puts adrenalin in the driver's seat as the factor preventing hypoglycemia.

Adrenalin release that occurs during a low blood glucose event has one other desirable side effect—it makes the patient nervous, shaky, and hungry. These symptoms of low blood glucose should drive you to eat and directly help correct the low. But, you guessed it, there is one more glitch in the system, particularly in patients with type 1 diabetes. The release of adrenalin can be lost in response to hypoglycemia (we will go into this more later) and so now we have a patient who cannot reduce internal insulin production, does not release glucagon due to a loss of communication between alpha and beta cells, and also does not have the backup hormone that causes some of the symptoms of hypoglycemia, plus biochemically driving the creation of new glucose production from the liver! With this critical failure, you are now extremely vulnerable to hypoglycemia, and cannot tell when you have a low glucose due to a loss of warning signals.

A couple of final hormones can help to a certain degree. Cortisol from the adrenal glands and growth hormone from the pituitary gland in the brain are released during hypoglycemia but are not important in an immediate response. Instead, they contribute to resolution of the low glucose if it persists for hours (like over the course of a night). So even though you may not be growing in height, you still make growth hormone and it has an additional function of helping you out during a prolonged period of low blood glucose.

The brain is in charge of your body's entire response to a low glucose concentration. The brain runs on glucose, but it can learn to burn breakdown products of fat during times of fasting. Without glucose, the brain stops working, and you pass out. On the way down to unconsciousness, electrical activity can become chaotic in the brain, leading to seizures. Given this near-absolute dependence on glucose for fuel, the brain directs the redundant set of backup systems described above. But there is one final trick for preserving the flow of glucose to your brain. In the face of repeated low blood glucose levels, the brain gets the signal to increase its efficiency in extracting glucose from the circulation. Small channels in the brain allow the movement of glucose into the brain. One line of thinking is that these channels increase in number if a patient is repeatedly below the normal glucose concentration. By "up-regulating" the number of these channels, the brain is able to suck more glucose out of the circulation at lower glucose levels, thereby preserving its own function. There are other theories as to how the brain is able to maintain normal glucose stores in the face of repeated hypoglycemia.

Here is the dark side of intensified diabetes management: If you push your therapy enough so that you are frequently experiencing blood glucose levels below normal, you may end up with a great A1C, but your brain is going to change its metabolism so that it can maintain a normal "brain glucose concentration" during subsequent hypoglycemia. This may sound like a great idea except that now, in the face of what should be a glucose level that triggers all of the defense mechanisms, the brain is satisfied that it has enough energy, and it doesn't respond to the low body-glucose concentration. In and of itself, this would be no big deal, but the ability to pull this trick off is not infinite. So there is a glucose concentration at which your brain cannot compensate, and it will finally have to shut down operation. The margin of safety from the point at which you are finally made aware of the low brain-glucose level and when you pass out becomes very narrow. After a person with this problem eats something to treat the reaction, it is still going to take minutes for the absorption to occur and there may not be enough time between when they finally get the signal to eat and when they lose consciousness. This is referred to as hypoglycemia unawareness. Mostly we see this in patients with type 1 diabetes, and so we will deal with prevention and treatment of the problem in that section below.

Complications of diabetes, particularly in small blood vessels, are directly linked to A1C both for patients with type 1 and type 2 diabetes. During the Diabetes Control and Complications Trial (DCCT), we demonstrated that better overall glucose levels would prevent eye and kidney disease, as well as reduce nervous system disease. Recently, a history of good glucose control was found to reduce the risk of heart attacks 15 years after the end of the trial. So one would be hard pressed to find a reason not to achieve as near normal glucose control as possible—except for those pesky low blood glucose levels! Although your brain is probably swimming from the review of the preceding facts, be thankful that the system was put together with as much backup built in, otherwise the general public, even without diabetes medications, would be experiencing hypoglycemia all the time!

Type 1 Diabetes

Some limitations exist in your response to a low blood glucose. Let's meet the challenge head on. First of all, in trials of intensified diabetes management, like the DCCT, 60% of the severe episodes of hypoglycemia (seizures/comas/episodes requiring the help of someone else) occurred between the hours of midnight and 4 AM. Measuring your blood glucose level immediately before you go to sleep *every night* is a key way of predicting which nights you are more vulnerable. If you are less than 100 mg/dL, you know this is going to be a night that you are going to need more of a snack, or even some liquid glucose plus a snack.

Given the fact that many patients who achieve near-normal A1C values become accustomed to glucose values of 75 mg/dL to 90 mg/dL, you cannot rely on the "I feel fine" factor. You would do something completely different with a blood glucose of 75 mg/dL than you would with 175 mg/dL, right? You might even skip the snack for 175 mg/dL.

I tell my patients that if their glucose is less than 80 mg/dL at bedtime, they should have 6 oz of juice or milk, plus their usual snack.

Snacks may be unnecessary for insulin pump–managed patients, since the programming can be set at the minimum amount to achieve a normal fasting value and reduce the risk of lows during sleep. If you are on a long-acting insulin, like Lantus (glargine) and Levemir (detemir), you are going to go through a period of the night when you have too much insulin in your system to meet your needs. To cover for this fact, you will need to have a small snack, in the neighborhood of 25 grams of starch (half of a peanut butter sandwich, a small container of yogurt, or one half cup of cottage cheese).

Let's say, instead, that you are at 250 mg/dL at bedtime. How long was it since your evening meal? If you eat late (within 2 hours of lying down), resist the urge to take more insulin — the dinnertime insulin is still working and you are likely to see a fall in your blood glucose in the next hours. If it has been 4 hours since you took insulin for your evening meal, then maybe you will need to do a "touch up." Realize, though, that you are not going to be awake to sense the onset of and excessive fall in glucose and so you may not want to be so aggressive.

Many patients use correction factors of 1 unit of insulin for every 50 to 75 mg/dL over a target of 150 mg/dL. So for a blood glucose of 250 mg/dL at bedtime, you might take 2 units of rapid-acting insulin to correct before morning (remember that you cannot mix any other type of insulin in the same syringe with Lantus if that is what has been prescribed for you). My advice is not to try and correct to 100 mg/dL. Shooting for this degree of tight control is asking for trouble over the night. Insulin replacement is not a perfect science and if you try to make it into that, you will eventually pay for it with a major low blood glucose during the night. An occasional fasting glucose of 150 mg/dL is not going to ruin your overall A1C.

This brings up one other topic that is worth mentioning. Insulin has the power to prevent complications. Power is addictive. I have seen more than my fair share of people who come to the conclusion that if they can tolerate a glucose concentration of 65 mg/dL and not have any symptoms, then they must be safe. They conclude that lower is better. One of my great teachers coined a phrase that is still true: "Hypoglycemia begets hypoglycemia." The more lows you have, the more lows you are going to have. Remember that you lose the symptoms of low glucose concentrations the more times you experience them.

As much as we strive to help patients reduce the number of high blood glucose levels they have, we also have to work equally hard to minimize the number of lows. The A1C is just the average blood glucose level, and you can get a "great number" with a lot of lows balanced against a lot of highs. When you interact with your diabetes team, do not forget that you are more than a number every 3 months—you have to consider your day-to-day control, both highs and lows.

I Am Not Drunk, I Have Diabetes

Alcohol deserves special mention in this section, especially for the patient with type 1 diabetes. Alcohol prevents the liver from making glucose. Insulin does the same thing in a different way, and the two added together can be double trouble. Drinking is part of growing up and so in my young patients, I understand that they are going to experiment—especially when they go off to college. Everything in moderation is a good motto for liquor and diabetes. Because judgment is impaired during hypoglycemia and also with alcohol intoxication, you can imagine the effect of the two of them together. I used to give patients cards that read "I'm not drunk, I have diabetes," since hypoglycemia can be mistaken for drunken behavior. I have gotten realistic enough to understand that humans will experiment in risk-taking behaviors even after having been informed of the danger—and I do not give out those cards anymore! If you are going to drink, then take precautions to have something near you to treat a reaction during the night. If I could get you to do it, I would have you wake up in the night and check a blood glucose. At least have a small additional snack before falling asleep—alcohol-associated hypoglycemia usually occurs hours into your sleep period.

Sex Is Exercise

While we are talking about hypoglycemia in the bedroom, let's also cover the risk of hypoglycemia after sex. Sex is exercise. You use muscles for this activity just as much as though you went to the gym or for a swim. The longer the duration of sexual activity, the greater the use of glucose to fuel the muscles in your legs, arms, and hips.

Exercise involves muscles using glucose. Every time you exercise, you should know what your glucose level is going into the activity. Some of my patients prefer to have a snack before exercise or sex in order to prevent hypoglycemia. The longer the exercise period, the more monitoring you should do and the more calories that you may need to ingest. A long bike ride on a Saturday could require frequent snack intake to keep you from getting too low.

Treating Hypoglycemia

Treatment of hypoglycemia is a simple task, as long as you have your head about you. The first few times it happens, you will feel the overwhelming urge to open the refrigerator door and inhale everything in front of you. Eating or drinking more than you actually need to correct the low blood glucose is not going to make you return to normal any faster! Your best bet is to drink 6 to 8 oz of your favorite juice. The goal is to treat your glucose back up to a normal value, not to drive it into the stratosphere.

It will take at least 10 minutes for your blood glucose to start to recover. To reassure yourself that you have stayed the same or started to go back toward normal, recheck your glucose often the first few times that you experience a low.

Liquid sugar is always going to be better than a solid, and so I suggest that patients buy and carry with them small boxes of juice. They do not require refrigeration and they have about 12 to 18 grams of sugar in them—just the right amount for one reaction. Thus the temptation to overdo the treatment is partially taken out of your hands. Alternatively, you might choose to have glucose tablets with you since they are also convenient and do not spoil. But remember that you will have to eat 3 to 5 tabs to get the right amount of sugar to treat the reaction.

Milk is one of the best treatments for a low blood glucose, but you have to be near a refrigerator, so it is not practical when you are away from home. About 6 oz of milk is sufficient, and because of the protein and fat in it, carbohydrate absorption is slowed down so you get a slower but more sustained return to normal.

Solid substances, other than glucose tabs, are always going to be slower to fix the low blood glucose because they have to be broken down from their solid form. I advise against candy bars and ice cream for the treatment of insulin reactions since you get a lot of calories along with the sugar. In the long run, all patients are going to have to fight the battle of weight gain, even patients with type 1 diabetes who are slender at the time of diagnosis.

Glucagon

In an emergency, there is nothing like an injection of glucagon to save the day. Although your body may not appropriately release glucagon during a low-glucose period, an injection of 1 mg, prescribed by your physician, is very powerful. The injection can be given in muscle or fat.

Generally, the patient's parent, significant other, or an appointed person will be the one administering it, because the time to use it is when you cannot swallow. If the brain does not have enough glucose, it cannot coordinate the muscles in the throat to do the swallowing action. Giving someone sugar by mouth at that point will cause part of the treatment to go into the lungs. If the person with you assesses that you are not capable of swallowing, then they need to get out the glucagon.

Some formulations of glucagon require that the liquid be mixed with the solid prior to injecting it. Give the person most likely to administer the glucagon an opportunity to become familiar with the type of glucagon you have been prescribed. It will take 15 to 20 minutes for your glucose to recover from this treatment, but that is faster than most paramedics can come to the rescue. It is probably preferable to most people to wake up to a familiar face rather than to that of a stranger hovering above them.

Losing Consciousness

If you have gotten such a low glucose that your brain's electrical activity is not working well, you may have a seizure or convulsion. Fortunately, you will not remember most of what happens, but it can be frightening to the person helping you to watch your arms and legs jerk uncontrollably. Direct your likely helper to turn you on your side so that if you drool, it goes out of your mouth and not down into your lungs. Besides not giving you sugar by mouth, also tell him/her not to put anything in your mouth. (In the old days, people thought that they needed to keep patients from biting their tongues when they were low. Putting a finger into someone's mouth experiencing a seizure is a great way to lose it!) Talking through this procedure ahead of an occurrence with the person most likely to treat you will prevent a great deal of chaos during an episode.

Brief periods of this severe kind of low are not likely to lead to brain damage. If glucagon is given, the effect of restoring the glucose to normal may be short-lived, and when you are able to do so, you should eat something. However, many people become nauseous after receiving glucagon, so I recommend crackers and water to keep it simple. These seem to be less likely to increase the nausea.

Hypoglycemia Unawareness

Considering all of the patient-driven tools we have discussed to protect against hypoglycemia and the redundancies in hormonal responses with which we have all been equipped, bad events still happen. Vigilance in monitoring your glucose concentrations is undoubtedly the key to knowing where you are going to be in the next hours. As cumbersome as testing frequently may be, it still represents the key method of preventing low blood glucose levels.

After accounting for unusual exercise, missed snacks, and alcohol consumption, 90% of the severe episodes of hypoglycemia in DCCT remained unexplained. Many of the investigators believed it was the development of hypoglycemia unawareness that explained much of the excess risk.

Patients who develop hypoglycemia unawareness, who are very careful to avoid subsequent low glucose concentrations for even short periods regain their symptoms of hypoglycemia. If you develop unawareness, try backing off on how tightly you are running your blood glucose levels. Set your target a little higher. You will not compromise your A1C control that much, but you will regain your ability to know when you are low and increase the safety for yourself and for those around you. Driving a car with a low blood glucose is obviously dangerous and can be substantially reduced by monitoring your blood glucose and then doing something about it!

Case #1: Type 1 Diabetes

Let's recap all of this information by reviewing the case of a patient I took care of who died tragically after living with diabetes for 26 years. This patient had rather severe diabetic gastroparesis, which means that food she ingested processed too slowly from the stomach into the small intestine where absorption should occur. This is a form of neuropathy that is fairly common in both type 2 and type 1 diabetes. When it happens, gastroparesis makes patients with type 1 diabetes particularly more vulnerable to low blood glucose levels, since insulin injected before the meal may get into the circulation more rapidly than the glucose from the food can be absorbed. Further, the recovery from hypoglycemia can be slow since even the rate of absorption of sugar from a liquid treatment is slow.

The patient in this story was a nurse who worked early morning shifts. She lived alone, and one morning she failed to come into work on time. She had experienced repeated bouts of low blood glucose levels that she had tried to prevent and treat appropriately, but because she had developed hypoglycemia unawareness, she often did not know she was very low. She always measured a bedtime glucose concentration, and sometimes would take a few extra units of rapid-acting insulin at bedtime if her glucose was too high (she used 1 unit for every 60 points above 150 mg/dL).

Because of the erratic absorption of the glucose from her diet, predicting where her blood glucose value was going to be at any time of the day or night was difficult. She had eaten a typical evening meal the night before this major episode of hypoglycemia and had taken 4 units of rapid-acting insulin, infused by her pump over 2 hours beginning at the time of the meal. (One way of managing the issue of getting too much insulin in the system before the food has a chance to be absorbed in such patients is to have them take the dose at or after the time of the meal, or, if one is using an insulin infusion pump, we recommend spreading the dose out over several hours.) At bedtime, 2½ hours after the meal, she found she was too high and took an extra 4 units of rapid-acting insulin. (This patient was a great record keeper and had written it down in her logbook.) Her background insulin was delivered by an insulin pump. Her most recent A1C was 7.0%.

When she failed to show up for work, her colleagues called her home, and one of them eventually went over to check on her. At 10 AM, she was found lying in bed taking short, shallow breaths every now and then. She could not be aroused. After having her blood glucose treated with emergency intravenous glucose by the paramedics, her blood glucose was over 200 mg/dL. Three months later, she had still not come back from her coma, developed pneumonia, and after a difficult course, she died.

This case represents a real risk of managing type 1 diabetes intensively. Admittedly she had a condition (gastroparesis) that further predisposed her to getting low, but she made one critical error: she took a large dose of insulin at bedtime. So she was heading into the most vulnerable time of the day with an already impaired ability to detect hypoglycemia, and now had a lot of insulin in her system.

Four units may not seem like much to some patients who have type 2 diabetes and who may take over 100 units of insulin per day, but the usual insulin replacement dose average in a 110-pound woman (this woman's real weight) is only about 40 units. An extra 4 units represents a 10% increase given at a time when she was not eating anything. (As it turns out, she did the math wrong with the correction factor and took 1.5 units more than she should have.)

One other important lesson is taught from this sad case: repeating or supplementing insulin doses within 4 hours of the injection of a previous rapid-acting insulin dose can lead to trouble. The final effect of the first dose is not known before the next dose is given. We walk a fine line between enough is good enough, and a bit more is dangerous.

Type 2 Diabetes

Remember that all of the preceding mentioned lines of hormonal protection are available to patients with type 2 diabetes, plus they have the capacity to shut down their own body's production of insulin in the face of falling blood glucose concentration. Therefore, it is much more difficult to cause severe hypoglycemia in these patients.

Some of the oral medications for the control of type 2 diabetes can cause hypoglycemia, particularly the sulfonylurea (SFU) medications (Glucotrol [glipizide], Glibenclamide [glyburide], and Micronase [glyburide] are examples) by causing the beta cells to pump out their insulin even in the face of a normal or low blood glucose.

The leading population at risk is generally the elderly. Because many older folks tend to eat a larger meal during the middle of the day and a lighter evening meal, they can run out of fuel during the night. The SFUs work for 24 hours and therefore increase the risk of hypoglycemia during sleep.

The other main class of medications, metformin and the thiazolidinediones (TZDs), do not drive the body to make more insulin and therefore have very limited, if any, ability to cause low blood glucose levels. But when combined with an SFU, hypoglycemia can be seen with metformin and/or a TZD. The risk of hypoglycemia with these combinations is probably a function of the baseline hemoglobin A1C being much closer to normal before the second medication is added.

Generally, when hypoglycemia occurs in someone with type 2 diabetes, it is not associated with loss of consciousness. The event still needs to be treated, but the more severe episodes seen in patients with type 1 diabetes are thankfully fairly rare. The newest classes of medications to become available to treat patients with type 2 diabetes are the injectable GLP-1 agonists (Byetta [exenatide] or Victoza [liraglutide]) and the oral DPP-IV inhibitors (Tradjenta [linagliptin], Januvia [sitagliptin], or Onglyza [saxagliptin]). Neither the injectable GLP-1 or oral DPP-IV have any capacity to cause hypoglycemia by themselves or when given with metformin or pioglitazone. But if these classes are given with an SFU, the risk of nonsevere hypoglycemia substantially increases during the first months of treatment. If you are on an SFU when these medications are added to your treatment, then the dose of the SFU should be reduced. One of the new strategies being used in treating patients with type 2 diabetes is to use only combinations of medications that do not produce hypoglycemia.

Case #2: Type 2 Diabetes

Severe hypoglycemia can and does occur when insulin treatment is added to any of the preceding therapies. To demonstrate this point, let me tell you the story of a woman with type 2 diabetes who was managed with metformin and SFUs. She was not at her target A1C, so the decision was made to add insulin to her treatment regimen. She measured her glucose every morning and then took her insulin before driving to the nursing home where she worked. Her routine was to eat breakfast after she got to work.

One morning she had a glucose concentration of 64 mg/dL at home, took her insulin, and about 40 minutes later was in a head-on accident with an 18-wheeler. The driver of the truck saw her slumped over the wheel as she swerved across the median into the front of his rig.

Her glucose concentration at the site of the accident was low, and on arrival to the emergency room it remained low. She now lives in a mentally compromised state in a long-term care facility. Some disconnect had occurred in her education about the use of insulin, eating, and driving.

Insulin is an important addition to the treatment of many patients with type 2 diabetes, and this case is a reasonably uncommon story, but nonetheless, severe hypoglycemia can also be associated with insulin use in both forms of diabetes.

Summary

While hypoglycemia can be a barrier to getting the best control over your blood glucose, most times it is a bother in your day that takes time away from being at your best. Prevention is the best strategy for managing hypoglycemia. If it cannot be prevented, then try not to overtreat it because you will set up the vicious cycle of yo-yoing up and down. Last, especially if you have type 1 diabetes, try to trust someone to be close enough to you that they can spot that your blood glucose is low, even if you are relatively unaware.

14

Preventing Heart Attacks and Strokes

Don't Get Off the Bus Before You Are Ready!

Introduction

Most people with diabetes (PWD) do not realize that heart disease or atherosclerosis is one of the more serious and common complications in PWD, as well as in the general public. Atherosclerosis is the process of the buildup of fat deposits in the arteries or blood vessels, making it more difficult for blood to pass through them. The end result is total blockage of the artery, leading to severe damage of the tissues of the heart and brain. The classic microvascular complications of the eye, kidney, and nerves are usually discussed and more often stressed in the diabetes literature, however, much less commonly than cardiovascular disease. Heart attacks, strokes, and clogging of the blood vessels of the legs (peripheral vascular disease or PVD), are classified as macrovascular complications because they involve the large (macro) arteries or blood vessels of the body. We now know that preventing and aggressively treating the risk factors for macrovascular disease is as equally important as addressing microvascular complications.

You may find it surprising that up to 80% of people with type 2 diabetes "get off the bus" because of heart attacks and strokes, and not from the classic microvascular complications. I hate to be so morbid, using words such as mortality or death; I like to use the phrase "get off the bus" instead. I hope this more gentle term does not take away from the seriousness of the problem. Heart disease and stroke are the leading killers of Americans, diabetic or not. **Figure 14-1** demonstrates how dramatic the situation really is. This figure shows the mortality (death rate) due to coronary artery disease in men and women with type 2 diabetes compared with the mortality rate in people without diabetes over time. The mortality rate is recorded as the number of deaths per 1000 people. Time zero indicates the time of diagnosis of diabetes in these people, who are in the neighborhood of 40 to 50 years of age. You can see that in only a few short years after the time of diagnosis, the death rate due to heart disease in PWD starts to significantly accelerate and separate from that of the people who do not have diabetes. Please notice that in nondiabetic individuals, the women have fewer heart prob-

Figure 14-1

Death Due to Heart Disease in People With Type 2 Diabetes

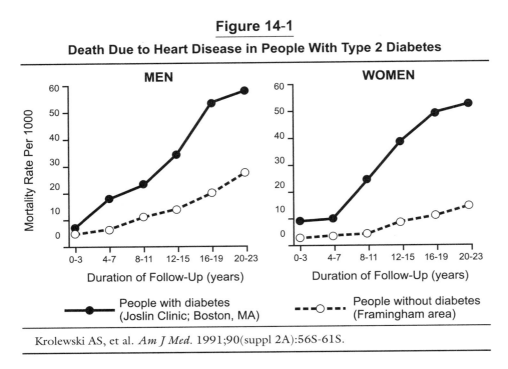

Krolewski AS, et al. *Am J Med.* 1991;90(suppl 2A):56S-61S.

lems compared with men. This fact is referred to as a "cardiovascular advantage" that nondiabetic women usually enjoy compared with nondiabetic men. However, now look at the death rate due to heart disease in the diabetic women compared with that in the diabetic men. It is the same, and the cardiovascular advantage is lost. The explanation for this phenomenon is unclear, but one thing is certain: Women with type 2 diabetes are at extreme risk for premature heart disease, especially after they reach menopause.

Another major problem is that PWD may have a diminished sensation of the early warning signs of heart disease (for example, chest pain). This can lead to a dangerous situation since treatment can be instituted early if a person goes to the emergency room or clinic with chest pain rather than sitting at home, unaware that heart disease is present (the medical term for this condition is silent ischemia). The reason for this lack of awareness of cardiac symptoms is unknown, but may be related to pain fibers being damaged by diabetes just as occurs with neuropathy in the feet. In a similar fashion to retinopathy and diabetic kidney disease, serious and advanced heart disease can be present without any symptoms. Unfortunately, when the first symptom (such as chest pain) finally occurs, it may be too late to intervene. Awareness of these potential problems by you and your caregiver is the key.

People with type 2 diabetes are normally diagnosed later in life and, therefore, are more likely to have heart disease just because of their advanced age. High blood pressure (BP) and high cholesterol levels also contribute to the increased risk of heart disease. People with type 1 diabetes do not develop heart disease until later in life because they are usually diagnosed with diabetes at a much younger age, although the incidence is still higher than in people of the same age without type 1 diabetes.

You must be aware of the risk factors for heart disease and stroke so that you can do everything in your power to prevent, detect, and aggressively treat them. This chapter will focus on the important information that you need to know to take control of the situation. Trust me—you do not want to be a cardiac cripple or a paralyzed stroke victim.

Risk Factors for Heart Disease and Stroke

You and your caregiver can modify several of the risk factors that contribute to heart disease. Unfortunately, you cannot change your age, gender, family history, or the fact that you have diabetes. However, it is important that you look at each one of these risk factors carefully and decide if you can improve your own situation. The more risk factors that you have, the more aggressive you should be with modifying the changeable ones. The risk factors are listed in **Table 14-1** and discussed below.

Table 14-1

Risk Factors for Heart Disease and Stroke

- Existing heart disease (atherosclerosis)
- A family history of heart disease (atherosclerosis)
- Age >45 years in men and >55 years in women
- Diabetes
- Tobacco smoking
- Severe weight problem
- High blood pressure
- Abnormal cholesterol levels

Existing Heart Disease or Atherosclerosis

If you already have had a heart attack or stroke, then your chances of having further problems are greatly increased. Now is the time to be the most aggressive to modify your risk factors. I have patients who have lived long and healthy lives after their first heart attack or stroke, because they did take the situation seriously.

Family History of Atherosclerosis

Heart disease is a hereditary condition. If anyone in your immediate family has had heart problems, you may be at greater risk. Your immediate family includes your siblings, parents, uncles, aunts, and grandparents. Sorry, but your healthy spouse will not help you out here. Having a family history of heart disease is a very important risk factor, and although we cannot change our family history, we can be aggressive with our treatment plan.

Age and Gender

Age and gender play important roles in determining risk status. If you are a man and older than 45 years or a woman older than 55 years, your risk of heart disease significantly increases. These numbers were determined from large epidemiologic observational studies in nondiabetic individuals. These age limits are used to calculate an individual's risk of developing heart disease, along with the other risk factors we are going to discuss. The medical profession uses these calculations (*Risk Assessment Tool For Estimating Your 10-Year Risk Of Having A Heart Attack*) to determine how aggressively a patient should be treated (*http://hp2010.nhlbihin.net/atpiii/calculator.asp*). The higher the risk, the more aggressive the approach. Go online and calculate your risk and if high, please discuss this with your caregiver.

Existing Diabetes

Obviously, you cannot change the fact that you have diabetes, but you can work on improving control of your diabetes. The phrase "metabolic syndrome" has been used to describe a cluster of cardiovascular risk factors associated with type 2 diabetes, such as elevated BP, abnormal cholesterol levels, increased propensity to form blood clots, etc; all of which help to explain the relationship of having diabetes and a higher risk of atherosclerosis.

Since the publication of the third edition of TCOYD, there have been three large studies (ACCORD, ADVANCE, and VADT) that all demonstrated that aggressive diabetes control did not have a significant impact on heart disease but it did on the microvascular complications such as eye, kidney, and nerve disease. These studies also highlighted the importance in individualizing the A1C goal for each individual and that older folks with a history of heart disease may be at risk for adverse events, such as serious hypoglycemia, if they are treated too aggressively.

Cigarette Smoking

I know that cigarette smoking is a tough habit to break, but it really is a killer in terms of causing heart attacks and strokes, especially in PWD. It is definitely one of the worst habits to have as a diabetic and one of the more difficult to stop (other than eating Oreos, Doritos, and Krispy Kreme donuts). It has been shown that there is a powerfully negative synergistic effect between smoking and diabetes. Even if you cut down your smoking by 50%, you will have done yourself a great favor. I will not dwell on this point, because I know you get grief from everyone around you if you currently smoke. Do anything you can, using any technique, to stop or reduce your cigarette consumption. Trust me—you do not want to be in need of a heart or lung transplant.

Severe Weight Problems

If you are 20% to 30% over your ideal weight, then you certainly do not need me to tell you that the excessive adiposity (fat) puts a tremendous strain on your heart. People with severe weight problems need a supportive health care team, including a clinical psychologist, to help them overcome emotional barriers and adhere to a weight-loss and maintenance program. It is not easy, and currently there is no magic pill for weight loss. However, two weight loss medications were recently approved by the FDA (Qsymia made by Vivus Pharmaceuticals and Belviq made by Arena Pharmaceuticals). We also have new diabetes drugs that may be very helpful for weight loss in PWD, such as Byetta, Bydureon, Victoza, and Symlin. A newer class of oral medications not approved at the time of this edition is the SGLT-2 inhibitors, such as dapagliflozin, canagliflozin, and remogliflozin, which lead to glucose control and modest weight loss. Our armamentarium for weight-loss products is increasing.

High Blood Pressure

High BP is an important modifiable risk factor. Keeping your BP in the normal range will help prevent macrovascular disease (heart attack and stroke), as well as microvascular disease (kidney failure and eye disease). Controlling your BP is discussed in *Chapter 14* and will be discussed further in this chapter.

Abnormal Cholesterol Levels

Abnormal cholesterol levels are common in PWD and are one of the main contributors to accelerating the atherosclerotic process. The cholesterol abnormalities seen in PWD are complicated and deserve a detailed discussion later in this chapter.

Controlling High Blood Pressure

Aggressive BP control is probably one of the more powerful interventions for reducing the incidence of heart attack and stroke. As mentioned earlier, I believe it is important that every person with high BP have a home blood pressure–monitoring device, just as every person with diabetes should have a glucose-monitoring device. You should also take several readings a week at different times and record them for you to analyze and discuss with your caregiver. You can pick up a blood pressure–monitoring device at your local pharmacy or larger discount store. Choose one that you feel comfortable using and one that has a good return policy. It is also important to bring your BP device with you on your office visit once or twice a year to have the staff check it for accuracy.

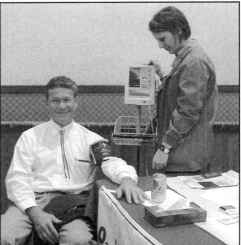

I am taking advantage of the free service of having my blood pressure taken as provided at a TCOYD conference in Amarillo, Texas.

It is imperative that you know how normal BP is defined. The American Diabetes Association currently recommends lowering BP to at least less than 130/80 mm Hg, and if you have evidence of protein in your urine (microalbuminuria) or your kidney function is already less than normal, your caregiver may want your BP even lower, for example, less than 120/80 mm Hg.

In general, there are some basic treatment strategies that I follow that may help you in working with your caregiver to tailor your program to effectively reach your BP goals. These general treatment strategies are listed in **Table 14-2** and discussed below.

Table 14-2

General Treatment Strategies for Treating High Blood Pressure in People With Diabetes

- Do not delay aggressive therapy
- Know your BP goals and values
- Know about the side effects of the drugs you take
- Design a regimen that is simple and easy to follow on a day-to-day basis
- Combining medications may be needed
- Avoid drugs that exacerbate your diabetes and other associated conditions

Do Not Delay In Starting Therapy and Be Aggressive

Once high BP is detected, there should be no delay in instituting aggressive therapy. Many doctors and patients wait too long before antihypertensive measures are undertaken. High BP does not normally cause any pain or discomfort, and because of this fact, therapy is too often delayed. Believe it or not, for some patients, it takes several years before the appropriate treatment regimen is in place. Do not let yourself go untreated.

Know Your Blood Pressure Goals and Values

You need to know what your BP runs on average during your daily activities. Your BP at the doctor's office may not be indicative of your true values. This is why you need to get a blood pressure–monitoring device and use it at home and other places such as work. This will allow you to determine whether your BP values are within the goal range most of the time. Remember that BP values fluctuate during the day, so repeated measurements are important in order to get an adequate overview of your BP. Although not commonly ordered, there are 24-hour ambulatory monitoring devices that measure your BP every 20 minutes during the day and every hour at night. The day-long readings are extremely helpful when determining what the BP is and to adjust the medications for the maximum effect.

Know About the Side Effects of the Drugs

It is your responsibility to know the side effects of the drugs with which you are being treated. Read package insert information and ask questions about the side effects. Some of the side effects you will be able to live with (especially because you knew about them ahead of time), and others will limit your use of a particular medication. Fortunately, we do have lots of choices.

Design a Regimen That Is Simple and Easy to Follow

Design a regimen that is simple and easy to follow on a day-to-day basis. Most people can take medications 2 times a day on a regular basis without forgetting. It is more difficult to take medications 3 times a day and almost impossible for most people to take drugs 4 times a day for an extended period of time. Most likely, you will be on blood pressure–lowering medication indefinitely. Many of my patients, including myself, take several BP medications in the morning and at bedtime. I use two little cups in which I put my BP pills. I prepare the two cups at bedtime so that after I wake up and brush my teeth, the second morning cup of pills is ready and waiting for me to swallow. When I travel, I use the little pill holder containers… now I am showing my age. I also keep a small supply of pills at work just in case I forget to take them at home. Everyone's habits and schedules are different, and you need to design a pill schedule that works easily for you. Even if you have the smartest doctor in the world and access to the best drugs, it is of no benefit to your health if your medication schedule is too complicated so that you forget to take the drugs regularly.

Combining Medications

The hypertension of diabetes is a tough condition to treat, and it is the rule, rather than the exception, that you may need more than one type of BP medication. I am on three different medications that work in different ways to control my BP. In addition, at least 60% of my patients with diabetes and hypertension need more than one medication to control their BP. Remember that it's not how many pills you take, but rather how well your BP is controlled. Most of the various antihypertensive medications can be used together safely with little or no side effects. Some of the common combinations will be discussed later.

Treatment Options

There are many different types of medications that are available to lower your BP. You need to become familiar with them so that you can carry on an intelligent conversation with your caregiver and play an active role in your treatment plan. **Table 14-3** lists the various categories of BP medications with a few examples of each type.

It is not really feasible or necessary to discuss in detail the pharmacologic therapy for high BP. There are entire medical textbooks written on this subject alone. Conversely, I feel it is important to discuss some of the therapeutic strategies for monotherapy (using only one drug) and combination therapy that are commonly prescribed for people with hypertension and diabetes. The main goal is to get the BP down to at least 130/80 mm Hg and to less than 120/80 mm Hg if there is evidence of protein in the urine that is indicative of kidney damage. If the BP goals are not reached with a single drug, then a second agent is added (not substituted) to the first one (combination therapy). It is not uncommon for PWD to need three and four different medications to control their BP. It is much better to have normal BP and be on four different types of medication than to have elevated BP and be on only one drug. It is sometimes difficult to get over that psychological block about "taking all of those damn pills."

Table 14-3
Blood Pressure Medications[a]

ACE Inhibitors
- Benazepril (Lotensin)
- Captopril (Capoten)
- Enalapril (Vasotec)
- Fosinopril (Monopril)
- Lisinopril (Prinivil, Zestril)
- Moexipril (Univasc)
- Perindopril (Aceon)
- Quinapril (Accupril)
- Ramipril (Altace)
- Trandolapril (Mavik)

ARBs
- Azilsartan (Edarbi)
- Candesartan (Atacand)
- Eprosartan (Teveten)
- Irbesartan (Avapro)
- Losartan (Cozaar)
- Olmesartan (Benicar)
- Telmisartan (Micardis)
- Valsartan (Diovan)

Direct Renin Inhibitor
- Aliskiren (Tekturna)

CCBs
- Amlodipine (Norvasc)
- Diltiazem (Cardizem, Cardizem CD, Cardizem LA, Cartia XT, Dilacor, Diltia XT, Tiazac)
- Felodipine (Plendil)
- Isradipine (DynaCirc)
- Nicardipine (Cardene)
- Nifedipine (Adalat)
- Nifedipine GITS (Procardia XL)
- Nimodipine (Nimotop)
- Nisoldipine (Sular)
- Verapamil LA (Calan SR, Covera-HS, Isoptin SR, Verelan)

Alpha-Blockers
- Doxazosin (Cardura)
- Prazosin (Minipress)
- Terazosin (Hytrin)

Centrally Acting Agents
- Clonidine (Catapres, Catapres-TTS)
- Guanabenz (Wytensin)
- Guanfacine (Tenex)
- Methyldopa (Aldomet)

Indoline Diuretic
- Indapamide (Lozol)

Thiazide Diuretics
- Chlorothiazide (Diuril)
- Hydrochlorothiazide (Esidrix)
- Methyclothiazide (Enduron)

Beta-Blockers
- Atenolol (Tenormin)
- Betaxolol (Kerlone)
- Bisoprolol (Zebeta)
- Carvedilol (Coreg)
- Metoprolol (Lopressor, Toprol-XL)
- Nadolol (Corgard)
- Propranolol (Inderal, Inderal LA)

Combinations
- ACE inhibitors and diuretics (Accuretic, Captozide, Lotensin, Monopril HCT, Prinzide, Uniretic, Vaseretic, Zestoretic)
- ARBs and CCBs (Azor, Exforge)
- ARBs and diuretics (Atacand HCT, Avalide, Benicar HCT, Diovan HCT, Endarbyclor, Hyzaar, Micardis HCT, Teveten HCT)
- Beta-adrenergic blockers and diuretics (Corzide, Inderide LA, Lopressor HCT, Tenoretic, Timolide, Ziac)
- CCBs and ACE inhibitors (Lexxel, Lotrel, Tarka)
- Other combinations (Aldactazide, Aldoril, Clorpres, Diupres, Dyazide, Hydropres, Maxzide, Minizide, Moduretic)

Combination to Treat Hypertension and Abnormal Cholesterol Levels
- Caduet (amlodipine/atorvastatin)

[a] Not all drugs in each category are listed.

ACE Inhibitors and ARBs

An angiotensin-converting enzyme (ACE) inhibitor or an angiotensin receptor blocker (ARB) is usually the drug of choice when initiating antihypertensive therapy; this is also discussed in *Chapter 14*. ACE inhibitors have been proven effective at preventing and slowing the progression of atherosclerosis, in addition to protecting the kidneys.

ACE inhibitors and ARBs have few side effects and are tolerated well. ACE inhibitors and ARBs can be taken once or twice a day and can be safely combined with other medications to reduce BP to the desired goal. There are two situations in which ACE inhibitors should be used with caution:

- In people who have a tendency to have high potassium levels in the blood
- In people who have a condition called renal artery stenosis.

ACE inhibitors can also cause a persistent, dry cough in a small percentage of people.

Direct Renin Inhibitor

Tekturna (aliskiren) is a relatively new type of blood pressure–lowering agent called a direct renin inhibitor. Tekturna reduces the effect of renin (a hormone in the kidney that in high levels will cause high BP) and the harmful process that narrows blood vessels. Tekturna helps blood vessels relax and widen blood vessels so BP is lowered. It can be added to all other blood pressure–lowering agents and has a very low side effect profile. It should not be taken by women who are pregnant or planning to become pregnant.

Calcium Channel Blockers

Calcium channel blockers (CCBs) also represent a commonly used class of antihypertensive medications for PWD. In general, they are well tolerated with few side effects and can be taken once or twice a day. Each CCB is slightly different from the others, so it is important for you to discuss with your caregiver or read about the one you are prescribed. They have a different mechanism of action than the other classes of medications, so they can have beneficial synergistic effects on your BP when combined with the other drugs, especially ACE inhibitors or ARBs. The combination of a CCB and an ACE inhibitor is probably one of the more commonly prescribed combinations. Women who are pregnant or trying to become pregnant should not take ACE inhibitors or ARBs as they have been shown to cause problems for the fetus.

Alpha-Blockers

Alpha-blockers represent another class of BP agents that seem especially well-suited for PWD. Once again, the newer drugs listed in **Table 14-3** have few side effects and can be taken once or twice a day at the most. Alpha-blockers can be added safely to other medications such as ACE inhibitors and CCBs. Alpha-blockers may also favorably affect your cholesterol levels.

It is important to take alpha-blockers exactly as prescribed, especially when you are initiating therapy, because they can cause dizziness upon standing (orthostasis). Most of the time, alpha-blockers are started at bedtime to avoid this problem, which dissipates in a few days.

Centrally Acting Agents

Centrally acting agents, such as clonidine, represent an older class of medications. However, they can be effective to get your BP under control. They are usually not used as first- or second-line therapy because they sometimes cause dry mouth and tiredness. A skin patch for clonidine is available, which may be better tolerated than the pills, and you only have to change the patch every 7 days.

Indoline Diuretic

Indapamide is an excellent additive medication to control the BP. It is a once-a-day drug with no side effects. It is normally not a first-line agent because it is not as potent at lowering the BP and therefore many physicians are not familiar with this drug. I frequently prescribe indapamide as the third-line agent, after ACE inhibitors and CCBs.

Thiazide Diuretics and Beta-Blockers

Thiazide diuretics and beta-blockers may slightly raise your glucose and cholesterol levels but when used in lower doses in addition to other blood pressure–lowering agents, they normally do not cause any noticeable changes. They were the workhorses of the 70s, 80s, and early 90s; however, they typically are not used as first-line therapy, but rather as additional medications to the newer drugs, such as the ACE inhibitors, ARBs, and CCBs. For example, some patients are put on a low-dose thiazide diuretic if there is a kidney problem or if fluid retention is present. I prescribe low-dose thiazide diuretics occasionally if the more standard drugs of choice are ineffective at getting the BP down to goal ranges. Furthermore, some of the beta-blockers have been formulated or designed to be more diabetic-friendly (carvedilol or Coreg is one of the beta-blockers that is diabetic-friendly). In general, thiazide diuretics and beta-blockers are effective at lowering the BP. Remember that the primary goal is to get the BP down, no matter how you do it!

Controlling Cholesterol Levels

Abnormal cholesterol levels are another major contributor to athero-sclerosis, leading to heart attack and stroke. Unfortunately, PWD are prone to cholesterol problems and suffer from clogging of the arteries that deliver blood to the heart, brain, and legs. Once again, like many other complications of diabetes, abnormal cholesterol levels are pain-less and do not cause symptoms. This can be a dangerous situation, as it leads to delayed and under treatment.

It is important to clarify what types of lipids or cholesterol exist and the goals of therapy (**Table 14-4**). There are basically three different types of cholesterol or lipoproteins that are normally measured in your blood in a lipid panel:

- The LDL (low-density lipoprotein or lousy cholesterol)
- HDL (high-density lipoprotein or good cholesterol)
- Triglycerides.

Table 14-4

Goals of Therapy for Cholesterol Levels in People With Diabetes

	Total[a]	HDL	LDL	TG
Heart disease present[b]	<200	>40 (men) >50 (women)	<70 (well below 100)	<150
No heart disease	<200	>40 (men) >50 (women)	<100	<200

Abbreviations: HDL, high-density lipoprotein (cholesterol); LDL, low-density lipoprotein (cholesterol); TG, triglycerides.

[a] The total cholesterol may be misleading in determining your risk of heart disease *(see text)*. All values are in milligrams per deciliter (mg/dL).
[b] Heart attacks, congestive heart failure, strokes, etc.

These are all forms of cholesterol, but differ in size, shape, density, and have different functions. You should have a lipid panel measuring the different types of cholesterol done once a year or more frequently if you are initiating or adjusting cholesterol medications.

Most diabetes specialists recommend that all PWD get their LDL value below 100 mg/dL if they have had no problems with their heart at all and below 70 mg/dL if they have had a heart attack or any type of cardiovascular disease in the past. One must fast to get an accurate fasting triglyceride value (nothing to eat past midnight with the blood drawn first thing in the morning before eating), which is used to calculate the LDL cholesterol. In reality, you do not have to fast for the total cholesterol and HDL, but they are usually all measured together at the same time anyway.

I use the word "abnormal" when discussing the cholesterol or lipid problems in PWD because it is not simply that the LDL levels are too high or that the HDL levels are too low. There are other characteristics of the different types of cholesterol or lipoprotein that increase the risk of atherosclerosis. For example, the LDL and HDL cholesterols get "oxidized" and "glycosylated" (glucose molecules stick to them), making them more dangerous in terms of causing heart disease. Lastly, it is important for you to know that your triglyceride levels correlate with your glucose control, so lowering your A1C will improve your lipid profile. (**Table 14-5**).

Table 14-5

Lipid Abnormalities Seen in People With Type 2 Diabetes

- Elevated triglyceride levels
- Low HDL levels (good cholesterol)
- "Abnormal" changes in the LDL (bad) and HDL (good) cholesterol structures:
  – Oxidized
  – Glycosylated

Get A Lipid Panel at Least Once a Year

A lipid panel will consist of four different values (total cholesterol, LDL, triglycerides, and the HDL). The total cholesterol value may be a misleading number in determining your risk of heart disease. The total cholesterol is made up of both the LDL and the HDL cholesterol levels. Since the HDL levels are normally low in PWD, the total cholesterol level is lower than it would be in people with high levels of this protective HDL or good cholesterol. Do not be lulled into a false sense of security if your total cholesterol level is less than 200. You may still have low HDL and abnormal LDL levels, thus putting you at extreme risk for heart disease. This is why you should get a lipid panel that includes the LDL, HDL, and triglyceride levels and not solely a total cholesterol level.

What do all of these different and complicated lipid abnormalities mean to PWD? Basically, in the simplest terms, we need to be aware of what our cholesterol levels are and work with our health care providers to reach our target goals of therapy. Unfortunately, there are millions of Americans, with and without diabetes, who have untreated abnormal cholesterol levels in the high-risk range. The reasons for this are many, although patient and physician ignorance and apathy play a big part. In addition, there are no symptoms of high cholesterol levels so they too often get ignored!

Treatment Options

Meal planning and an exercise program are two of the more potent nonpharmacologic ways to improve your cholesterol levels and are discussed in detail in *Chapter 5* and *Chapter 6*. However, it is important to emphasize that PWD sometimes have tough-to-treat cholesterol levels, just as they have tough-to-treat high BP. Diet and exercise will rarely bring abnormal cholesterol levels down into the normal range. Even though oral medications may be needed to reach your cholesterol goals, you must maintain some type of dietary and exercise program. I am not asking you to lose 30 pounds, eat cardboard, and run marathons. I know that lifestyle changes must come gradually, in small incremental steps. In addition, you can improve your cholesterol levels, especially your triglyceride levels, just by lowering your blood glucose values into a more normal range.

I classify abnormal cholesterol levels into three basic categories when I consider pharmacologic therapy:

• Elevated LDL cholesterol
• Elevated triglyceride/low HDL levels
• Elevations in both LDL cholesterol and triglyceride levels and a low HDL level.

This inverse relationship of high triglyceride levels being associated with low HDL levels is a common abnormality in people with type 2 diabetes. Even though low HDL levels are of concern, there is no medication specifically designed to raise HDL levels. However, a secondary benefit of the other medications used to treat high LDL and triglyceride levels is to raise HDL levels modestly. The drugs commonly used to treat high LDL and/or triglyceride levels are listed in **Table 14-6**.

Most diabetes experts agree that the class of drugs called the statins is the most efficient, safe, and effective way to lower LDL levels. The statins work by blocking the key step in cholesterol production in the liver. There are few side effects and they can be taken once a day, usually at bedtime. The statins may also raise HDL levels 5% to 10%. These drugs have been used in millions of people worldwide for over 25 years and are super safe and effective. The statins are responsible for prevent-

Table 14-6
Drugs to Treat Abnormal Cholesterol Levels

Drugs to Treat High LDL Cholesterol Levels

- The "statins:"
  - Rosuvastatin (Crestor)
  - Fluvastatin (Lescol, Lescol XL)
  - Atorvastatin (Lipitor)
  - Pravastatin (Pravachol)
  - Lovastatin (Mevacor, Altocor)
  - Simvastatin (Zocor)
- Niacin or nicotinic acid:
  - Many over-the-counter preparations (nonprescription vitamin)
  - Niacin extended-release (Niaspan) is a newer niacin formulation that is better tolerated
- Bile acid sequestrants:
  - Colestid (colestipol)
  - Questran (cholestyramine)
  - Welchol (colesevelam)

Cholesterol Absorption Inhibitor

- Zetia (ezetimibe)

Combination Drugs

- Lovastatin/niacin ER (Advicor)
- Vytorin (ezetimibe/simvastatin)

Drugs to Treat High Triglyceride Levels

- Lopid (gemfibrozil)
- Tricor, Lofibra, Triglide, Antara (fenofibrate), Trilipix
- Niacin extended-release (Niaspan) is a newer niacin formulation that is better tolerated
- Omacor (omega-3-acid ethyl esters)

Combination Drug to Treat Hypertension and Abnormal Cholesterol Levels

- Amlodipine/atorvastatin (Caduet)

Abbreviation: LDL, low-density lipoprotein (cholesterol).

---

ing a ton of folks from getting off the bus due to heart disease and stroke.

An LDL-lowering medication called Zetia (ezetimibe), which works by blocking the absorption of cholesterol that comes from food, is now available. It has very few, if any, side effects and works well with statins to help people get their LDL levels to goal. A combination pill called Vytorin (ezetimibe/simvastatin) is also available, as well as several others. Please see the following section on combination medications.

Niacin can raise blood glucose levels and cause headaches and flushing. Niaspan is a slow-release niacin preparation that is better tolerated than the over-the-counter niacin preparations. Bile acid sequestrants, such as Questran and Colestid, which come in a powder that you mix with fluids, commonly cause stomach upset and constipation and can interfere with the absorption and effectiveness of other drugs or medications that you take in the same time period. Welchol is similar to

Questran and Colestid but comes in a pill form and is better tolerated. It is also approved for the treatment of type 2 diabetes and lowers glucose values as well. It is the only medication to date that is formally approved by the FDA for diabetes and cholesterol problems.

High triglyceride levels are best treated with a class of medications called fibric acid derivatives, such as Lopid (gemfibrozil), Tricor (fenofibrate), or Trilipix (fenofibric acid), all of which have very few side effects and are well tolerated. When the triglycerides are initially high (>400 mg/dL), one can see a dramatic drop in the triglyceride levels of up to 40% and a 10% to 25% increase in the HDL levels (when triglyceride levels drop, the HDL levels usually go up and vice versa). I want to emphasize that if your glucose control is poor, it will be difficult to bring the triglyceride levels to normal. Trilipix is the only drug in this class that is approved to use with statins. Niacin also lowers triglyceride and raises HDL levels, however, as mentioned above, has several side effects and raises the blood sugar levels.

If one of my patients has both LDL and triglyceride elevations, I decide which abnormality is of the greater magnitude. I normally prescribe a statin when the LDL is the predominant abnormality ,and Lopid, Tricor, or Trilipix if the triglyceride problem looks more out of range (>400 mg/dL). It is not uncommon that I prescribe Trilipix in addition to a statin, or a statin in addition to one of the triglyceride-lowering drugs, depending on which one I started first. Some statins, such as Lipitor (atorvastatin), Zocor (simvastatin), and Crestor (rosuvastatin), can have a significant impact on triglycerides as well when used in higher doses, and there may not be a need for a second drug.

Combination Blood Pressure and Cholesterol Medications

A combination pill that contains two different BP or cholesterol medications is becoming more and more popular, and there are several benefits. First of all, you do not have to swallow multiple pills and you get the dual action of two different types of BP and cholesterol medications that have been proven to work well together. Last, you will only have one co-pay and every type of savings can add up, especially if you are on a low fixed income. In addition, there are combination pills that have BP medications combined with a statin. **Table 14-3** and **Table 14-6** list the combination BP/cholesterol products currently available.

What About Aspirin Therapy?

There is no question that anyone who is at risk for heart disease should take one aspirin a day with rare exception. The evidence in the medical literature is overwhelmingly positive in support of aspirin therapy to prevent heart attack and stroke in people with and without diabetes. Aspirin is an old and inexpensive over-the-counter medication that is often overlooked and under-utilized. The exact dose that one needs has not been determined and ranges from 75 to 325 mg/day. I recommend a baby aspirin that contains 81 mg in men >50 years of age or women >60 years of age and having at least one additional major risk factor, such as a prior heart attack or stroke. I buy my enteric-coated aspirin (easier on the stomach) at big discount stores in large quantities. An aspirin a day helps to keep the heart attack away!

Case Presentation

Steve Edelman (yes, this really is my story) is a 57-year-old white man with a 42-year history of type 1 diabetes, diagnosed at the age of 15 in 1970. My current degree of control is good, with a glycosylated hemoglobin (A1C) usually between 6.9% and 7.4%, although my most recent one really sucked… too embarrassed to tell you. I was found to have protein in my urine in 1987 and was started on an ACE inhibitor. During the next few years, a CCB and indapamide were added to control my BP to less than 120/80 mm Hg, documented by my home blood pressure–monitoring machine and occasional 24-hour ambulatory-monitoring device. I am on three different drugs just to keep my BP normal, but this will reduce my chances of having a heart attack, stroke, or kidney failure.

My high cholesterol levels were first diagnosed in 1992. Grandparents on both sides of my family had heart attacks at an early age (before the age of 60). I do not smoke cigarettes (only an occasional good cigar, and I don't inhale) and have not experienced any problems with my heart (knock on wood!). My lipid panel before treatment was as follows: total cholesterol 260, LDL 171, HDL 76, and triglycerides 65. Current risk factors for atherosclerosis include diabetes, family history of heart disease, high BP, and high LDL cholesterol levels. I have four major risk factors for the development of atherosclerosis; however, I have a high level of the protective HDL, which counteracts some of the other risk factors. At least I am not postmenopausal!

My doctor started me on a statin with the goal of getting my LDL at least under 100. The triglycerides are normal and the HDL level is at a beneficial level. I also started taking one enteric-coated aspirin a day (81 mg). I am now on 40 mg of Lipitor (a statin drug) and my LDL went down to 71, my triglycerides stayed about the same at 70; however, my HDL rose to the 90s.

I was also advised to get a cardiac stress test before starting a strenuous exercise program to make sure that I had no underlying asymptomatic heart disease. It is not uncommon for PWD to not feel the classic chest pain that usually precedes a heart attack as discussed earlier. I also get a cardiac stress test once a year to be on the safe side.

Summary

Heart attack and stroke unfortunately account for a tremendous amount of death and human suffering in PWD. Atherosclerosis is also one of the biggest and most potent reasons why Americans "get off the bus." One of the main problems in diagnosing and treating PWD in a timely manner is the fact that both high BP and abnormal cholesterol levels may not cause any major symptoms unless it is the final event, such as a heart attack or stroke (chest pain and paralysis). This is why both high BP and abnormal cholesterol levels, two of the biggest and most modifiable risk factors for heart disease, have been called the silent killers.

The bottom line is that many of the major risk factors for atherosclerosis discussed in this chapter can be modified to reduce the chances of a stroke or heart attack. You need to be knowledgeable, not only about practical and realistic lifestyle modifications, but also about the most effective and well-tolerated medications to lower your BP and cholesterol levels. In addition, by simply taking one 81-mg aspirin a day, you may significantly reduce your chances of having a heart attack or stroke. These are the types of important issues that you need to discuss with your physician. Make sure you know your goals of therapy and that you reach and maintain those goals over the long term. It may be a struggle to attain acceptable BP and cholesterol values; however, maintenance of these levels will be relatively simple. Trust me, you do not want to have a heart attack or stroke!

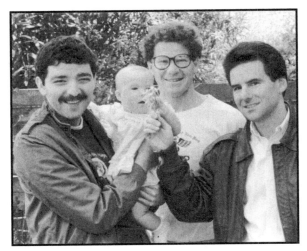

My buddy, Ken Facter, holding my daughter, Talia. Dr. Jamie Wolosin is on the right.

15

Preserve the Life of Your Diabetic Kidneys

Prevention, Early Detection, and Aggressive Management—Avoiding Dialysis and Transplantation

Introduction

Diabetic kidney disease is a scary thing. To think about being on dialysis or needing transplantation from a cadaver or living donor is depressing. Unfortunately, diabetic kidney disease causes a tremendous amount of grief and misery for people with diabetes and their loved ones. Diabetes is one of the leading causes of kidney failure in the world.

I will always remember quite clearly when I studied physiology during medical school in 1978. The professor was citing statistics from old textbooks about the high death rate in people with diabetes. He stated that 50% of people with diabetes die from diabetic kidney disease within 20 years after the initial diagnosis of diabetes. At the time, I was 23 years old with 8 years of diabetes behind me. I told myself that I would at least do everything in my power to prevent the development and progression of kidney disease.

In 1982, I discovered that my blood pressure was elevated for the first time and I did not want to take drugs. To me, it was a sign of weakness and vulnerability. The only medication that I regularly took at that time was insulin. This period in my diabetic life was emotionally significant because it marked the first time that I needed medication for a complication of diabetes. Even though I already had retinopathy, I did not need daily drugs after I received laser treatments. I finally slapped myself around and

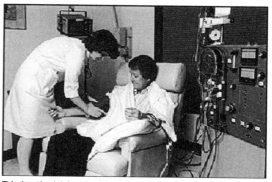

Diabetic kidney disease is preventable and treatable. Avoid end-stage renal disease and dialysis by taking control of your diabetes.

said, "Who are you fooling and what are you accomplishing by avoiding an important therapeutic modality to preserve the life of your kidneys?"

The message I have for you in this chapter is: Diabetic kidney disease is preventable and it is treatable once present. Through years of clinical research, we now know of several techniques to prevent the onset and delay the progression of diabetic kidney disease. In addition to aggressively treating kidney disease, screening methods for early diagnosis of this problem have been developed. This information is vital to all people with diabetes to avoid end-stage kidney disease (requiring dialysis or transplantation).

Definition

What is diabetic kidney disease, and why do diabetics develop kidney problems? Stating it simply, diabetic kidney disease is the failure of the kidneys to function properly due to poorly controlled blood glucose and elevated blood pressure over an extended period of time. Diabetic kidney disease is also referred to as diabetic nephropathy in the medical literature. The kidneys are important and vital organs responsible for filtering and cleaning our blood. The kidneys are also responsible for maintaining electrolyte balance (sodium, potassium, chlorine, carbon dioxide, etc) and normal fluid levels in our body. Years of chronically elevated blood glucose levels damages the vital filtering structures of the kidneys. Diabetic nephropathy is called a microvascular complication, because it involves very small blood vessels that feed oxygen and other nutrients to the kidneys as well as the eyes and nerves. This is why the term microvascular complications refers to the kidneys (nephropathy), eyes (retinopathy), and nerves (neuropathy).

Poorly controlled blood pressure, which can be an early manifestation of kidney disease or can be present because it runs in your family, is also very damaging to the kidneys. If left untreated, high blood pressure will greatly accelerate the decline of kidney function. It turns out that high blood pressure also contributes to acceleration of diabetic eye disease or retinopathy. There are many other medical reasons why a person's kidney might fail but for PWD, high blood pressure and high A1C values over the years are the two most important causative factors.

Inadequate screening for the early signs of diabetic kidney disease, thus delaying proper treatment, is also a serious problem. Remember, high blood pressure and early kidney disease do not occur with any noticeable symptoms, which makes screening of utmost importance. Sensitive tests are now available that can detect kidney disease at an early stage when the damage may be reversible with aggressive treatment.

The information and advice in this chapter are simple, straightforward, and relatively easy to follow. It is vitally important that you preserve the life of your diabetic kidneys.

Prevention

Prevention of diabetic kidney disease by maintaining tight glucose control has been convincingly proven by the Diabetes Control and Complications Trial (DCCT) as well as by several other large reputable studies in people with type 1 and type 2 diabetes.

The DCCT conclusively demonstrates the importance of glucose control in preventing the onset and delaying the progression of the classic microvascular complications of diabetes (eye, kidney, and nerve disease) in patients with type 1 diabetes. The importance of glucose control in patients with type 2 diabetes is now widely accepted by physicians as it is in those with type 1 diabetes. The majority of diabetes specialists and other caregivers who are interested in diabetes feel that the duration and severity of hyperglycemia will dictate the rate and extent of microvascular complications, such as eye, kidney, and nerve disease, in all patients with diabetes no matter what type of the disease is present.

If you have high blood pressure from any cause, you may be able to prevent the onset of diabetic kidney disease just by aggressively treating the blood pressure to keep it in the normal ranges or even lower! In addition, it may be possible that two types of blood pressure medication called an angiotensin-converting enzyme (ACE) inhibitor and an angiotensin receptor blocker (ARB) (discussed later in this chapter) can prevent the onset of kidney disease if started early enough. We know that they prevent the progression of kidney disease once you have it, but their role in prevention is not known for sure. The indications to start either of these two types of medication are discussed later in this chapter.

Early Detection

Diabetic kidney disease has a natural history similar to type 2 diabetes in that it takes years to develop and deteriorate to an end-stage situation. The big problem is that in the early stages, when aggressive therapy can prevent the progression of diabetic kidney disease, there are no symptoms that can be recognized. If you and/or your health care provider are unaware of the screening methods to pick up early problems, by the time you feel poorly from the late stages of kidney disease, you have missed a golden opportunity to catch things early and prevent progression of this potentially devastating complication.

Microalbuminuria

The first measurable laboratory abnormality in the course of diabetic kidney disease is the presence of albumin in the urine in small amounts, which is referred to as microalbuminuria. Albumin is a protein that is normally found only in small amounts in the urine. The prefix micro refers to the amount (small) of albumin in the urine. People with microalbuminuria have a high likelihood of experiencing decreasing kidney function if left untreated over a period of years.

The important thing to remember is that once microalbuminuria is present, there are therapeutic maneuvers to retard the progression of diabetic kidney disease. Remember that there are no symptoms of kidney disease in the early stages. This is why screening is so important—so that aggressive management can be started in a timely fashion. This is the key to preventing the need for transplantation or dialysis!

You are responsible for getting tested for the presence of microalbuminuria and obtaining aggressive therapy if needed. The test for microalbuminuria is now readily available, but that was not always the case. I will always remember the day when I got a call from a representative of an insurance company in 1991 from which I was seeking to get life insurance. He said, "Dr. Edelman, I regret to inform you that your application for life insurance was denied because the urine sample we received from you had several thousand milligrams of albumin in it." I was shocked, because I knew this was an indication of fairly advanced kidney disease—way past the microalbuminuria stage. This was another huge wake-up call for me.

If you have type 1 diabetes, you should be screened for microalbuminuria once a year beginning 5 years from the time of your diagnosis of type 1 diabetes. People with type 2 diabetes should be screened every year from the time of diagnosis because the diagnosis of type 2 diabetes may have been delayed for many years. There are several different screening tests for microalbuminuria, which occasionally involve a timed urine collection for albumin, typically for 24 hours. Your physician can also measure a ratio of the albumin in the urine to the creatinine (another substance that goes up with kidney disease) in the blood (**Table 15-1**). The purpose of showing **Table 15-1** is not for you to completely understand or memorize all of the medical jargon but for you to be aware of the different ways that your kidney function can be evaluated. The albumin-to-creatinine ratio has become the most popular test, because you do not need to do the tedious 24-hour urine collection, and it is fairly accurate. If you do perform a 24-hour urine test, the large urine collection jug must be kept in the refrigerator. (Remember to label it carefully!)

Table 15-1
Definitions of Urinary Albumin Excretion Rates

	Urinary AER (mg/day)	Urinary AER (mcg/minute)	Urinary Albumin (mg) to Creatinine Ratio
Normoalbuminuria	<30	<20	<30
Microalbuminuria	30-300	20-200	30-300
Macroalbuminuria	>300	>200	>300

Abbreviation: AER, albumin excretion rate.

Several new home test kits for microalbuminuria have now been developed. This fantastic advance will really improve the awareness and access to early testing and hopefully appropriate therapy (Google home microalbuminuria test kits to get more information). One can also be screened with simple and quick urine dip test strips that measure microalbuminuria in the urine (Micral test strips). These test strips are much different from the older strips. The older strips tested only for gross protein or macroalbuminuria, not microalbuminuria. This older method is too insensitive to pick up small amounts of albumin or protein in a timely manner. If the Micral test is negative, you can be rescreened in 1 year. However, if the screening test is positive or even marginally positive, I recommend getting a albumin-to-creatinine ratio or 24-hour collection for better quantification of protein spillage. Certain situations, such as strenuous exercise, may make your microalbuminuria test positive even though you do not have diabetic kidney disease. Hence confirming the presence of microalbuminuria with at least one additional test is suggested, especially before starting aggressive therapy.

I also feel it is important to repeat yearly microalbuminuria testing, even if you are being treated aggressively. If the microalbumin level continues to increase despite aggressive therapy, that will warrant a closer look by your physician for additional fac-

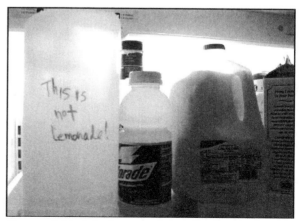

Be careful to label your urine collection jug!

tors that might hasten the decline of your kidneys. Some of these factors include making sure that your blood pressure control over a 24-hour period is adequate, using a special computerized monitoring device and examining any other medications that you are taking that may damage the kidneys. In addition, if your glucose control is not ideal, this should be an important area of focus.

If your doctor has already informed you of evidence of excessive protein in your urine (another way of saying macroalbuminuria or much more than a little protein in your urine), you are past the microalbuminuria stage. You now need to have regular urine tests to measure how much protein or albumin is in your urine and institute very aggressive therapy to retard the progression. In addition, most routine laboratory tests include a value called GFR or glomerular filtration rate, which is another excellent indicator of your kidney function.

It is also extremely important to realize that the presence of microalbuminuria or protein in the urine may be a marker for additional abnormalities other than the development of end-stage kidney disease. Microalbuminuria is also associated with the presence of diabetic retinopathy or eye disease, high cholesterol levels, and heart disease.

Blood Pressure Screening

Proper blood pressure screening is also an important tool in picking up signs of early kidney disease. If you have or are at risk for the development of kidney disease, obtain an accurate home blood pressure monitoring device so that you can take your own readings on a regular basis. It is important to measure your blood pressure at home during your normal daily activities and not

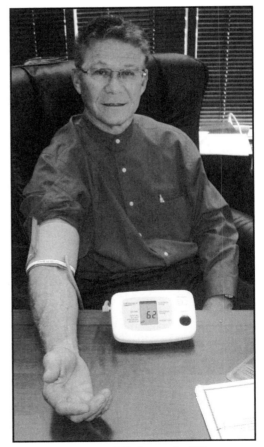

Get your own cuff. Pulse only 62!

only in a doctor's office. Home blood pressure monitoring allows for an accurate indication of what your blood pressure values are on the average. Home blood pressure monitoring devices are inexpensive and can be found at most pharmacies, department stores, or medical supply stores. Select one that you feel comfortable using and that has a good warranty. My blood pressure monitor fits quickly and easily on my wrist and appears to be very accurate. It is important to bring your home blood pressure device to your doctor's office once or twice a year so that one of the staff can compare the readings on your machine with the gold-standard method of manually pumping up the sphygmomanometer and listening to the pulse in your arm with a stethoscope. If the values are not within 10% of each other, your machine should be calibrated. If you go to the supermarket or drug store to get your blood pressure checked, be aware that they are not always accurate. Anyone with high blood pressure or hypertension should have their own machine at home, just as every person with diabetes should have their own home glucose monitoring device at home.

Aggressive Management

Diabetic kidney disease is treatable. You can truly make a difference in your risk of developing end-stage renal disease requiring dialysis or transplantation. Four therapeutic strategies have been well proven to prevent the progression of diabetic kidney disease. One other strategy has not been well proven (cholesterol reduction); however, it may be of therapeutic benefit and will be discussed (**Table 15-2**).

Table 15-2

Therapeutic Strategies to Prevent or Retard the Progression of Diabetic Kidney Disease

Proven Therapeutic Interventions
- Glucose control
- Blood pressure control
- Use of angiotensin-converting enzyme (ACE) inhibitors or an angiotensin receptor blocker (ARB)
- Low-protein meal plan

Unproven Therapeutic Interventions
- Cholesterol reduction (especially low-density lipoprotein [LDL] cholesterol)
- Antioxidants

Glucose Control

As previously discussed, the DCCT conclusively demonstrated that intensive glucose control can retard the progression of diabetic kidney disease already present in individuals with diabetes. It does not matter if you have type 1 or type 2 diabetes; glucose control is crucial. Follow the suggestions throughout this book, with the help of your caregivers, to achieve the best control that is possible for you. Get that glycosylated hemoglobin (A1C) value into a near-normal desirable range.

Blood Pressure Control

Aggressive blood pressure control, along with glucose control, is probably one of the more powerful interventions to reduce the progression of diabetic kidney disease. Please do not take this last statement lightly. It is super important!

The treatment of diabetic hypertension could be the topic of an entire book, but it deserves a few comments here and is discussed further in *Chapter 14*. First of all, it is important that "normal blood pressure" be correctly defined. Blood pressure goals have been defined differently and have been recently changed by several organizations (World Health Organization, American Heart Association, American Diabetes Association, etc). The American Diabetes Association currently recommends treatment to at least less than 130/80 mm Hg. Many kidney experts say that if you have evidence of protein or albumin in your urine, your average blood pressure should be less than 120/80 mm Hg (**Table 15-3**).

The top number in a blood pressure reading refers to the systolic blood pressure and represents

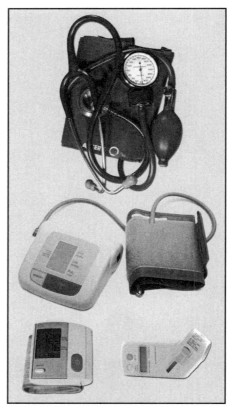

Blood pressure readings can be obtained using various monitoring devices. The "gold standard" is a stethoscope and sphygmomanometer *(top)* as typically used in your doctor's office. Home monitoring devices can be arm cuffs *(center)*, wrist cuffs *(bottom, left)*, or a finger cuff *(bottom, right)*.

Table 15-3

Goals for Blood Pressure Control

No Evidence of Protein or Albumin in the Urine
- Systolic blood pressure less than or equal to 130 mm Hg
- Diastolic blood pressure less than or equal to 80 mm Hg
  Medical jargon: ≤130/80 mm Hg

Persistent Protein or Albumin in the Urine
- Systolic blood pressure less than or equal to 120 mm Hg
- Diastolic blood pressure less than or equal to 80 mm Hg
  Medical jargon: ≤120/80 mm Hg

the pressure when the heart is working its hardest to pump out blood to the rest of the vital organs of the body. Of particular interest is that of the many organs in the body, the kidneys receive 25% of the "cardiac output," which demonstrates how important the kidneys are. The bottom number refers to the diastolic blood pressure and represents the pressure when the heart is resting, filling up with blood before the next systolic beat. The abbreviation mm Hg refers to millimeters of mercury, the universal unit of measuring blood pressure. When your blood pressure is too high, it puts a very large strain not only on your heart and blood vessels but also on your kidneys, brain, and eyes. Elevated blood pressure over the years leads to heart attacks, strokes, and accelerated eye and kidney disease. I have heard many experts say that controlling the blood pressure is as important as controlling the glucose values, and they have lots of clinical research evidence to back them up. Instead of debating which one is more important, how about just spending our efforts on controlling both of them?

Use of Angiotensin-Converting Enzyme Inhibitors

Angiotensin-converting enzyme (ACE) inhibitors represent an entire class of blood pressure–lowering medications. ACE inhibitors have proven effective in preventing and slowing the progression of diabetic kidney disease in terms of reducing albumin (protein) spillage into the urine and lowering blood pressure. ACE inhibitors have also been shown to benefit the kidneys of both type 1 and type 2 diabetics who have microalbuminuria, even when the blood pressure is normal. In this scenario, ACE inhibitors are given in low doses so that the blood pressure does not get too low (this is a rare problem in people with diabetes). In summary, ACE inhibitors protect the kidneys from further decline in function. You need to know if you are a candidate for taking an ACE inhibitor. **Table 15-4** lists some commonly used ACE inhibitors.

An ACE inhibitor is generally considered the first drug of choice for the treatment of hypertension of diabetes but should be used with caution in two types of patients:

- People who have a tendency to have high potassium levels in the blood—This usually occurs in people who have had diabetes for a long time and already have some damage to the kidneys.

Table 15-4

Commonly Used ACE Inhibitors

- Benazepril (Lotensin)
- Captopril (Capoten)
- Enalapril (Vasotec)
- Fosinopril (Monopril)
- Lisinopril (Zestril, Prinivil)
- Moexipril (Univasc)
- Perindopril (Aceon)
- Quinapril (Accupril)
- Ramipril (Altace)
- Trandolapril (Mavik)

Abbreviation: ACE, angiotensin-converting enzyme.

- Patients with a condition called renal artery stenosis—Renal artery stenosis basically means clogging (stenosis) of the arteries that deliver blood to the kidneys (renal means pertaining to the kidneys)
- Women who are pregnant or are trying to become pregnant should not take ACE inhibitors or ARBs as they have been shown to cause problems for the fetus.

How do you know if you have one of these two conditions? It is easy to find out if you have a tendency for high potassium levels in your blood. Potassium levels are commonly measured in most laboratory blood screening tests, and you should have several such measurements in your medical chart. If not, then you can get a simple blood test for potassium that does not require fasting. The symbol for potassium (which may be on your laboratory report) is K^+. Renal artery stenosis is more difficult to detect, although it is not too common. Usually, if you have stenosis or clogging of your renal or kidney arteries, you most likely will also have problems with other arteries in your body, such as your coronary (heart), cerebral (brain), and lower-extremity arteries. If you have any concerns or questions, simply ask your doctor about these issues. Last, some people may develop a persistent, dry cough while taking ACE inhibitors. This dry cough occurs in approximately 5% of people who take ACE inhibitors. The problem goes away when the ACE inhibitor is stopped, and then an ARB is normally substituted.

Use of Angiotensin Receptor Blockers

Angiotensin receptor blockers (ARBs) work in a similar manner as ACE inhibitors, and have been shown to protect the diabetic kidney as well. If for any reason you are not able to take an ACE inhibitor, then substituting for an ARB is a great alternative. Many caregivers use ARBs as first-line therapy for people with diabetes and hypertension, which is perfectly appropriate. **Table 15-5** lists the commonly used ARBs.

The bottom line is that all diabetics, with few exceptions, should be taking an ACE inhibitor or an ARB if there is albumin or protein in the urine and/or if the blood pressure is high. Even if your blood pressure is normal and you have microalbuminuria, you should still be taking an ACE inhibitor or an ARB. If your blood pressure is truly normal and you have absolutely no evidence of protein or albumin in your urine, then you do not need an ACE or ARB. Saying this, I know of physicians who put all of their patients with diabetes on an ACE or ARB no matter what. I am not at this stage in my recommendations yet, but since they are safe with few side effects, I do not have any huge objections.

Table 15-5

Commonly Used ARBs

- Azilsartan (Edarbi)
- Candesartan (Atacand)
- Eprosartan (Teveten)
- Irbesartan (Avapro)
- Losartan (Cozaar)
- Olmesartan (Benicar)
- Telmisartan (Micardis)
- Valsartan (Diovan)

Abbreviation: ARB, angiotensin receptor blocker.

Low-Protein Meal Plan

Diets high in protein have been shown to induce and accelerate kidney disease in animal and human studies. Based on the results of several clinical trials, it is recommended that people with diabetic kidney disease should restrict their protein intake to 0.8 grams per kilogram of body weight per day or about 10% of their total daily calories. I tell my patients that this is the equivalent of a small or medium amount of protein only once a day. There is also additional evidence that vegetable protein, such as beans and tofu, may be better than animal protein, and that white meat may be better than red meat. This may relate to the fact that red meat has more fat in it than do other sources of protein.

If you are a "steak and potatoes" type of eater, you should start thinking about reducing the amount of meat in your diet long before any evidence of diabetic kidney disease is present. Big changes in one's lifestyle must come slowly. I grew up eating meat at least 2 times a day. My family always had some type of red meat or chicken for dinner. My lunches usually consisted of a peanut butter and diet jelly or a cold-cut sandwich. In addition, I often had eggs for breakfast. This type of diet is at least 1.2 grams per kilogram of body weight per day or about 20% of my daily calories. I have now slowly adapted to a low-protein diet that I enjoy. I usually now have a toasted English Muffin with a small amount of peanut butter for breakfast, a veggie or white meat (chicken or tuna) sandwich for lunch, and a pasta dish or large salad for dinner. When I have a veggie lunch, then I have some protein with dinner. When I go out to eat, I satisfy my meat cravings by usually ordering the ribeye or 10-oz filet (medium rare, of course). Occasionally, I have days when I eat a lot of protein, and other days, none at all. Trust me—I do not turn down a huge slab of roast beef with white, creamy horserad-ish sauce at a banquet dinner. The key is to practice moderation in the diet, allowing yourself to enjoy what you eat so that sticking to your diet comes naturally, and is not a daily emotional fight or guilt-ridden process. We are not what we eat but how much we eat! Please refer to *Chapter 5* for further discussion on meals.

Cholesterol Reduction

Although not as well proven as the above therapeutic strategies for aggressively treating diabetic kidney disease, there is accumulating evidence that by lowering the cholesterol levels, especially the LDL (or bad cholesterol) level, the progression of kidney disease is reduced. The "statins" are the most effective class of medications for reducing your LDL cholesterol level. They are easy to take (once a day, usually at bedtime) and have little or no side effects (**Table 15-6**).

Reduction of LDL cholesterol has been strongly proven to reduce heart disease in people with diabetes and can only be beneficial. If it turns out that one can also reduce the decline of kidney function by lowering cholesterol levels, then by doing so I will have done both my patients and myself an extra service. I do not recommend taking any cholesterol-lowering medication if your LDL cho-

Table 15-6

"Statin" Medications Available for Lowering Cholesterol[a]

- Atorvastatin (Lipitor)
- Fluvastatin (Lescol)
- Lovastatin (Mevacor, Altocor)
- Pitavastatin (Livalo)
- Pravastatin (Pravachol)
- Rosuvastatin (Crestor)
- Simvastatin (Zocor)

[a] Discussed in detail in *Chapter 14.*

lesterol level is at the desired goal. Normal cholesterol levels and statin therapy are discussed in *Chapter 14.*

Case Presentation

Mary is a 24-year-old woman who was diagnosed with type 1 diabetes at age 12. She is currently on a long-acting insulin analogue (Lantus [glargine]) once a day given at bedtime and a fast-acting insulin analogue (Apidra [glulisine]) before meals. She checks her blood glucose sporadically when she "feels" it is high, with most of the morning blood glucose levels greater than 180 mg/dL, and she had a recent A1C of 8.6%. Her last dilated eye examination was 2 months ago and showed early diabetic retinopathy or eye disease. She reports that both feet are a little numb and tingle at night. She continues to exercise regularly, running 5 to 10 miles per week, and is at her ideal body weight. She is following a high-protein diet that she read about in a sports magazine several years ago. She does not smoke.

Over the course of the past year, her blood pressure has risen from a baseline of 110/70 mm Hg to 135/80 mm Hg. A urinary albumin-to-creatinine ratio measured 4 months ago was 50 mg/g (normal range <30, see **Table 15-1**). She takes no medication other than insulin.

Case Discussion

This woman is a poorly controlled type 1 diabetic who is at significant risk for the development of end-stage diabetic complications. She has microalbuminuria, which is the first clinical sign of diabetic kidney disease, and her blood pressure is elevated compared with her usual baseline. Many physicians would consider 135/80 mm Hg as normal, but compared with her usual blood pressure of 110/70 mm Hg, it is definitely high. In addition, her glucose control is not adequate, and she also has evidence of eye and nerve disease from poorly controlled blood glucose levels. Mary has evidence of all three major microvascular complications, and this should be a huge wake-up call for her and her physician.

Treatment of this patient's early diabetic kidney disease required a multifaceted approach, including improved glucose control, dietary changes (such as reduced daily protein intake), and aggressive treatment of her high blood pressure with an ACE inhibitor or an ARB. She agreed to:

- Test her blood glucose more regularly
- Consider getting a continuous glucose monitoring device
- Follow a low-protein diet
- Start taking an ACE inhibitor.

I encouraged her to keep a close eye on her blood pressure levels at home with a blood pressure cuff. If her blood pressure is not close to 120/80 mm Hg, adding a second blood pressure medication will be warranted for sure.

Summary

Diabetic kidney disease is preventable and treatable. The two most powerful and proven methods of preventing diabetic kidney disease is to maintain strict glycemic control and blood pressure control from the time of diagnosis. Early detection is of vital importance in order to initiate aggressive treatment early. Yearly microalbuminuria testing is currently the most sensitive technique for detecting early kidney damage, and it is also a marker for other conditions, including heart disease. Once the presence of microalbuminuria and/or high blood pressure has been detected, aggressive therapy with a number of proven strategies should be instituted as soon as possible. These strategies include:
- Glucose control
- Blood pressure control
- Use of ACE inhibitors or ARBs
- A low-protein meal plan.

You can make a difference in your life and the life of your diabetic kidneys. You can prevent the need for dialysis or transplantation.

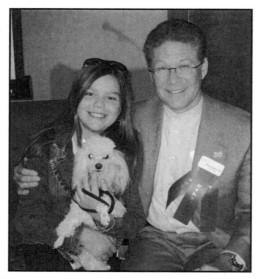

Young woman with type 1 diabetes and her low glucose alert service dog.

16

For Your Eyes Only

Don't Lose Sight of the Problem

by Steven V. Edelman, MD
and Paul E. Tornambe, MD

The Main Message

Diabetic retinopathy is the result of microangiopathy, abnormal sorbitol pathways, glycosylation of the retinol basement membranes, and possibly the oxidation of cellular and molecular structures of the orbital layers—we scared you, didn't we? We are not going to make you read a chapter on the pathophysiology of diabetic retinopathy. You can get this type of information from any medical textbook on diabetes. We would rather tell you the most important sight-saving information that you should know as a person living with diabetes.

Get a dilated eye examination at least once a year by an eye specialist who is very familiar with diabetic eye problems! This is the main message of this chapter. Just by getting your eyes carefully examined annually, you can lessen or prevent your chances of going blind or becoming visually impaired. If everyone with diabetes took this simple advice, the incidence of blindness would be a fraction of what it is today. Today, diabetic retinopathy is unfortunately the leading cause of blindness in the United States.

The American Diabetes Association recommends a dilated eye examination once a year but does not specify who should administer the examination. The person who may be making sight-saving decisions about your eyes could be an ophthalmologist, an endocrinologist or diabetes specialist, a primary care physician, a nurse practitioner, or an optometrist.

Traditionally, an ophthalmologist with a special interest in diabetic eye disease or retinopathy should be the person looking after your eyes, especially if you already have documented problems. Although it is true that there are some optometrists and other caregivers who are capable of picking up the early signs of retinopathy, many do not have this type of expertise. I send all of my patients to an ophthalmologist who has the most experience with diabetic retinopathy like my co-author and good buddy. Early detection and aggressive treatment are the keys to avoiding serious problems.

It is important to pick up the early changes in the eye that are a result of diabetes because there are many measures that one can take to prevent the progression to blindness (**Table 16-1**). Remember—there are no symptoms of diabetic retinopathy until it is at an advanced stage when aggressive therapy may not be effective in saving your vision. This is why regular screening is so important.

Table 16-1

Measures That You Can Take to Prevent Blindness Once You Have Diabetic Retinopathy

- Get your blood glucose level under the best control possible
- Make sure that your blood pressure is in the normal range
- Visit an ophthalmologist with a special interest in diabetic retinopathy as often as prescribed (at least once a year)

An Eye Doctor's "Bird's-Eye" View

Diabetes is a disease of small blood vessels. The eye contains many small blood vessels, so the eye is frequently involved in diabetes. The eye is an organ of vision. Like the photographer's camera, light enters the eye from the front through the cornea (like the camera lens) and the picture is taken on a fine membrane (like the film) called the retina. The information is then transferred to the brain by way of the optic nerve. The retina contains millions of nerve fibers that are nourished by very small blood vessels. These blood vessels become involved in diabetes.

Sadly, most diabetics go blind for one reason: they are brought to the attention of the eye specialist too late. The National Eye Institute (NEI) sponsored an extensive study of diabetic retinopathy, results of which were published in 1976. The study proved that with appropriate and timely laser treatment, the risk of severe visual loss from diabetes can be reduced by 70%.

There are two forms of diabetic retinopathy: a background form and a proliferative form. In type 1 diabetes, retinopathy can begin as early as 5 years after the diagnosis of diabetes is made. Therefore, a teenager who has had diabetes for 5 years must be evaluated at least yearly by an eye-care specialist to check for diabetic retinopathy. For people with type 2 diabetes, screening should start at the time of diagnosis since it is possible that the diabetes has been around for years before the diagnosis.

In background diabetic retinopathy, the retinal blood vessels leak fluid and sometimes bleed. If the leakage develops close to the area of central vision, reading vision will be compromised (**Figure 16-1**). The NEI trial has proven that laser treatment can stop the progression of

Figure 16-1

Compromised Reading Vision With Proliferative Diabetic Retinopathy

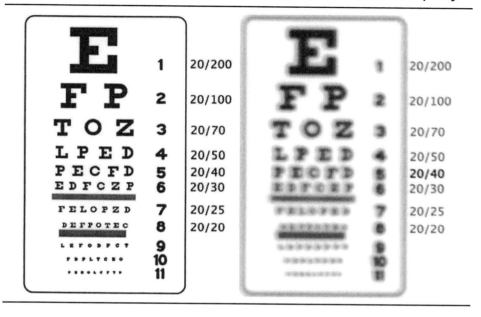

diabetic retinopathy. However, as the person with diabetes gets older, other blood vessels start to leak, and several laser treatments may be required over a lifetime. This is why we advise that people with type 2 diabetes have an eye examination as soon as diabetes is diagnosed as they may have had borderline disease for years and the eyes might already be affected.

Proliferative diabetic retinopathy is a more rapidly progressive form of diabetic retinopathy. As the small blood vessels in the eye fail to carry oxygen to the retinal tissue, the tissue releases VEGF. This substance tells the body to make blood vessels so more oxygen can be brought to the retina. Unfortunately, the blood vessels that the body makes inside the eye are weak and fragile, and they tend to break and bleed easily. Again, laser treatment is effective in directly cauterizing these vessels, and it also improves oxygenation to the retina, which prevents VEGF production. If laser treatment is not applied, the blood vessels continue to bleed, scar tissue forms, and the retina is torn as the scar tissue contracts. The retina will then separate from the back of the eye (retinal detachment) and die, resulting in blindness.

Vitrectomy is an operation developed in the 1970s, which, using space-age technology, can remove the blood and scar tissue and restore the retina to its proper position. Again, if instituted early enough, blindness can be prevented. During vitrectomy surgery, instruments less than 1 mm in diameter are inserted into the eye. The blood is vacuumed out of the eye and the scar tissue is removed with microscopic forceps and scissors. Laser can then be applied internally to stop the bleeding. The operation can take several hours but is usually done on an outpatient basis. It is effective in more than 90% of cases.

Currently, medications are being developed to inject into the eye in order to prevent scar tissue formation, stop bleeding, and treat swelling of the macula called diabetic macular edema. We will see more pharmacologic manipulation of disease within this next century. VEGF inhibitors are just the beginning. Long-lasting steroid implants are available which can last 3 months to 3 years and are aimed at treating diabetic macular edema. We will also likely define the gene(s) that causes this disease and will either manipulate the gene or produce the substance that the gene doesn't make to prevent the complications of diabetes.

For the time being, there are three things you can do to minimize the damage to your eyes caused by diabetes: First, if you think you do not have diabetes but have a family history of diabetes or are experiencing symptoms of thirst, frequent urination, and weight loss, you may have diabetes. Early detection and appropriate treatment will significantly reduce the incidence of diabetic complications. If you have diabetes, make sure your first- and second-degree relatives get regular screening. Second, if you have diabetes, make every effort to control it tightly. The National Institutes of Health completed a very important study that proved, beyond a doubt, that tight blood glucose control reduces the incidence of blindness, heart disease, and peripheral neuropathy. Third, get a dilated eye exam by someone who knows what he/she is looking for at least once a year! Tight blood glucose and blood pressure control, close medical supervision, and regular dilated exams will decrease the complications of diabetic eye disease. Just do it!

Diabetic Retinopathy and Laser Therapy

Diabetic retinopathy is caused by years of excessively high blood glucose or sugar levels. Glucose sticks to and damages many of the structures of the body; however, certain organs are more susceptible to the adverse effects of prolonged hyperglycemia, including the eyes, kidneys, heart, and nerves. The specific structure of the eye that is damaged is called the retina, which is one of many important layers that make up the eye. Diabetic retinopathy results in the development of new blood vessels in an attempt to supply more oxygen-rich blood to the damaged retina; however, these new blood vessels are fragile and break easily. When these abnormal blood vessels break, they bleed into the center of the eye (vitreous hemorrhage). The vitreous is normally full of clear fluid and when blood inappropriately enters this liquid cavity, it becomes cloudy red and vision is severely impaired. If the bleeding stops either on its own or by laser therapy, the blood will slowly sink to the bottom of the eye like the oil in salad dressing, and vision will slowly improve over weeks to months.

One of the biggest advances in diabetes therapy has been the development and availability of laser therapy for the treatment of retinopathy. This type of laser therapy is very different from the corrective laser surgery that allows people to be glasses-free. Laser therapy alone is responsible for preventing severe visual impairment and blindness in millions of Americans. Laser therapy must be done in the early stages of retinopathy, before the abnormal blood vessels break and long before there are any noticeable eye symptoms. The basic concept behind laser therapy is that when the ophthalmologist aims and shoots a laser beam into your eye, the energy generated works to coagulate (or seal up) the leaky blood vessels. Laser therapy is also used to purposefully destroy the outer areas of the retina in order to reduce the body's adaptive drive to deliver blood to those areas. In this manner, the number of abnormal vessels will decline, reducing the chance for a bleed or vitreous hemorrhage. The outer areas of the retina are mostly responsible for peripheral vision and are not vital to maintain adequate sight. In addition, night vision may be diminished after extensive laser therapy. Reduced peripheral and night vision is a small price to pay to prevent total blindness.

Exciting New Developments for the Eye

It is also exciting that new medications are being tested and developed that may help prevent the progression of microvascular complications, including retinopathy.

A new set of drugs may change the way we manage diabetic retinopathy. At the time of this writing, doctors are learning how to use these drugs called VEGF inhibitors (Avastin [bevacizumab], Lucentis [ranibizumab], Macugen [pegaptanib sodium], Eylea [aflibercept]). VEGF (which stands for vascular endothelial growth factor) stimulates abnormal blood vessels to grow into the eye (proliferative diabetic retinopathy) and VEGF also stimulates normal blood vessels in the eye to leak (diabetic macular edema). At the moment, these drugs must be injected into the center of the eye, sometimes more than once. In the case of proliferative retinopathy, a single injection has been shown to dramatically stimulate complete regression of the new proliferative vessels in 5 days (**Figure 16-2A** and **16-2B**). After a month or two, the drug wears off and the blood vessels return. This treatment "buys time" for the patient and doctor to apply laser treatment or perform a vitrectomy operation more safely with less chance of bleeding. Interestingly, sometimes an injection of this drug in one eye improves the disease in the fellow eye. We do not know exactly what the reason is for this crossover effect. Laser is still necessary, but in severe cases, this treatment will give retina surgeons a better chance to save more advanced cases. New lasers have been developed that apply a pattern of spots rather than a single shot. This has the advantage of delivering evenly spaced laser spots of the same intensity. This permits more precise delivery of laser energy and perhaps less loss of peripheral vision. It is also much more comfortable to the patient and the treatment may be done in less time, frequently without the need for anesthetic injections. New imaging devices are now available which permit a widefield view of the retina. This new technology now permits doctors to evaluate all areas of the retina at the same time rather that piecing together many smaller views in a collage. This is particularly valuable when doing fluorescein

Figure 16-2

Use of VEGF Inhibitors With Proliferative Diabetic Retinopathy

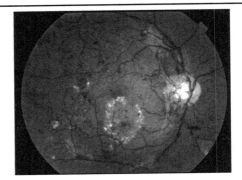

A. Note blood vessels on the optic nerve of this eye prior to treatment with Avastin

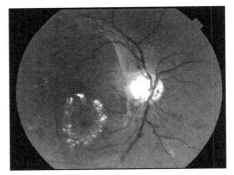

B. Five days after injection of Avastin into the eye, the blood vessels on the optic nerve have regressed completely

Abbreviation: VEGF, vascular endothelial growth factor.

angiography, for now we can image all vessels at once over several minutes. This technology precisely shows the surgeon where the most diseased tissue lies, so that laser can be targeted only to the most poorly perfused tissue leaving healthier tissue alone. This also minimizes loss of peripheral and night vision following laser treatments.

Drugs to Treat/Prevent Diabetic Retinopathy

Diabetic retinopathy may be defined as normal blood vessels, which have been damaged and now leak fluid, lipid, and blood (background diabetic retinopathy) or the development of new abnormal fragile blood vessels, which "break" and can bleed significantly (proliferative diabetic retinopathy). What causes diabetic retinopathy? Well, elevated blood glucose in diabetes leads to the overaction of a protein called PKC beta. PKC beta plays an important role in damage to small blood vessels that can lead to increased vascular permeability (leakage). This prevents enough oxygen and nutrients from getting to retinal tissue. Lack of oxygen releases another protein called VEGF, which makes blood vessels leak even more and stimulates the proliferation of abnormal fragile blood vessels, which then bleed. A new class of drugs taken orally inhibits the action of PKC B, thus damage to the blood vessels is minimized and retinopathy is less likely to develop and advance. In recent clinical trials, these drugs have decreased the incidence and severity of swelling in the retina (macular edema) but did not prevent eyes from developing proliferative diabetic retinopathy. However, as mentioned earlier, another class of drugs called VEGF inhibitors, which are injected into the eye, cause a dramatic regression in proliferative diabetic vessels. Thus we have drugs that alter the course of diabetic retinopathy. This is just the beginning of new drugs, which will allow us to pharmacologically treat and possibly prevent diabetic retinopathy!

People with diabetes should also be aware that Avandia could cause macular edema and decreased vision. If patients taking Avandia have ankle edema and decreased vision, they should consider stopping Avandia. The same swelling noted in their legs can develop in their macula.

The Story of My Eye Problems

I (Steve Edelman) distinctly remember when I first developed eye problems. It was in the fall of 1983, after 12 years of living with diabetes. A classmate of mine, John, was a big burly guy who gave me the biggest bear hug of my life after one of our successful intramural softball games. Several hours later, I noticed my vision was blurry and the straight lines of one of my textbooks looked wavy. Another close classmate, Patty, drove me to an ophthalmologist; after a brief examination, he told me I had diabetic retinopathy. Patty cried and I started worrying about going blind. This was the first dilated eye examination of my life. My primary care doctor had never sent me for a dilated eye examination. Remember that in 1983, the Diabetes Control and Complications Trial (DCCT) was just getting started and many physicians were uninformed about any preventive strategies.

Unfortunately, the retinopathy progressed. One morning in March of 1986, I awoke unable to see out of my left eye. All I could see was a dense red haze. After several months of waiting for the blood to sink, I received laser therapy. It was difficult to work long hours as an endocrinology fellow and be handicapped and distracted during every waking minute of every day. I was able to read and study only with the aid of a big magnifying glass. A big red blob that moves around in your visual field is hard to ignore.

Over the next several years, I had three more eye hemorrhages, but I thank my lucky stars that they did not occur at the same time. One of the bleeding episodes was during a family vacation in Germany. I was really a lot of fun during that trip! After what seems like a zillion dilated eye examinations and over 2000 laser zaps to each eye, my eyes have stabilized and I have not had a hemorrhage since 1993 (knock on wood). At my last visit with Dr. Tornambe in May of 2012, my eyes were stable. My vision was slightly worse and apparently the deterioration was due to the extensive laser therapy I had many years ago. Some of the advances discussed above will reduce the need for extensive laser burning of the retina and subsequent vision loss.

I consider myself lucky to have good vision as I write this book. I am able to drive and carry on a normal visual life. In exchange, I am happy to live with reduced peripheral vision and poor night vision. When I go into a dark movie theater, it is pitch black to me for a long time as my eyes are slow to adapt. I use large monitors that I hook up to my laptop and wear special glasses for reading and working at the computer. Many of my eye problems could have been avoided if I had been educated and motivated to become more actively involved in my own care as a young adult.

Summary

The bottom line is that it is your responsibility to get a dilated eye examination at least once a year, preferably by someone familiar with the complications of diabetes in the eyes. This person must be an ophthalmologist if you already have eye problems. Get your blood glucose and blood pressure under control, both of which have major effects on your eyes. You can prevent blindness. Don't lose sight of the problem!

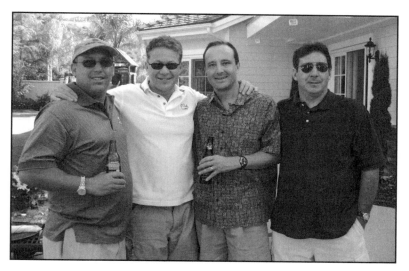

Me and my buddies *(from left to right)* Mike Spinazzola, me (Steve Edelman), Rob Merkin, and Bob Weinberger.

17

Be Sweet to Your Feet

by Ingrid Kruse, DPM

Introduction

Foot problems, including foot ulcers, are a major cause of disability in people with diabetes. Even today, diabetes remains the leading cause of foot and leg amputation in the world. Techniques to prevent amputations range from the simple, but often neglected, foot inspection to complicated vascular reconstructive surgery.

In order to take an active role in preventing foot problems, you must first understand why foot problems occur so frequently in people with diabetes. The main reason is nerve damage (neuropathy) but blood flow problems (vascular disease) and poorly controlled diabetes also contribute to the problem. Luckily, all of these are treatable and, more importantly, preventable problems.

Neuropathy

Neuropathy, or nerve damage, will affect approximately 50% of people who have had diabetes for more than 25 years. High blood glucose levels over long periods of time are highly correlated with the development and progression of neuropathy; tight blood glucose control has been shown to reduce the incidence of neuropathy. The Diabetes Control and Complications Trial (DCCT) showed that neuropathy could be prevented in almost 70% of the cases where patients had excellent glycemic control.

Neuropathy typically starts in the toes with some tingling and numbness but can progress up the leg to where people are numb all the way up to their knees. It may also affect the fingers and hands but this is less common. The ability to feel pain is one of our body's main warning systems. It informs the brain that something is wrong somewhere... to ignore pain is never a good thing. Anyone who has forced himself or herself to keep exercising despite being injured or has ignored a toothache knows that things typically get worse when you do that sort of thing.

When you lose the ability to feel pain, an alarm bell will not go off and you will become prone to injury that may go undetected for quite a while. Here is a typical scenario that I have seen many times: Let's say you have developed some numbness in your feet due to diabetes. You are out walking or shopping, and inadvertently you step on a nail. Your nerves won't feel the injury and can't warn you by giving pain signals. By the time you get home, you will have a wound in your foot and probably some blood on your sock. If you happen to notice the blood when you take off your shoes, you will discover the wound and can take steps to prevent infection by cleansing it and apply-

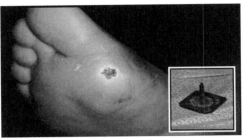

Puncture injury sustained when stepping on a nail or tack.

ing a dressing to the wound. However, if you did not notice the blood, or even worse, if you continue wearing the shoe with the nail sticking through it into your foot, you may soon have an infected foot ulcer. This is exactly why the daily foot inspection (discussed in detail later in the chapter) is so important and one of your best preventive measures, especially when you already have some nerve damage.

The nerves that are typically affected in diabetic neuropathy are the smallest ones: pain, temperature, fine-touch, and pressure nerves.

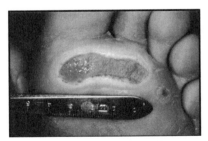

Blistering injury resulting from temperature insensitivity.

It is not uncommon for people to burn themselves and not realize it. Something as simple as sitting too close to an open fireplace with your feet propped up and reading a book, or walking barefoot outside on hot pavement, or using hot water bottles on your feet can all have disastrous consequences.

When your feet are numb, you can also fracture (break) a bone without knowing it. Your foot, ankle, and leg will become very swollen and warm; this is called a Charcot's joint. It may take a long time for your doctor to figure out what is going on since there are many reasons for swelling in the feet and legs. The big distinction here is that we're talking about just one foot and leg being swollen, not both. It is important to see your health care provider or podiatrist immediately if this should happen and make sure you get an x-ray to check for fractures. Treatment of Charcot's joint includes taking measures to reduce the tremendous swelling and then keeping the joint protected to let it heal. This means avoiding any kind of weight on it and usually involves the use of a cast or protective brace. Protecting the foot from bearing weight is of utmost importance even if you don't feel any pain when walking; these fractures need to heal. Sometimes a bone stimulator and medication are used to facilitate healing the fractures. If you continue walking around on an acute Charcot's joint, your foot will become distorted and deformed over time, making it impossible to fit into regular shoes.

Acute Charcot's joints are often missed by doctors since they are not that common, so it is important that you know about them and their presentation.

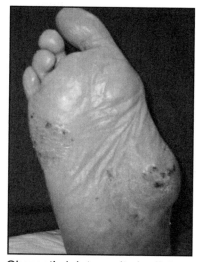

Charcot's joint results in distortion of the foot over time.

Diagnosis

How can you tell whether you have neuropathy and how much damage is present? A simple, painless, and quick way to find out is to have your physician check your feet with the 5.07 Semmes Weinstein monofilament or 10-gram monofilament (**Figure 17-1**). Depending on whether you can feel the pressure from those little nylon filaments on your feet allows you to find out if you have so-called "protective sensation"; that is, enough feeling in your feet to know when some injury occurs. The doctor may also do vibration testing with a tuning fork (which tends to show up earlier than other signs), check reflexes, temperature sense, and pinprick sensation.

Other causes of neuropathy, such as vitamin B_{12} deficiency, should also be excluded before making the diagnosis of diabetic neuropathy.

Painful Diabetic Neuropathy

In some patients with neuropathy, the predominant symptom of their neuropathy is not numbness but pain. This is called painful diabetic neuropathy (PDN). In this situation, the nerves are not damaged to the point where they are unable to feel anything but rather they are irritated and hyperactive, firing all the time and giving your brain pain messages for no good reason. This type of pain is typically worse at night and the most common symptoms include burning pains, sharp shooting pains, stabbing pain, electric shock pain, tingling sensation, cramping pain, hot or cold sensations, feeling tightness in the toe joints or ankles, and hypersensitivity to even light touch, such as bed sheets or socks.

These symptoms can be explained by the predominant nerves that are affected by neuropathy, as mentioned before: pain, temperature, fine-touch, and pressure nerves.

Treatment and Prevention

This neuropathic pain is difficult to treat and patients rarely have complete resolution of their pain. It is usually considered successful if a medication can decrease the pain by 50%. Also, the typical medications used to treat neuropathy take 4 to 6 weeks before they have any effect since the doses need to be increased very slowly in order to prevent side effects. Always consult your doctor before taking any type of medication.

The majority of the medications used to treat PDN fall into two categories: antidepressants and antiseizure medications. Commonly used drugs include amitriptyline, imipramine, and

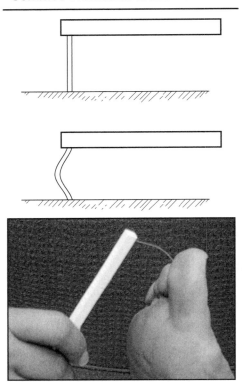

Figure 17-1

Semmes Weinstein Monofilaments

Applying a nylon filament mounted on a holder perpendicularly to the surface of the skin (top) with sufficient force (10 grams) to cause the filament to bend (bottom) for a duration of approximately 1.5 seconds will determine the existence of neuropathy. Research has shown that a person who can feel the force of the filament will not develop ulcers associated with neuropathy.

desipramine, which are tricyclic antidepressants (TCAs) and Neurontin (gabapentin), which is an antiseizure medication. There are now two medications on the market that were specifically approved by the FDA for the treatment of PDN. One of them is Lyrica (pregabalin), a second-generation gabapentin that is more potent and causes less sedation (drowsiness) than gabapentin. However, patients on pregabalin must be carefully monitored for possible side effects and adverse events. The typical dosage is 300 mg to 600 mg per day, given in divided doses either 2 or 3 times daily. The other drug specifically approved for neuropathic pain is Cymbalta (duloxetine), an antidepressant. Typical dosage is 60 mg to 120 mg per day. Side effects include nausea, dizziness, and somnolence (feeling like a zombie). Patients taking Cymbalta should have their liver enzymes monitored.

In Europe, alpha lipoic acid (an antioxidant) has been used quite successfully by giving it as an intravenous infusion, which showed not only improvement of symptoms but also nerve function. The antioxidant is also available in pill form as a nutritional supplement in the United States but there are no studies done on whether this is as effective as the intravenous therapy.

There are also topical agents (applied directly to the skin) available to treat PDN. One of them is capsaicin cream, a hot chili pepper extract that needs to be rubbed into the entire painful area 4 times a day; one must use gloves while applying it to avoid getting a burning sensation in the fingers. This may make it logistically difficult for some people to do. The other is the 5% lidocaine patch that was approved by the FDA for treatment of PDN. It has the advantage of having no side effects, therefore, it is safe to use and has shown improvements in pain as well as quality of life in patients with PDN. The patch is simple to apply: peel off the sticky portion and apply to the area where it hurts. Another option is 5 % lidocaine gel, which may be easier to use on the bottom of your feet where the patch can slide around too much. There are also non-medication treatment options for painful peripheral neuropathy such as acupuncture and electro-acupuncture, as well as infrared light therapy and the TENS unit (transcutaneous nerve stimulation). A last resort may be surgery (surgical decompression of the nerves) but again, there are not enough studies available to recommend this as a treatment option at this time.

In summary, PDN is a difficult complication to treat. It requires a lot of discussions between doctor and patient to figure out the best medication approach. People diagnosed with PDN need to remember that it typically takes 4 to 6 weeks for any of these agents to start working, and by that, we anticipate on average a 50% improvement in pain. Having falsely high expectations will only lead to frustration.

Our best strategy for combating neuropathy is still strict glycemic control. As mentioned before, not only does this prevent the onset of neuropathy, it has also been shown to slow down the progression of neuropathy by almost 60%! If you only have a little bit of numbness in your toes and really optimize your blood glucose readings, you can stop the neuropathy at this very early stage and prevent any of the problems that accompany nerve damage.

Taking control of your diabetes will indeed prevent complications!

Vascular Disease

Blood flow problems, or vascular disease, is the second most important reason why people with diabetes have foot ulcers that fail to heal and result in amputations. Arteries are the blood vessels that carry blood from the heart to various parts of the body (including the feet) as opposed to veins, which carry the blood back to the heart.

Arteries are usually soft and pliable structures but in diabetics can become rigid and stiff due to excess calcium deposits, which make it difficult for them to push the blood along. Furthermore, blockages can develop in the artery itself (called atherosclerotic plaques), eventually shutting off the circulation through that vessel and thus compromising the circulation to the foot. This is in essence how blood flow problems develop. Once you have a situation where the flow of blood is impaired, this also means that oxygen, nutrients, and even medications (such as antibiotics) do not get delivered where they should go. In a foot in which an ulcer and perhaps an infection is present, it will be almost impossible for the wound to heal.

Fortunately, we have made great progress in restoring the circulation to the feet of patients with vascular disease. Bypass surgery can be performed from an area above the blockage all the way down to the foot with great success. More recently, surgeons have started placing stents in the arteries to bypass them, which is a much less invasive surgery and is more easily tolerated by the patient. The above procedures have saved many limbs in people with diabetes.

Having your circulation assessed is an important part of the foot exam. This may simply require checking the pulses, but if they are absent, it may be necessary to do further testing in the vascular laboratory using a Doppler device and other techniques. These are painless tests that give your physician a lot more information about the status of your circulation.

What are the risk factors for developing blood flow problems and is there anything you can do to prevent vascular disease? The incidence of vascular disease goes up with the number of years you have had diabetes, just as it does for neuropathy. It also increases with age in general, and unfortunately, we cannot do anything about those factors. Other risk factors, such as smoking, high cholesterol levels, and high blood pressure, can be addressed and treated. This will then contribute to keeping your blood flowing!

Immunity

I would like to mention a little bit about your immune system. It plays a crucial role in fighting infection and can be adversely affected by poor blood glucose control. If your blood glucose frequently rises above 250 mg/dL, the immune cells (white blood cells) that travel through your bloodstream to the feet in order to fight infection become sluggish and don't move well in a forward direction. Also, their ability to engulf and gobble up the invading bacteria is impaired, and the infection starts raging out of control. Even in a person with well-controlled diabetes, blood glucose commonly goes up when an infection is present. Therefore, you may need to temporarily take extra insulin or a higher dose of oral medications in order to bring it back down. Testing blood glucose frequently is important whenever you are ill. Make sure you discuss with your caregiver how to make adjustments in your medications when you have an infection.

The Daily Foot Inspection

Daily foot inspection is probably the single most important screening tool for preventing serious foot problems in people with diabetes! It is best done just before you go to bed, since most injuries occur not while sleeping but rather during the day:

1. Wash feet daily with mild soap and dry carefully, especially between the toes, in order to prevent athlete's foot infections.
2. Athlete's foot infection between the toes looks like a crack in the skin or whitish, moist-looking skin. It can also look like little blisters or bumps in the arch area or dry, peeling skin on the bottom of the foot. It may or may not itch. Treat athlete's foot with creams such as Lamisil, Clotrimazole, or Tinactin, and remember to use the cream both in the morning and at bedtime.
3. Inspect for blisters, cuts, scratches, or bruises. Check for cracks in the skin, commonly in the heels. Use moisturizers after bathing.
4. If you have trouble reaching your toes, use a long-handled hand mirror or have a family member or friend assist you.
5. Check your shoes for foreign objects, torn linings, or things sticking through the bottom before you put your feet in them.
6. Always wear socks, but avoid socks with holes or mends.
7. Shoes should fit your feet in both length and width, don't go up a half size in length when the shoe is too narrow. Remove the

insole of your shoe (good athletic shoes have removable insoles) and place your foot on top of it to see if it is wide enough or make a tracing of your foot on a piece of paper and then place the shoe on top of it. Never try to break in shoes; they should fit perfectly at the time of purchase. Choose a soft leather upper or try athletic shoes and buy them at the end of the day when your feet tend to be more swollen than in the morning. The first time you wear new shoes, wear them only for 1 hour and only around the house. Then inspect your foot for blisters or red areas and slowly increase the wearing time. Medicare will pay for shoes and protective insoles if you are at risk for developing a foot ulcer. See your podiatrist for a prescription.

8. Trim your nails straight across with a slightly rounded edge. If you have neuropathy, vision trouble, or difficulty trimming them yourself (for example, if you have thick fungus nails), see a podiatrist! Please avoid all types of "bathroom surgery," like trying to fix an ingrown nail yourself—the results can be disastrous!

9. Do not walk barefoot, even in the house, because of danger of stepping on pins, needles, tacks, glass, or other items on the floor.

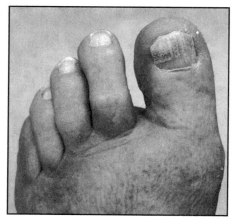

Trim toe nails straight across with slightly rounded corners. Thick, fungus nails should be attended to by a podiatrist!

10. Make the daily foot inspection a regular part of your daily routine, just like brushing your teeth.

Troubleshooting

What should you do when you find a blister or cut on your foot at the time of the daily foot inspection? Cleanse the area with an antiseptic; hydrogen peroxide is a cheap and effective antiseptic that you can buy in any drugstore. Inspect the wound for foreign objects, which should be removed. Also be sure to check your shoes, the culprit could be inside.

Apply an antibiotic ointment (such as Neosporin) and cover with gauze and tape, not just a band-aid. If there is any redness around the wound or if there is an odor or pus coming from the wound, you have an infection and need to be seen by your physician for wound cultures, antibiotic pills, and possibly x-rays. Do not ignore a foot infection; it will get worse. If you have neuropathy and experience fever, chills, nausea, vomiting, or your blood glucose is running unusually high, always check your feet—these may be your only warning signals when an infection is present in your foot.

Advanced Wound Care Technologies

There are now many new products and technologies available to assist us in healing diabetic foot ulcers. Negative pressure wound therapy (Wound Vac) is very helpful in deep or large wounds and produces faster wound healing than standard wound care. Also, the bioengineered skin substitutes (Apligraf, Dermagraft), which were derived from neonatal foreskin tissue (no jokes, please), contain living cells that are designed to be absorbed into the wound and help heal wounds faster by recruiting stem cells, producing growth factors, and stimulating new blood vessel growth. This is especially helpful in so-called "chronic wounds" or "stalled wounds."

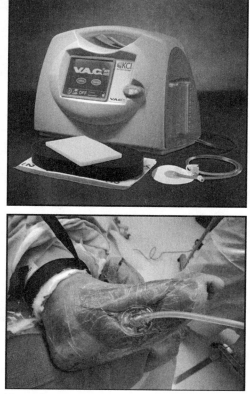

Summary

Neuropathy and vascular disease are common complications of diabetes but do not have to lead to amputations. Early diagnosis, halting the progression of neuropathy by strict glucose control, and checking your feet daily for injuries will help you minimize problems and treat them effectively. Addressing factors regarding your circulation, such as high cholesterol, blood pressure, and smoking, will keep you from developing serious vascular disease. This cannot be stressed enough—controlling your diabetes is

Negative pressure wound therapy, KCI— Wound Vac.

of the utmost importance, not only for preventing these complications but also for ensuring that your immune system is functioning at its optimum level and is ready to protect you from infection and aid in healing.

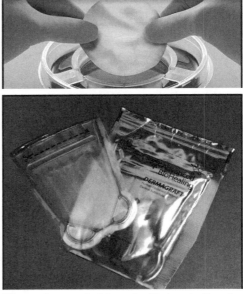

Bioengineered skin substitutes Apligraf *(top)* and Dermagraft *(bottom)*.

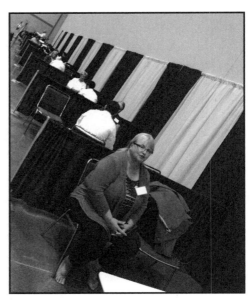

TCOYD participants get their feet examined in Des Moines.

18

Diabetes Can Affect Your Musculoskeletal System

Stiff Hands, Trigger Fingers, and Aching Joints

by Rachel Peterson Kim, MD
and Steven V. Edelman, MD

Introduction

The musculoskeletal system is quite commonly affected by diabetes. The term "musculoskeletal system" refers to your joints, muscles, tendons, ligaments, and bones. Diabetes can cause a number of changes in the musculoskeletal system, which is usually a surprise to people with diabetes as well as to their caregivers. These changes can result in a variety of symptoms and conditions of which you should be aware. Some musculoskeletal conditions are unique to people with diabetes, whereas others are the same as those seen in people without the disease; however, they may occur at a higher frequency among people with diabetes. Importantly, many of these conditions are treatable, but you must first recognize and identify them, which has traditionally been the main problem. This chapter will review some of the more common musculoskeletal problems seen in people with diabetes.

Hands

The hands are commonly affected in diabetes. This can be quite problematic, as our hands clearly play an integral role in our daily personal and professional life. Diabetes can affect the hands in a number of ways.

Diabetic Cheiroarthropathy (Limited Joint Mobility Syndrome)

The syndrome of limited joint mobility (also known as diabetic stiff-hand syndrome or diabetic cheiroarthropathy) is very much what it sounds like. There is limitation of joint movement, especially of the small joints of the hands, with a decreased ability to bend and/or straighten the fingers. The fourth and fifth fingers are typically affected first. It is generally a painless condition. The "prayer sign" observed in this condition is an inability to flatten the palms together completely, with a visible gap remaining between the opposed palms and fingers (**Figure 18-1**). Over time, the skin of the hands often becomes thickened, waxy, and tight, especially on the back of the hands. Limited joint mobility syndrome (LJMS) occurs in both type 1 and type 2 diabetes, and the risk increases with increasing hemoglobin A1C values as well as with increased duration of diabetes. Nearly half of adults with type 2 diabetes have some evidence of LJMS. LJMS is difficult to treat and generally irreversible. Optimizing control of blood glucose is advised. Physical and occupational therapy with passive stretching of the palm may be of benefit. When LJMS affects the feet, it may also be associated with an increased risk of foot ulcers.

Flexor Tenosynovitis

Flexor tenosynovitis (FTS), or trigger finger, is a frequent musculoskeletal complication of diabetes, and occurs more commonly than in the general population. Affected people complain of a catching sensation, or locking, of the finger(s). FTS is caused by a thickening and fibrosis of the tendon sheath that limits movement of the flexor tendon of the affected finger(s). It is often painful, and there may be a nodule that can be felt on the palm at the base of the affected finger. The finger may actually become stuck in a flexed or bent position, requiring the use of the other hand to straighten it out (**Figure 18-2**). Trigger finger is more common in long-standing diabetes (**Figure 18-3**), and the risk of developing flexor tenosynovitis goes up as A1C levels increase. A local steroid injection may be adequate treatment, at least temporarily, but sometimes minor outpatient surgery is required for trigger finger. Treatment with local steroid injection may be less effective in patients with diabetes compared with those without diabetes.

Figure 18-1

The "Prayer Sign" of Diabetic Cheiroarthropathy

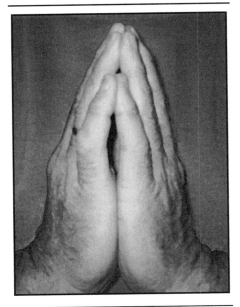

Diabetic cheiroarthropathy limits the ability to bend or straighten the fingers. Predictive of other diabetic complications, this syndrome tends to correlate with the duration of diabetes. This is Dr. Edelman's hands.

Dupuytren's Contracture

Dupuytren's contracture results from a thickening, shortening, and fibrosis of the connective tissue (fascia) just under the skin of the palm. The result is a pulling downward of the fingers (particularly the third and fourth fingers in people with diabetes). Bands, bumps, or nodules are often felt along the palm. The frequency of Dupuytren's contracture is higher in people with diabetes and increases with the duration of diabetes, and is also associated with the presence of peripheral neuropathy in type 2 diabetes. Dupuytren's has a variable course. For mild cases, passive stretching of the digits and palms a few times a day is recommended (you can use a tabletop). For more advanced cases in which function is affected and/or there is significant pain, steroid injections may be tried but are not very effective in longstanding cases. Surgery may be done for extreme cases, but the recurrence rate is high. More recently, injection of collagenase has been tried with some significant improvement seen and is an (expensive) alternative to surgical treatment of Dupuytren's.

Figure 18-2

The Trigger Finger of Flexor Tenosynovitis

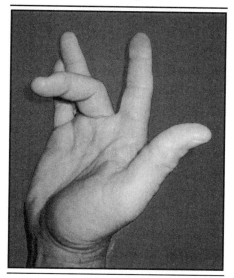

Flexor tenosynovitis is a catching sensation or locking of the finger(s) associated with pain and sometimes requiring use of the other hand to straighten the affected digit.

Carpal Tunnel Syndrome

Carpal tunnel syndrome (CTS) is seen in up to 20% of people with diabetes and people with diabetes are at three times higher risk of developing CTS than people without diabetes. CTS is due to compression of the median nerve as it passes through the wrist into the hand. In people with diabetes, this compression may be due to structural changes in the connective tissue of the wrist caused by high blood glucose. The finding of CTS is related to the duration of diabetes. Affected people often notice a burning pain, pins-and-needles sensation, or loss of sensation in the thumb, index, and middle fingers as well as half of the ring finger. The pain may radiate up the forearm and may be worse at night. It is usually made worse by activities such as driving, holding a newspaper or book, typing, or using a knife and fork. There may be associated loss of dexterity or weakness of the hand. If CTS is not severe, initial treatment consists of using wrist splints. Anti-inflammatory medications may also be tried (such as ibuprofen). Local steroid injection of the carpal tunnel is another option. For severe or refractory cases, carpal tunnel release surgery may be performed.

Shoulders
Adhesive Capsulitis

Adhesive capsulitis (frozen shoulder) has been reported in roughly 20% to 25% of people with diabetes, and is five times more common in people with diabetes than those without diabetes. In this condition, the capsule that surrounds the shoulder joint becomes thickened and stiffened, contracting down around the head of the humerus and resulting in restricted range of motion of the shoulder joint. Affected people notice stiffness, decreased movement, and sometimes pain in the shoulder. The cause of this stiffening and contraction of the shoulder joint capsule is not well understood. It is generally reversible and responds well to appropriate treatment. Treatment typically involves gentle stretching and range-of-motion exercises, often through physical therapy. Pain-relieving medications and/or steroid injections into the joint may also be used. Another treatment modality sometimes used is shoulder manipulation under anesthesia (MUA) by an orthopedic surgeon. It is a noninvasive procedure where general anesthesia is given, then the surgeon moves the shoulder through its range of motion. Occasionally, arthroscopic capsular release is required.

Figure 18-3

**Trigger Finger
Coupled With Arthritis**

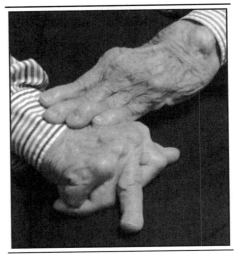

A patient with a long history of type 1 diabetes and arthritis, displaying trigger finger in all of her fingers except the middle one in her right hand.

Reflex Sympathetic Dystrophy

Reflex sympathetic dystrophy (RSD) or "shoulder-hand syndrome" is another shoulder condition seen in people with diabetes. Typical symptoms include severe pain or a burning sensation in the affected arm from the shoulder down to the hand. However, it may affect other parts of the arms or legs as well. There may be associated swelling, skin changes such as shiny skin, changes in hair growth, and color or temperature changes of the affected area. Increased sensitivity to temperature and touch may also be seen. Trauma may precipitate RSD, but the cause is not always known. Anti-inflammatory medications, other pain relievers, and oral steroids have been used in conjunction with physical therapy for this condition. Sympathetic nerve blocks (blockade of some of the nerves of the sympathetic nervous system that supply the affected area) with an injection of numbing medication, usually performed by an anesthesiologist, may also be helpful.

Feet

People with diabetes must be meticulous about foot care. Injuries to the feet often go unnoticed in people with diabetes due to underlying peripheral neuropathy and the associated decreased sensation in the feet. For this reason, inspecting your feet on a regular basis is critical to prevent infections that may develop silently without any symptoms.

Diabetic Osteoarthropathy

Diabetic osteoarthropathy (also known as Charcot's joint or neuropathic arthropathy) is a chronic, severe, destructive form of arthritis associated with loss of sensation in a joint from underlying diabetic peripheral neuropathy. The foot is most commonly affected. This condition is quite rare, affecting approximately one in 700 people with type 1 or type 2 diabetes. Although the exact cause is uncertain, it is postulated that repeated inadvertent microtrauma to the joint, which goes unnoticed due to the underlying neuropathy and decreased sensation, results in laxity, instability, and degenerative changes with resulting deformity. Usually there is no history of overt trauma or injury, such as falling off a curb. There may be skin changes overlying the affected area, including redness, swelling, bruising, and ulcers. The diagnosis is confirmed with x-rays and/or MRI. Treatment includes immobilization and avoidance of weight-bearing ("offloading") on the affected area, appropriate shoes, and possibly bisphosphonate therapy. Surgery is usually avoided in most cases.

Muscles

Diabetic muscle infarction (loss of adequate blood supply to an area of muscle, with resultant death of tissue) is a rare condition. It occurs spontaneously, without a history of trauma, and tends to affect people with a long history of poorly controlled diabetes. This condition is seen more commonly in people using insulin who also have other microvascular complications, such as neuropathy, nephropathy (kidney disease), or retinopathy (eye disease). Typical symptoms include the abrupt onset of pain and swelling of the affected muscle groups, such as the thigh (most commonly affected) or calf. Investigations such as MRI are done to exclude other conditions, such as tumors, muscle infection or abscess, blood clots, localized muscle inflammation, or infection of the underlying bone. Muscle biopsy may be needed to confirm the diagnosis. The cause of diabetic muscle infarction is not well understood at this time. Treatment consists of rest and pain relief, as well as antiplatelet and/or anti-inflammatory medications. Routine daily activities may be painful but are not thought to be harmful. Physical therapy may cause worsening of spontaneous diabetic muscle infarction. The condition tends to slowly resolve over weeks to months in most cases.

Case Presentation

Steve is a 57-year-old physician who has been living with type 1 diabetes for over 40 years (yes, it is me again). In 1997, I started to develop a catching sensation in my right middle finger as I opened and closed my fist. This catching sensation developed into a painful locking of my finger when I bent it, and I had to use my left hand to unlock it. I developed a nodule on the upper part of my palm just below where the middle finger leaves the palm. I am also unable to align my palms and fingers together so that there is no gap between them (you can basically drive a truck through my gap). Those are my hands in the trigger finger and positive prayer sign photos (**Figures 18-1** and **18-2**).

I have both the syndrome of limited joint mobility and a trigger finger. For my trigger finger, I saw an orthopedic surgeon who injected the joint with steroids that helped for a few weeks but really screwed up my blood glucose for a few days. Eventually the problem got so painful and debilitating that I had hand surgery; it was an outpatient procedure lasting about 30 minutes (I required only local anesthesia with numbing medication).

The surgery involves simply cutting a cylindrical sheath in which the finger tendon travels back and forth when you flex your finger. With a trigger finger, the sheath gets too narrow or is swollen; the tendon slides through fine when you flex your finger but gets stuck when you try to straighten it. By cutting the sheath, the blockage is fixed (**Figure 18-4**).

I eventually went through the same situation with two more surgeries. My left thumb started to lock up last year, but when I had to take anti-inflammatory drugs for several months for a knee problem, the triggering went away... at least for now.

Summary

Diabetes does commonly affect the musculoskeletal system in a variety of ways. These conditions can have a significant impact on the quality of daily life of people with diabetes. However, many of these complications are treatable, with resultant improvements in quality of life and more independence in activities of daily living. Become aware of the possible ways in which diabetes may affect your musculoskeletal system, and discuss these symptoms with your primary care physician or rheumatologist.

Figure 18-4

Surgical Procedure to Relieve Trigger Finger

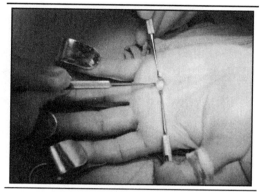

Steve Edelman's hand is shown here with the sheath being isolated so that the surgeon could cut it, relieving the trigger finger.

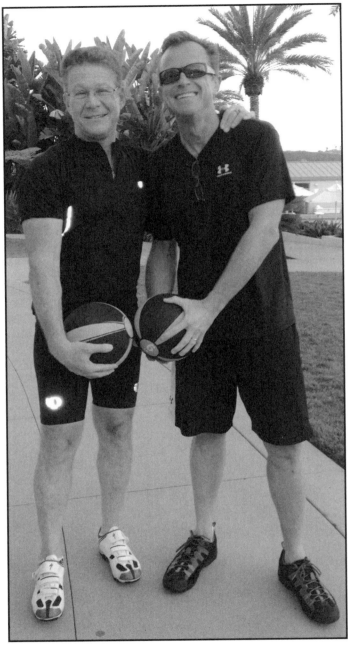

Juan Frias and Steve Edelman exercising at the gym.

19

Diabetes Can Affect Your Digestive Track

From Your Mouth, to Your...

by James D. Wolosin, MD

Introduction

Gastrointestinal (GI) disorders are common and those individuals affected by diabetes are certainly not immune to these problems. The medical term "GI" or "GI tract" refers to those areas of the body from your mouth and throat, past your stomach and small intestine, and ending with the colon (large intestine) and rectum (**Figure 19-1**). The liver, gallbladder, and pancreas are also considered to be part of the GI tract as they are closely linked with digestive function.

Any discussion of GI manifestations of diabetes should first deal with the reality that most of us will experience, at some time in our life, common nondiabetic-related problems with our GI tract, whether it be ulcer disease, gallstones, irritable bowel syndrome, food poisoning, or some other malady. Up to 75% of people visiting diabetes clinics will report significant GI symptoms. Common complaints may include constipation, abdominal pain, nausea, vomiting, and diarrhea. Treatments provided in these situations are often no different between diabetics and nondiabetics. Nonetheless, it is apparent that in both the short and long term, poorly controlled diabetes can lead to specific GI problems.

Figure 19-1

Diagram of the Gastrointestinal Tract

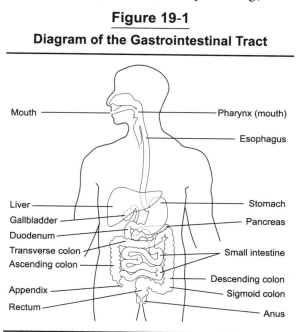

Mouth

Pharynx (mouth)

Esophagus

Liver

Stomach

Gallbladder

Pancreas

Duodenum

Transverse colon

Ascending colon

Small intestine

Descending colon

Sigmoid colon

Appendix

Rectum

Anus

As with other complications, the longer you have diabetes and the poorer the glucose control, the more severe the GI problems may be. Many GI complications of diabetes seem to be related to abnormal function of the nerves supplying the gut. Just as the nerves in the feet may be affected in the condition known as peripheral neuropathy, involvement of the intestinal nerves may lead to enteric neuropathy. This neuropathy may lead to abnormalities in intestinal motility (movement), sensation (pain), and secretion/absorption (digestion of foods). The purpose of this chapter is to familiarize you with the GI problems that you may experience living with diabetes (**Table 19-1**).

Table 19-1

Gastrointestinal Problems in Diabetes

- *Mouth*: thrush
- *Throat*: thrush and reflux or heartburn
- *Stomach*: ulcers, gastroparesis (delayed stomach emptying)
- *Small intestine*: bacterial overgrowth, delayed emptying, and celiac sprue
- *Large intestine or colon*: neuropathy
- *Pancreas*: exocrine insufficiency
- *Liver:* fatty liver
- *Diabetic medications that may affect the stomach*: sulfonylureas, Glucophage, Glyset, and Precose

Throat and Stomach
Esophagus

The esophagus is the muscular tube that connects the mouth with the stomach and serves as an active conduit through which food is propelled. As we age, abnormalities of esophageal movement or motility become more common; the medical term for this is presbyesophagus or esophagus of the elders. This may be more common in diabetes, but it tends to cause only minor symptoms in most people. The most common esophageal problem seen in people with diabetes is yeast infection or candidiasis. Yeast loves sugar. When blood glucose levels are consistently high, yeast can grow in numerous areas, including the mouth, esophagus, intestine, vagina, and skin. Treatment is usually easy as there are numerous medications available to treat this including nystatin (various manufacturers and brand names) and Diflucan (fluconazole). When acid backs up into the esophagus from the stomach, heartburn occurs. This is no more common in diabetics than nondiabetics unless there is a component of delayed emptying of the stomach. Up to 30% of the general population experiences some degree of heartburn or gastroesophageal reflux disease (GERD). Treatment of GERD may include changes in diet/lifestyle, medications, elevation of the head of the bed, and occasionally surgery. Numerous effective medications are available including Zantac (ranitidine), Pepcid (famotidine), Prilosec (omeprazole), Aciphex (rabeprazole), and others.

Delayed Stomach Emptying (Gastroparesis)

After eating, the stomach distends with food and digestive acid, then slowly contracts to mix, grind, and digest the meal. This involves a delicately coordinated process called peristalsis during which waves of muscular contractions force the food toward the outlet of the stomach. The contractions are coordinated with opening of the pylorus or "exit valve" of the stomach. The end result is gradual emptying of the stomach. In individuals with a long-standing history of diabetes, damage to the nerves supplying the stomach (eg, the vagus nerve) and damage to the stomach muscles can lead to gastroparesis or impairment in stomach emptying. This can be very difficult to deal with because erratic stomach emptying leads to unpredictable food absorption and blood glucose levels that are difficult to control. This is particularly true in people with diabetes treated with insulin where low blood glucose may occur following a mealtime injection of insulin followed by slow emptying of food from the stomach. Gastroparesis may cause bloating, distention, abdominal pain, nausea, or vomiting. Food and acid may back up into the esophagus (bottom part of the throat), leading to symptoms of heartburn and regurgitation. Fatty foods and very fibrous foods normally exit the stomach slowly and may be poorly tolerated in people with diabetic gastroparesis. Consumption of frequent small meals may provide some symptomatic relief. It is important not to stuff yourself at any meal.

Medications such as Reglan (metoclopramide) stimulate the stomach (gastric) nerve endings damaged by long-standing diabetes and may improve delayed stomach emptying. Erythromycin is an antibiotic that has unique properties that stimulate stomach motility and may be beneficial in select individuals. Propulsid (cisapride) may also help accelerate stomach emptying but is now only used in special circumstances because of cardiac side effects. Motilium (domperidone) is another agent that accelerates emptying of the stomach and is better tolerated than Reglan; however, it is not available in the United States (it is available in Canada and Mexico). Botox injections into the pylorus have been used successfully in some cases to enhance stomach emptying. Finally, a gastric pacemaker has recently been introduced that may help some individuals with diabetic gastroparesis. Newer agents that enhance stomach emptying will hopefully be available in the near future. Most important, careful attention to blood glucose control is essential.

Ulcer Disease

Ulcer disease is a common problem in people with or without diabetes and affects up to 10% of the population at some time during their life. Acid irritation of the stomach or esophagus leads to heartburn, indigestion, and a burning sensation in the upper abdomen (dyspepsia). Ulcers can occur either in the stomach or duodenum (the first part of the small intestine). *Helicobacter pylori*, the bacteria responsible for many ulcers, is no more common in people with diabetes than in the general population. In fact, diabetes itself does not increase one's risk of developing ulcers. Individuals with ulcers and ulcerlike symptoms are treated in the same fashion whether or not they have diabetes. Treatment is geared toward suppression of gastric (stomach) acid secretion with H_2 blockers (Tagamet [cimetidine], Pepcid [famotidine], Zantac [ranitidine], and Axid [nizatidine]) or the more potent proton pump inhibitors (Prilosec [omeprazole], Aciphex [rabeprazole], Protonix [pantoprazole], Nexium [esomeprazole], Prevacid [lansoprazole], Dexilant [dexlansoprazole], and Zegerid [omeprazole/sodium bicarbonate]). This allows the acid-irritated lining of the intestine to heal. If *H pylori* is present, you will need to be treated with antibiotics as well. Nonsteroidal anti-inflammatory medicines like aspirin, Motrin/Advil (ibuprofen), Aleve (naproxen), and others are well known causes of ulcers and gastritis. If you are on these medications and are having stomach problems, you need to speak to your doctor as they may need to be stopped.

Yeast Infections of the Gastrointestinal Tract

People with diabetes may develop yeast infections in the GI tract, especially when blood glucose is running high. When yeast infections occur in the mouth, it is called oral thrush and is characterized by a thick white coating of the tongue and throat, along with pain and burning in the mouth and throat. The infection may extend further down the throat and cause intestinal bleeding, heartburn, and difficulty swallowing. This type of extensive yeast infection is usually diagnosed with an endoscopic examination of the upper GI tract. Treatment is highly effective and is focused on the eradication of the yeast infection with medicines such as nystatin, Nizoral (ketoconazole), and Diflucan (fluconazole). Controlling the blood glucose is of utmost importance since the yeast loves a sweet environment. That is why women with poorly controlled diabetes experience vaginal yeast infections so frequently.

Small Intestine
Bacterial Overgrowth Syndrome

In some cases of long-standing diabetes, the enteric nerves supplying the small intestine may be affected, leading to abnormal motility of the small intestine. This leads to slowing of food transit through the intestine and some stagnation. This may result in an overgrowth of naturally occurring bacteria, leading to symptoms such as abdominal discomfort, bloating, diarrhea, and weight loss. Individuals who have had prior intestinal surgery may be at increased risk for this. The diagnosis of this condition may be difficult as it is hard to culture the contents of the small bowel accurately. Various breath tests may be helpful in diagnosing this condition, but more frequently, physicians may try a course of treatment with antibiotics to see if this helps. While just about any antibiotic can be helpful in lowering the bacterial count in the intestine, a newer antibiotic called Xifaxan (rifaximin) has certain unique advantages in treating this condition. It is a nonabsorbable antibiotic (active only in the intestine) and has a very broad spectrum of activity against the bacteria in the intestine. In addition, medications that promote more rapid motility in the small intestine may be of benefit in clearing out the overgrowth of bacteria.

Diabetic Neuropathy of the Small Intestine

At times, damage to enteric nerves may lead to a chronic abdominal pain syndrome similar to the pain that may occur in the feet of people with peripheral neuropathy. This condition may be difficult to treat but will sometimes respond to pain medications and tricyclic antidepressant medications, such as Elavil (amitriptyline). Tricyclic antidepressants act on the sensory nerves to decrease pain sensation and increase pain tolerance. Other medicines with possible benefit include Tegretol (carbamazepine), Dilantin (phenytoin), Lyrica (pregabalin) and Neurontin (gabapentin), but these medications have a higher incidence of side effects. Narcotic-type medications can relieve the pain of neuropathy but they should be used with caution as they can easily become habit forming and the pain becomes accentuated when the medications are not taken.

Celiac Disease

Celiac disease (also known as celiac sprue) is a rather uncommon disorder of digestion that is caused by a reaction to gluten, a protein commonly found in wheat, barley, rye, and sometimes oats. Although it may occur in up to 0.5% of the general population, the disorder is more common in type 1 diabetics, and approximately 6% may be affected.

Why this occurs is uncertain. There is clearly a genetic or inherited component to the condition and up to 10% of first-degree relatives of a patient with celiac disease may also be affected.

Celiac disease is not considered a true food allergy, but when people with this condition consume gluten, their immune system is activated, leading to damage to the lining of the small intestine. Because the body's own immune system is triggering this damage, celiac disease is considered to be an autoimmune condition. The type of damage that occurs to the small intestine is unique and leads to changes that can be easily identified by a biopsy of the small intestine. There is flattening and inflammation of the characteristic fingerlike projections coating the lining of the small bowel (villi). When this damage occurs, food and nutrients cannot be absorbed properly and inadequate absorption occurs (malabsorption). This leads to multiple symptoms, including diarrhea, bloating, abdominal pain, weight loss, and fatigue. Stools may become grey and oily in appearance due to inadequate absorption of fats. Lack of proper nutrition may lead to anemia, vitamin and protein deficiency, and thinning of the bones (osteoporosis). In children, growth retardation is a frequent problem. A rare skin condition called dermatitis herpetiformis may occur in conjunction with celiac disease.

Unfortunately, the symptoms of celiac disease are nonspecific and are similar to those seen in more common conditions such as irritable bowel syndrome. This frequently leads to a delay in the diagnosis of celiac disease. When this condition is suspected, the first testing should include a blood test for immunoglobulin A tissue transglutaminase antibody (TTG IgA). This blood test is relatively accurate in diagnosing this condition. In addition, a biopsy of the small intestine may be advised. All of these tests may become negative or normal if a gluten-free diet is eaten.

The only treatment for celiac disease is to avoid consumption of all gluten. Unfortunately, gluten is present in a large amount of the food that we consume. Wheat, rye, and barley are very common and are present in foods such as grain, pasta, cereal, cakes, and bread. Gluten is commonly used as a thickener and is present in many gravies and sauces. The good news is that many foods are gluten-free, including fresh meat, fish, and chicken, as well as fruits and vegetables. Over the past 10 years, awareness about gluten sensitivity has increased and there are now specialty stores that supply gluten-free breads and pastas. Many foods are labeled as gluten-free in stores. There is a large amount of information available on the Internet as well *(www.celiac.org, www.csace liacs.org)*.

Gluten intolerance is actually much more common than celiac itself. This occurs when an individual experiences symptoms of digestive upset, gas, bloating, and other problems after wheat or gluten consumption. The exact cause of this is uncertain but it is likely related to poor or incomplete absorption of wheat and gluten products. The celiac blood tests are normal, small intestine biopsies are normal, and there is no damage to the lining of the intestine. This is also different from wheat allergy where individuals typically develop rashes or wheezing with ingestion of wheat products. Symptoms resolve rapidly when gluten is withdrawn from the diet.

Celiac disease is a relatively uncommon cause of intestinal problems that occurs more frequently in individuals with type 1 diabetes. Patients with diabetes who are experiencing intestinal problems should be screened for celiac disease. A simple blood test can determine whether there is a concern for this very treatable condition.

Colon or Large Intestine

There is limited information available regarding the effects of diabetes on the colon (or large intestine). Neuropathy may affect the nerves of the colon, leading to some decrease in motility. Constipation is one of the more common GI complaints seen with neuropathy of the colon. Proper evaluation must first ascertain that there are no structural abnormalities of the colon, such as mechanical blockage. Fiber supplementation with bran or psyllium products (Metamucil, Citrucel, Konsyl), as well as a high-fiber diet, increases the water content of the bowel movement and may relieve constipation. Mild laxatives, such as milk of magnesia, Dulcolax (bisacodyl), or Miralax (polyethylene glycol) will often help as well. Amitiza (lubiprostone) is a prescription medication that brings more water into the colon and softens stool successfully. All of these medications can be taken on a regular basis if needed.

Diabetic Diarrhea

As many as 20% of people with a long-standing history of diabetes may experience frequent, unexplained diarrhea. Diabetic diarrhea is a syndrome of unexplained persistent diarrhea in people with a long duration of diabetes. This may be related to problems in the small bowel or colon. Abnormally rapid transit of fluids may occur in the colon, leading to increased bowel movement frequency and urgency. In addition, abnormalities in the absorption and secretion of colonic fluids may develop, leading to increased bowel movement volume, frequency, and water content. Diabetic diarrhea may also be due to neuropathy, leading to abnormal motility and secretion of fluid in the colon. In addition, there are a multitude of intestinal problems that are not unique to diabetes that can cause diarrhea, the most common of which is the irritable bowel syndrome.

Evaluation and treatment of diarrhea is similar in people with or without diabetes. If the basic medical evaluation of diarrhea is unable to target a specific cause for the diarrhea, then treatment is tailored toward providing symptomatic relief with antidiarrheal agents such as Lomotil (diphenoxylate/atropine) and Imodium (loperamide). Fiber supplementation with bran, Citrucel, Metamucil, or high-fiber food items may also thicken the consistency of the bowel movement and decrease watery diarrhea. In addition, antispasmodic medicines such as Levsin (hyoscyamine), Bentyl (dicyclomine), and Donnatal (belladonna/phenobarbital) may decrease stool frequency. Finally, in severe cases, injections of a GI hormone (Sandostatin [octreotide]) have been shown to significantly decrease the frequency of diabetic diarrhea. Antibiotic treatments may be of benefit if bacterial overgrowth is present. Probiotics are live bacteria that, when ingested, may promote intestinal health. There are a vast array of probiotics available over the counter and sometimes it is worthwhile trying these. The bottom line is that you need to work with your caregiver to find the most effective treatment strategy that works best for you. Tighter control of blood glucose may be beneficial in this situation.

Pancreas

The pancreas is the organ that secretes insulin, the hormone that helps to control the blood glucose levels in the body. This is called the endocrine function of the pancreas. However, the pancreas also has an exocrine function (ie, secretion of digestive enzymes directly into the intestinal tract to aid in the breakdown and absorption of carbohydrates, proteins, and fats). Up to 80% of individuals with type 1 diabetes will have some degree of impairment in pancreatic exocrine function, but this is rarely significant enough to lead to any clinical problems with digestion. The pancreas has a tremendous reserve, and a modest reduction in pancreatic enzyme secretion rarely leads to difficulty in food breakdown or absorption. The exocrine function of the pancreas may also be affected in some patients with type 2 diabetes but to a lesser extent. The symptoms of pancreatic exocrine insufficiency include watery diarrhea, floating bowel movements in the toilet bowl, and cramping after eating. The treatment is simply to take pancreatic enzyme pills with each meal. The results of therapy are usually quite good. In individuals who have had chronic problems with inflammation of the pancreas or have had surgical removal of the pancreas, diabetes may ensue due to a lack of insulin secretion from the gland. Insulin therapy is generally required in these situations.

Liver

We have entered a new era in which obesity has become much more prevalent and with it has come an epidemic of diabetes. One of the very first abnormalities that arise in the metabolic syndrome that is associated with obesity and adult-onset diabetes is the development of nonalcoholic fatty-liver disease. This syndrome is associated with obesity, elevated cholesterol/triglycerides, and insulin resistance. Fat is deposited within the liver and leads to abnormalities similar to alcohol-related liver disease. While up to 25% of the American public have this condition, only a small percentage (less than 5%) go on to the more advanced stage of nonalcoholic steatohepatitis or NASH. These numbers are much higher in obese individuals and those who have type 2 diabetes. NASH is associated with progressive liver disease and may even advance to cirrhosis or liver cancer.

Fatty liver has become one of the more common causes of abnormal liver tests. Common symptoms include right-upper abdominal pain and fatigue. Treatment usually is centered on weight loss and good control of blood glucose levels. Medicines such as Actos (pioglitazone) and Avandia (rosiglitazone) may help lower elevated insulin levels in type 2 diabetes and may lead to improvement in the fatty-liver syndrome. Glucophage (metformin) may also be of benefit in treating fatty liver but further research is needed before this can be recommended as a routine treatment. Recent studies have suggested that vitamin E supplementation may also be of benefit in fatty liver syndromes.

Fatty liver is often one of the first signs that an individual is developing diabetes and can be a wake-up call to change one's lifestyle to help prevent the development of diabetes.

Gallstones

Diabetic patients seem to have an increased incidence of gallstones and other gallbladder problems, but these problems, much like fatty infiltration of the liver, are primarily related to the obesity associated with type 2 diabetes and not the diabetes itself. Obesity leads to secretion of bile (the fluid that goes into the gallbladder) by the liver that is oversaturated with cholesterol. This bile tends to form tiny cholesterol crystals in the gallbladder that eventually grow into gallstones. Gallstones are also common in the general population, with a 15% lifetime risk.

People without diabetes with gallstones have traditionally been advised to avoid surgery for gallstones (cholecystectomy) unless symptoms of gallbladder disease develop. Typical symptoms include intermittent right-upper abdominal pain, nausea, and jaundice (skin and eyes turn yellow). In the past, people with diabetes have been instructed to have surgery for gallstones whether or not they had symptoms because of a concern for an increased risk of complications, such as infection or rupture of the gallbladder. However, more recent experience with modern medical and surgical care would indicate that this is not the case. Thus people with diabetes and gallstones should be managed in a fashion similar to nondiabetics. Surgery is generally recommended only for those individuals whose gallstones are causing symptoms.

Gastrointestinal Side Effects of Medications Used to Treat Diabetes

Patients with diabetes are treated with a wide range of medications designed to control blood glucose and, although most are well tolerated, some may have significant GI side effects. Any discussion of the GI complications of diabetes would be incomplete without mentioning the potential side effects of some of these medications. Insulin itself is generally well tolerated and free of any significant GI side effects. This topic is also discussed earlier in the chapter on oral agents.

Sulfonylureas

Orinase (tolbutamide) and Diabinase (chlorpropamide), which are older sulfonylurea drugs, may be associated with nausea, vomiting, diarrhea, and loss of appetite, although this occurs in less than 5% of patients. Newer, second-generation sulfonylurea drugs, such as DiaBeta (glyburide), Micronase (glyburide), and Amaryl (glimepiride), are rarely associated with intestinal problems; nausea, diarrhea, and abdominal pain occur in less than 2% of patients.

Glucophage

Glucophage (metformin) may be associated with significant intestinal symptoms, such as diarrhea, loose stools, nausea, gas, and appetite suppression, in up to 20% of patients. These symptoms tend to occur shortly after the medication has been started and improve with time. Starting with a low dose of medication and slowly increasing it may minimize symptoms. Intestinal symptoms are rare in patients taking the medication long-term. Occasionally, a metallic taste in the mouth may occur.

Precose and Glyset

Precose (acarbose) and Glyset (miglitol) act to lower blood glucose levels by preventing the breakdown and absorption of dietary carbohydrates. GI side effects are common due to the malabsorption of carbohydrates and the presence of undigested sugars in the small intestine. These include gaseousness, diarrhea, and abdominal discomfort. Slow titration is important to reduce these side effects (see *Chapter 7*).

Incretins (Byetta, Bydureon, and Victoza)

Byetta, Bydureon, and Victoza are in a relatively new class of drugs for diabetes called incretins discussed in *Chapter 7*. They are impressive agents because they not only improve blood sugar levels but also lead to weight loss at the same time. They induce satiety, which is the feeling of being full or satisfied, so people lose significant amounts of weight. All of these agents can cause nausea when initiating therapy, which is why they are started at a lower dose, then titrated to a higher dose over time. Most of the time, the nausea is mild and goes away with time, usually in just a few days or weeks. Very rarely does someone need to stop the incretin because of severe nausea, but it can happen and at the current time is not possible to predict who will or will not get severe nausea.

Summary

So what can you do to help prevent the GI problems that may sometimes develop with diabetes? First and foremost, take care of yourself and use common sense. Tight control of your blood glucose will help prevent the complications of enteric neuropathy and worsening of your bowel function. Eat sensibly and follow a low-fat, high-fiber diet. Avoid overeating, weight gain, and obesity since these are independent risk factors for the development of some GI problems, especially gallstones and fatty liver. Obesity is a major contributing factor associated with type 2 diabetes and a low-fat, low-calorie diet along with exercise may lead to better blood glucose control and subsequently to a decreased incidence of long-term complications. Pay careful attention to your diet and try to avoid any food items that tend to precipitate symptoms. Fatty foods in particular may delay emptying of food from your stomach and will contribute to bloating, nausea, and vomiting in some individuals. Stress management is important as emotional factors will often affect GI motility and exacerbate intestinal problems. Remember, GI problems are extremely common both in the general population and in individuals with diabetes. Many of these problems are readily treated by primary care physicians, diabetologists, and gastroenterologists. Do not hesitate to discuss these problems with your physician, especially if the problems are persistent or are associated with other significant health-related conditions.

20

Caring for Your Teeth and Gums

An Imperative Task for People With Diabetes

by Mayssoun S. Khoury, DDS,
Cyndee R. Fena, RDH, MT,
and Steven V. Edelman, MD

Introduction

Diabetes is strongly associated with many inflammatory conditions. Among these is periodontal disease, which is considered the sixth major complication of diabetes. According to a previous Surgeon General report, "The mouth reflects general health and well-being." A dentist can readily detect undiagnosed diabetes in the presence of gum infection, abscessed teeth, and several dental cavities in a person who regularly practices good oral hygiene.

This chapter will clarify the way diabetes affects the gums and the teeth, the bidirectional relationship between diabetes and periodontal disease, discuss the additional oral problems associated with diabetes, and explain various effective measures that help prevent and treat such problems.

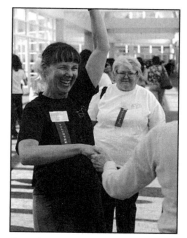

Cyndee Fena had an infectious enthusiasm for life and was our head volunteer at TCOYD. Unfortunately, she passed away from a severe hypoglycemic reaction in 2006.

How Can Diabetes Affect Gums and Teeth?

The mechanism by which diabetes affects the gums and the teeth is through the following changes:

- Change in the function of the immune cells: the white blood cells ability to fight infection is impaired.
- Changes in the saliva: high content of sugar in the saliva, and the reduced saliva flow rate.

These changes acting together contribute to the occurrence of periodontal disease.

What Is Periodontal Disease?

Periodontal disease is a painless process that damages the supporting structures of the tooth (gums, underlying bone, and ligament tissue that fasten the tooth to the jaw bone). It is estimated that over 80% of the adult population in the United States has periodontal disease during their life.

Periodontal disease causes more loss of teeth than tooth decay and is considered more serious because it is almost symptom-free until its destruction becomes severe. Once you have this condition, it is almost impossible to eradicate it with preventive procedures only. However, early detection and continued treatment can slow down the destructive process.

Periodontal disease is called plaque disease because plaque is the main reason for this condition to appear. What is plaque? Plaque is a thin coat or layer which comes from saliva and forms on the tooth surface and traps many bacteria. Fortunately, it can be removed by proper brushing and flossing.

When a person with poorly controlled diabetes does not brush or floss thoroughly, plaque starts to build up on the surface of teeth. With the help of nutrients from the high content of sugar in saliva and the host food, the bacteria begin to grow. In a few days, the plaque can turn into calculus (a hard substance that gathers under the gum line). As plaque continues to form over the calculus, the gums become red, sore, swollen, and bleed easily from brushing and flossing. This first stage of periodontal disease is called gingivitis. With gingivitis, there are often no pain signals to alert the person with diabetes. Gingivitis can be treated completely by effective oral hygiene procedures, but if left unchecked, it can become quite serious.

If gingivitis is neglected, periodontal disease progresses, the inflamed gums pull away from the surface of the crown and root of the tooth, forming a pocket where bacteria accumulate and destroy the ligament tissue and the bone; this is when periodontitis occurs. At the final stage, the supporting structures are eroded; the tooth becomes loose and is eventually lost.

Table 20-1 lists periodontal disease signs and symptoms of which you should be aware.

Bidirectional Relationship Between Diabetes and Periodontal Disease

Diabetes reduces the body's resistance to infection. This explains why periodontitis is a common problem in individuals with diabetes, especially among people with poorly controlled diabetes. Moreover, recent research implies that chronic periodontal disease may be a risk factor for developing diabetes by allowing bacteria to enter the bloodstream and activate the immune system. These active cells produce inflammatory signals that have destructive effects throughout the body, including the pancreas. Periodontitis can also complicate the management of blood glucose levels.

This bidirectional relationship requires treatment of two chronic diseases (diabetes and periodontitis). This critical task can be accomplished by increasing awareness on the part of people with diabetes (PWD), physicians, dentists, dental hygienists, and diabetes educators.

Table 20-1

Signs and Symptoms of Periodontal Disease

- Gums bleed from brushing and flossing
- Teeth look longer due to receding gum lines, and they become sensitive
- Bad breath or bad taste forms in the mouth caused by pocket formation
- Teeth become loose and separate
- The person's bite changes when teeth close against one another
- The fit of dental appliances may change (partial dentures)

Additional Oral Problems That Can Occur in People With Diabetes

In addition to periodontal diseases, there are other oral problems that can affect PWD, including the following:

- *Dry mouth (xerostomia)*: Many individuals with poorly controlled diabetes experience dry mouth as a result of salivary gland dysfunction or the dehydration effect of the diabetes process itself. It can also be a side effect of medications that are often prescribed for PWD (drugs used to treat high blood pressure, swelling of legs, neuropathy, and depression). Dry mouth predisposes patients to an increase of plaque accumulation (which enhances the development of dental cavities and periodontal diseases), decrease of taste sensation, difficulty in swallowing, and inflamed painful oral mucosa.

  The appropriate management for dry mouth caused by diabetes is to improve glucose control. **Table 20-2** outlines additional suggestions for dry mouth management.

- *Oral fungal infection (candidiasis)*: As a result of high blood glucose levels, the reduced saliva flow rate and the high content of sugar in saliva create an attractive environment for fungal infections, especially among those who wear dentures (due to improper cleaning of the dentures), those who smoke, and those who are often required to take antibiotics.

Oral fungal infection produces white patches in the mouth that may be sore or may turn into ulcers. Any oral ulcer that does not heal within 2 weeks should be seen and examined by a dentist.

The management of oral candidiasis requires good oral hygiene. This includes:
– Gently cleaning the involved tissue
– Applying topical antifungal agent
– Properly cleaning dentures
– Avoiding smoking
– Improving glucose control.

Table 20-2

Dry Mouth Management

- Visit the dentist at least twice a year, depending on tendency for plaque accumulation and the status of the peridontal tissue)
- Apply good oral hygiene care
- Use fluoride toothpaste
- Wash the mouth with antibacterial mouth rinse (alcohol-free)
- Use moisturizer on the lips regularly
- Drink a lot of water (avoid drinks containing caffeine)
- Avoid spicy, sugary, and salty food
- Use artificial saliva or saliva stimulants
- Chew sugar-free gum

- *Decrease of taste sensation*: a symptom often affecting individuals with diabetes, and may result from:
  – Change in salivary chemistry
  – Dry mouth
  – The presence of oral fungal infection.
- *Delay of wound healing*: individuals with poorly controlled diabetes do not heal quickly after oral surgery, because the blood flow to the treatment site can be slow. This problem can be eliminated by improving glucose control and applying good oral hygiene care.
- *Oral neuropathy*: although a rare complication of diabetes, is often manifested by numbness or burning sensation in the mouth or on the tongue and lips (similar to neuropathy in the feet). This condition is usually worse in individuals with poor diabetes control.
- *Halitosis (bad breath)*: another common condition in the general public as well as in PWD. Diabetes leads to several abnormalities that can cause the development of oral malodor, such as ketoacidosis (which produces a very distinct acetone fruity sweet odor) and dry mouth. Also, gingivitis and periodontitis are considered common causes of halitosis.

Identifying the cause of halitosis helps to develop the appropriate treatment plan. If the bad breath originates from poor diabetes control, then we should look first into improving the glucose control. If the bad breath originates from periodontal disease, then we should start treating this inflammatory condition by promoting improvement of oral hygiene and tongue brushing. **Table 20-3** lists the additional oral problems associated with diabetes.

How Can You Keep Your Teeth and Gums Healthy?

To keep their teeth and gums healthy, individuals with diabetes should follow the general guidelines listed in **Table 20-4** and discussed below:

- *Control blood glucose level.* Periodontitis is a common problem among people with poorly controlled diabetes because of the bidirectional relationship between diabetes and periodontal disease. The person with diabetes should be aware of the signs and symptoms of these two conditions and understand that neglecting oral health will eventually develop oral infection that might interfere with management of diabetes.

- *Avoid smoking (if you are a smoker).* Tobacco is one cause of periodontal disease. Smoking can be associated with gum recession, pocket formation, and the loss of bone and teeth. This explains why smoking cessation programs are essential for the successful treatment of periodontal disease.

- *Eat a well-balanced diet.* Nutrition is important for the maintenance of oral tissues, and the nutritional factor is related to preventing infection and enhancing wound healing.

Table 20-3

Additional Oral Problems Associated With Diabetes

- Dry mouth
- Oral fungal infection
- Decrease of taste sensation
- Delay of wound healing
- Oral neuropathy
- Halitosis

Table 20-4

General Guidelines to Keep the Teeth and Gums Healthy

- Control diabetes
- Avoid smoking
- Eat a well-balanced diet
- Apply good oral hygiene (effective brushing, flossing, and mouth rinsing; if you wear dentures, clean them properly)
- Visit your dentist at least twice a year for professional teeth cleaning, cavity control, monitoring, and possible periodontal treatment

- *Apply good oral hygiene.* Oral hygiene is considered the cornerstone of prevention. Since every mouth is different, your dentist needs to personalize an oral hygiene regimen for you. The general guidelines in basic oral hygiene are the following:
  - *Brush your teeth twice daily.* Brushing removes plaque and food particles from the sides of the teeth and stimulates the gums. It is advisable to use a soft or extra-soft toothbrush positioned at a 45-degree angle so it can scrape under the gums as you brush away from the gum line while applying gentle force. Once you finish brushing, you should brush your tongue gently to freshen your breath. Change your brush every 3 months. Soak your brush once a week in hydrogen peroxide or an antiseptic mouthwash to clean it of bacteria. Unless your dentist recommends a certain type of toothpaste, use whatever kind you enjoy, but it should contain fluoride. Many individuals prefer electric toothbrushes. Ask your hygienist about the proper way of brushing using a powered toothbrush.

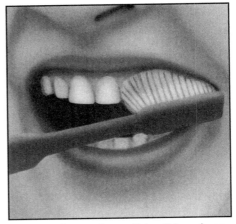

Use a soft to extra-soft toothbrush positioned at a 45-degree angle to your teeth when brushing.

  - *Floss at least once daily* (**Figure 20-1**). It has been shown that after teeth are brushed, 40% of the tooth is still unclean. Flossing finishes the job that brushing starts. It removes plaque and food particles from between the teeth and around the gums. The proper flossing method is as follows: Take an 18-inch piece of dental floss and be sure to move along the floss (or to a new place on the floss) for every new area you are cleaning so you are not transferring plaque and bacteria into other areas. Keep

Figure 20-1

Proper Flossing Technique

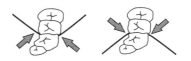

Wrap floss around half of the tooth, maneuvering the floss through the space while scraping the plaque off from the gums to the top of the tooth. Repeat for each tooth sharing a space.

your fingers close to the teeth, and gently maneuver the floss through the space between them. Wrap the floss around half of the tooth and scrape the plaque off from the gums toward the biting surfaces of the teeth. When choosing dental floss, you should always consider your specific oral condition. For example, ribbon floss can be used to clean around dental implants. For individuals who have periodontitis with deep pockets that dental floss may not be able to reach, it is advisable to use a WaterPik irrigation device in conjunction with tooth brushing.

- *Be careful with mouthwashes.* Some contain fluoride to protect the teeth from decay and some have an antibacterial effect to control gingivitis. Be careful with mouthwashes that have a high content of alcohol, since these can be hard on your gums (alcohol can sometimes make the gums blister and peel). Unless your dentist suggests a specific mouthwash or toothpaste, you should choose oral care products that display the American Dental Association's Seal of Acceptance. It is advisable to wash your mouth twice daily for 30 seconds each time.

- *Clean dentures properly (if you wear them).* Dirty dentures are sources of bacteria and fungi which may cause unpleasant odor and localized or systemic fungal infection. Patients are advised to take good care of their dentures and the soft underlying tissues, and to visit the dentist once a year to check the fit of the dentures and to detect and treat any oral problem.

• *Have your teeth cleaned regularly.* You should visit your dentist at least twice a year. The frequency of cleaning may increase 3 to 4 times a year if you are diagnosed with periodontal disease and your diabetes becomes out of control. If after periodontal probing your dentist finds that you have periodontal disease and gum treatment is necessary, consultation with your physician is desirable. You may need antibiotics before any future dental treatment because you are more susceptible to infection after cleaning, especially if your blood glucose

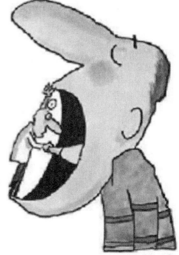

Visit your dentist at least twice a year.

level is not under control. Since your ability to fight off infections is compromised by high blood glucose levels, it is important to get your glucose level under control prior to any dental appointment. If your gum infection is severe, you may need to make a change in your insulin or medication dosage to better control your diabetes.

To decrease the risk of an episode of low blood glucose (hypoglycemia) in the dental office, appointments should be scheduled after meals, preferably in the morning. Depending on your type of diabetes, be cautious when scheduling an appointment during your lunch break or late in the day (before dinner) when your blood glucose level may become low, especially if your dental procedure interferes with eating. You should bring your own glucose meter to your appointment so that you can check yourself if needed. Avoid long appointments. If several procedures must be done to complete your dental work, spread them out over several visits. This is especially helpful in individuals with type 1 diabetes on a multiple-injection insulin regimen and who have had hypoglycemic episodes in the past. **Table 20-5** lists some important precautions to take when visiting the periodontist, dentist, or hygienist.

Table 20-5

Precautions to Take When Visiting the Dentist

- Make your appointment at an appropriate time, especially if you are on insulin therapy
- Bring your glucose meter to your appointment
- Get your blood glucose under adequate control prior to your dental appointment if possible
- Avoid long appointments, especially if you are on insulin therapy

Questions Your Dentist May Want to Ask You

Your dentist needs to be provided with important information about your diabetes at each appointment to avoid any potential problems:

- Do you take any oral medications and/or insulin to control your diabetes?
- How much, what kind, and how many times a day do you take oral diabetic drugs and/or insulin?
- When have you last eaten today? What was your last glycosylated hemoglobin (A1C) value, and when was it taken?
- What other medical conditions do you have?

Having this information available before your appointment will make it go faster and easier. Print it out on a sheet of paper to leave with your dentist to review and put in your chart.

Case Presentation

Steve Edelman is a 57-year-old man who has lived with type 1 diabetes for the past 42 years. He is a busy physician and was told by his dentist that he had periodontal disease. The dentist pushed a thin metal probe along his teeth next to his gums and measured how far the probe penetrated (the probe, when it penetrates deeply, indicates periodontal disease). Steve's blood glucose control was adequate (A1C 7.2%), although he did not floss regularly (usually only during the week preceding and just after his dental appointment!). Steve always seemed to become motivated after his appointment to floss regularly, but that lasted no more than 4 or 5 days. His usual time to floss was at bedtime and although he had good intentions, Steve was usually too tired and told himself he would do it the next night, which never happened. After extensive periodontal work, lots of time at the dental office, and a huge bill that was not covered by his dental plan, Steve decided to change his ways.

Steve finally learned how to brush his teeth correctly. He also flosses regularly after dinner instead of at bedtime. Steve keeps an extra toothbrush, mouthwash, and dental floss at work and in his car for those days that he feels really motivated. His breath has improved and his dentist noticed a marked improvement in his periodontal disease. He also has his teeth cleaned 3 times a year instead of twice a year.

Summary

As the Surgeon General's Report on Oral Health states, good oral health is integral to general health. The mouth reflects general health and well-being. Therefore, taking control of your teeth and gums is important. Like so many complications of diabetes, periodontal disease can creep up on you slowly until the condition is fairly severe. Preventive measures include regular proper brushing, rinsing, and especially flossing your teeth. It seems that the major challenge is to develop good dental habits that you can perform regularly on an ongoing basis and not just a few days before your scheduled dental appointment.

Q: What does the dentist of the year get?
A: A little plaque.

21

Taking Care of the Skin You're In

Dry Skin, Rashes, and Other Skin Disorders That Affect People With Diabetes

by Janet M. Trowbridge, MD, PhD

There are a number of skin conditions that affect people with diabetes. They have impressive polysyllabic names like necrobiosis lipoidica diabeticorum, diabetic dermopathy, and acanthosis nigricans, and are best diagnosed and treated by a dermatologist. **Table 21-1** lists some dermatologic conditions that affect people with diabetes.

This list is by no means comprehensive. Ironically, dermatologists sometimes get the first clue that diabetes might be affecting a person. That's because, ultimately, the skin is a canvas on which the body's inner workings are projected. The skin is an amazing organ.

In fact, your skin is your body's largest organ. It is a critical part of your body's immune system. Since uncontrolled diabetes can lead to poor immune function, the skin's myriad of functions can be impaired. So while you care for your heart and kidneys and lungs, you should also remember to take care of your packaging. Your skin is your first line of defense against a very harsh world.

Table 21-1

Some Skin Conditions Associated With Diabetes

- Xerosis (dry skin)
- Yeast and fungal infections (candidiasis/tinea)
- Acanthosis nigricans
- Necrobiosis lipoidica
- Eruptive xanthomas
- Scleredema diabeticorum
- Neuropathic ulcers
- Diabetic dermopathy
- Granuloma annulare

Think about it! Your skin has to protect you from extreme changes in temperature and humidity. Your skin is also front and center for mechanical trauma such as abrasions and burns. Finally, skin breaks are the portal by which a plethora of organisms can enter and cause a great deal of damage. The environment is full of bacteria, fungi, and viruses just waiting for the chance to break though the skin's barrier and set up shop. We call these "opportunistic infections." Many organisms, especially yeast and fungi, are plentiful in our environment and usually don't get the chance to cause much trouble. That's why wound prevention and especially foot wound prevention is so critical. As a dermatologist, I see a lot of feet, and a common complaint from patients with diabetes (as well as the general public) is toenail and foot fungus.

Toenail Fungus (Onychomycosis) and Athlete's Foot (Tinea Pedis)

The name says it all, almost, because in addition to fungal growth, we also see yeast and bacteria in this setting (**Figure 21-1** and **Figure 21-2**). The concept is that microtrauma creates a warm, moist inviting environment (think Miami!) for potential pathogens. Once fungi sets in, the nail becomes yellow, thickened, brittle, and difficult to cut. The skin on the foot and between the toes can become scaly, inflamed, and itchy, resulting in tissue breakdown. This is a set up for a wound. The best treatment is—you guessed it—prevention. Regular podiatric care is a must. Never, ever try to cut, file, or otherwise do battle with nail fungus. An easy means of prevention is keeping feet dry, wearing cotton socks, and keep toenails trimmed short.

Figure 21-1
Athlete's Foot (Tinea pedis)

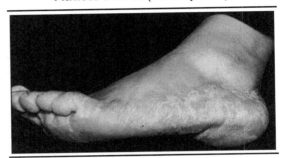

Figure 21-2
Toenail Fungus

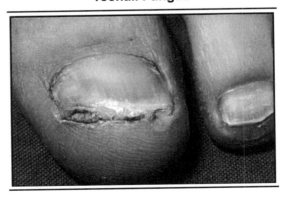

Treatment

An agent such as urea, which is available with a prescription (one brand is Carmol-40), is great for keeping the nail thin and pliable. It is also good to use in combination with topical antifungals if fungus gains a "foothold." I have people alternate the urea with an antifungal solution or cream. There is even a clear antifungal nail lacquer on the market.

This regimen is also great for scaly, itchy feet. We call it a "moccasin" distribution and it is incredibly common. You can alternate an antifungal cream such as Lamisil, which is available over the counter, with the urea. Despite what you see in television and magazines ads, oral antifungals are not a panacea for fungal infections. The cure rate is far from 100%! Because many of these agents have side effects like liver damage and because they can interact with other more critical medications, I try to avoid them.

Fungus and Yeast Elsewhere (Think Other Moist, Warm Regions)

The body has other warm, moist real estate too. And under the right circumstances, yeast and fungus will move in. What does fungus look like? Affected areas are usually round, red, and scaly. The outer borders look raised and are redder than the center that may even start to look like normal skin (**Figure 21-3**). It is often very itchy and tends to spread slowly over time.

Yeast, or candida, is pinkish and moist appearing. It favors what are called "intertriginous areas," basically areas where skin touches skin, such as the genitals, groins, armpits, and the skin under the breast (**Figure 21-4**) or belly. A telltale sign that an itchy area is yeast is the presence of little red pustules studding the edge of the affected area. Thrush refers to yeast in the mouth (**Figure 21-5**).

Figure 21-3

Fungal Infection on the Body (Tinea corporis)

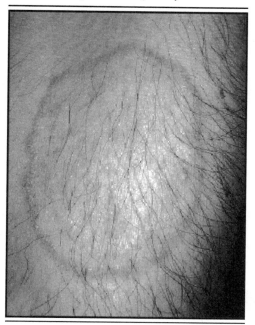

Bolognia JL, et al. *Dermatology.* New York, NY: Elsevier; 2003. *www.dermtext.com.*

Treatment

Prevention is the cornerstone. Keeping moist areas as dry as possible is the key. Patting dry and air-drying after bathing and using drying powders, such as Zeasorb or Zeasorb-AF (AF stands for antifungal), can help. Wearing cotton clothing is also helpful. As with all skin issues in a diabetic, you must be certain to seek out help if you suspect you have an infection because this might signal that your diabetes is poorly controlled. If so, you are poorly equipped to fight off yeast and fungus. An over-the-counter topical antifungal/antiyeast such as clotrimazole or ketoconazole is often sufficient. However, in some cases, a physician may prescribe an oral medication, such as fluconazole, itraconazole, or terbinafine.

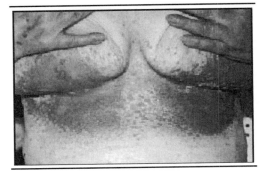

Figure 21-4
Inframammary candidiasis

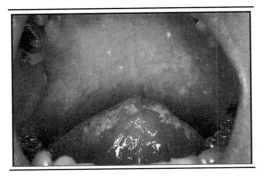

Figure 21-5
Thrush or Oral Yeast Infection

Acanthosis Nigricans

I mention earlier that sometimes dermatologists are the first to diagnose diabetes and this is one of the tip-offs. Brown color and a velvety textural change of skin around the face, neck, underarms, (**Figure 21-6**, *top*) and groin is most commonly found in association with diabetes and obesity. The elbows, knees, toes, and fingers (**Figure 21-6**, *bottom*) may also be affected. The changes can very subtle or extreme. I see this a lot in practice. It often precedes the other telltale signs of the disease. Why this happens is not entirely clear. The most common explanation holds that high levels of insulin lead to these skin changes.

Treatment

Weight loss is often a good way to stop and even reverse these skin changes Controlling diabetes might also help. However, there are no guaranteed fixes for this one. The use of keratolytics, such as urea and ammonium lactate, might decrease the thickness of the skin. Retinoids might also help. In general, this is mostly a cosmetic concern. So here I am saying it again: Prevention is the key. If diabetes runs in your family, be on the lookout for this one. I am seeing many, many children in the office these days as part of the epidemic of diabetes and obesity in kids.

Granuloma Annulare

Granuloma annulare (GA) is groups of brown to reddish bumps that are arranged in rings. It can appear anywhere on the body and may not have any associated symptoms. Lesions can resolve spontaneously and may even regress after being biopsied. The association of GA with diabetes is not absolute. Like acanthosis nigricans, GA can be a marker for diabetes. The condition can be localized to a single or few lesions or it may be generalized, that is, spread over a large area of the body such as the trunk.

Treatment

Localized GA is treated with potent topical steroids such as clobetasol for a limited period of time. We can also inject steroid directly into lesions in the hopes of stopping the inflammatory process that leads to its development. When GA is generalized or widespread, it can be tricky to control. A dermatologist will prescribe systemic medications aimed at aborting inflammation, such as prednisone or dapsone, or even antibiotics thought to exert anti-inflammatory effects.

Figure 21-6

Acanthosis Nigricans

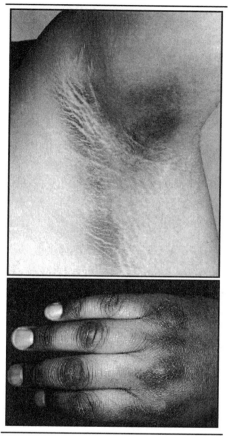

Diabetic Dermopathy or "Shin Spots"

Diabetic dermopathy refers to the brown to dull red, round, often indented spots on the shin that occur after minor trauma (**Figure 21-7**). Shin spots probably represent impaired skin barrier and repair functions discussed previously. Other than being unsightly, they are not dangerous. There is no treatment other than—you guessed it—not getting them in the first place. Long pants and compression stockings (if you suffer from poor circulation) can help, as can glucose control and being careful!

Necrobiosis Lipoidica Diabeticorum

Figure 21-7

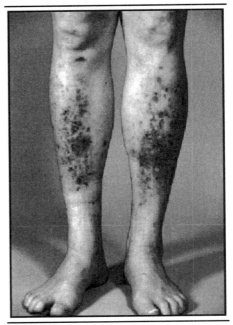

Diabetic Dermopathy (Shin Spots)

How's that for a name? Most dermatologists call this NLD because pronouncing it all at once can be difficult and it sounds rather serious. NLD refers to yellowish to orange areas on the shins or legs (**Figure 21-8**). They are firm to the touch and may be shiny and slightly depressed with raised borders. NLD is not usually painful or otherwise symptomatic. The skin appears thin and sometimes tiny blood vessels are visible. These areas are very fragile and may bleed and ulcerate under minimal trauma. In general, the lower leg heals poorly and these are particularly difficult to treat. A small proportion of chronic ulcers may progress to a type of skin cancer called squamous cell carcinoma. NLD is more three times more common in women than men.

Treatment

High-potency topical steroids such as clobetasol have been used successfully to treat early NLD. Injecting steroid directly into the area is also sometimes helpful. Topical retinoids have also been used. Oral medications such as aspirin, dipyridamole, and pentoxifylline are also worth a try. These treatments are based on the concept that NLD is caused by microvascular damage (like many of the other manifestations of diabetes), so making the blood thinner and blood elements such as platelets more slippery, better flow can be accomplished and perhaps healing can proceed. Once NLD has taken hold, it is imperative that the utmost care be taken to avoid injuring these highly fragile areas.

Eruptive Xanthomas

Xanthomas are cholesterol deposits in the skin. They often occur suddenly in crops and without warning. Red to yellowish papules can occur anywhere on the body (**Figure 21-9**). They may be itchy but commonly cause no symptoms other than shock at their sudden appearance. This is skin condition that leads dermatologists to diagnoses diabetes. A common scenario is for an apparently healthy person to walk into the office, present an elbow, hand, or buttock, and say, "This just popped up." Eruptive xanthomas are caused by uncontrolled glucose and lipids. They occur in people without diabetes too. Blood tests after fasting will reveal the culprit!

Treatment

Treatment includes bringing the glucose and most often triglycerides under control with diet and medication. Xanthomas will regress once this is accomplished usually leaving no scars unless the areas have been scratched or picked.

The Big Itch and How to Prevent and Tame It

The most common complaint of people with and without diabetes is itchy skin. A sudden increase in pruritus or itch may signal worsening liver or kidney function and should be brought to the immediate attention of your health care provider. Once an internal cause has been ruled out, managing the itch most commonly precipitated by dry skin is a stepwise approach.

The bad news is that itchy skin can be an annoying and chronic condition that left untreated can lead to damaged skin from constant itch-

Figure 21-8

Necrobiosis Lipoidica Diabeticorum

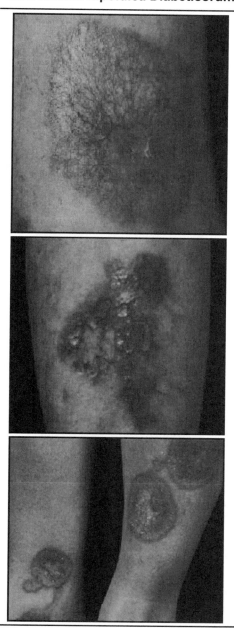

Figure 21-9
Eruptive Xanthomas

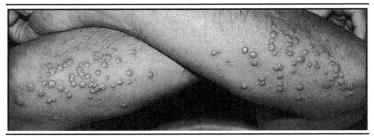

ing and rubbing. *And damaged skin leads to infection!* Also, the more you scratch, the more you will itch! There is something peculiarly satisfying about scratching an itch. That's because we have nerve endings in our skin that once stimulated by the scratch, send our brain a positive message. Resisting the urge to scratch can be very difficult.

The good news is there are a variety of simple strategies you can follow to "beat the itch."

1. Moisturize, Moisturize, Moisturize! Moisturize from within and without. Drink water. Use a humidifier. Apply a moisturizer daily. There are many, many moisturizers on the market. Pick one you will use. It need not be fragrant or fancy. Frost yourself! Some of my favorites are by Neutrogena, Cetaphil, CeraVe, and Eucerin, but I am always trying new brands. For tough spots such as feet and elbows, your doctor might prescribe compounds containing urea (see Carmol above-use 20% for skin) or lactic acid. AmLactin contains the latter agent and is available without a prescription. A great moisturizer is called Aquaphor. It is basically high-test Vaseline. Putting it on at night under your jammies is an easy way to grease up worry free at night. Crisco and olive oil work well too but are not recommended if you have pets.

2. Avoid hot showers, excessive sun, synthetic clothing, and powerfully chlorinated hot tubs and pools. Resist the urge to become pruny. It also helps to skip the post-bathing towel rub. Drip dry and grease up while there is still a little moisture on your skin. Soak, then grease!

3. Do not scratch. Scratching leads to skin damage and guess what? More itching. Put down the back scratcher and pick up the moisturizer. Products like Sarna and Eucerin Calming Cream can help soothe and relieve the itch. If prevention fails, your doctor can prescribe an antihistamine or other medications designed to treat the itch, especially if it is preventing you from getting rest.

Remember, it is important to keep in mind that intractable itching can be a sign of serious disease such as liver or kidney problems or even malignancies. So, if you have frosted, hydrated, and generally babied your skin barrier and the itching persists, seek the advice of a medical professional.

Summary

In closing, I'd like to remind you that many skin disorders are associated with diabetes but most are harmless. Most are preventable and many are reversible with good glucose control and careful skin care. In terms of cosmetic concerns, the field of laser and light dermatology is advancing fast, so we may be able to magically erase acanthosis and necrobiosis lipoidica in the near future.

Finally, please remember that your skin is your largest organ. Give it the care and attention you reserve for your finest garment and you will be rewarded with a strong, supple gorgeous wrapper.

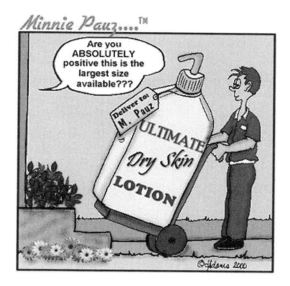

22

Obstructive Sleep Apnea

It Can Take Your Breath Away

by Aaron B. Morse, MD, FCCP

What's a Chapter on Sleep Apnea Doing in a Book About Diabetes?

Obstructive sleep apnea is a very common disorder affecting a large percentage of the population. Most people with sleep apnea snore and complain of daytime sleepiness and fatigue, but sleep apnea can do a lot more than make you feel lousy during the day. It can kill you.

Like diabetes, it is often seen in people who are overweight. It is common in diabetics, with several studies suggesting an incidence of 20% in type 2 diabetes. Also, like diabetes, it can contribute to a number of cardiovascular problems, so the combination of sleep apnea and diabetes is particularly dangerous. There is evidence that sleep apnea can make diabetes worse, and treating sleep apnea may, in some cases, improve diabetic control. When you finish reading this chapter, you will know everything you ever wanted to know about sleep apnea but didn't know what to ask, and you will be better able to take control of your health.

How Does Sleep Apnea Occur?

Basically, the soft tissues in the throat relax and block the throat when we breathe. This sets off a panic response in the brain resulting in unconscious arousals from sleep as well as repetitive drops in blood oxygen level. All of the problems that occur with sleep apnea come from these events, which can occur hundreds of times per night without any awareness on the part of the individual.

The process begins during inspiration when we actually suck the tongue and soft tissues into the throat. Snoring represents partial closure of the throat, where the soft tissues vibrate and make noise. Snoring, however, is not a disease, but a social problem. While it can produce sleep disorders in bed partners, it does not affect the person who snores. Many people who snore are completely unaware of it and may even deny it, though they chase others out of the room. The human throat, however, is a soft, floppy tube, which allows this obstruction to occur (**Figure 22-1**).

It turns out that humans are unique in the animal kingdom in being susceptible to sleep apnea, because we need this floppy tube to speak. Without it, we would be barking at each other. The downside is the risk for sleep apnea. (How about a bit of trivia: The only exception is the English Bulldog who, unfortunately, can get sleep apnea and still can't speak).

You will see that this simple event precipitates multiple physiologic, metabolic, and cardiovascular consequences. Sleep is supposed to be a time of quiet for the brain and the body. While the exact purpose of sleep is unknown, we do know that brain waves slow and become more regular. Pulse, blood pressure, respiratory rate, and metabolic rate also drop.

A sleep study on a person with sleep apnea demonstrates multiple changes happening at the same time: Airflow stops, oxygen level drops, heart rate speeds up, brain waves quicken, and the brain briefly awakens. Blood pressure can shoot up to high levels during apneas. This is like being strangled all night long... 30, 40, or 50 times per hour or more! For people with severe sleep apnea, breathing and sleeping become mutually exclu-

Figure 22-1

What Happens During Upper Airway Obstruction

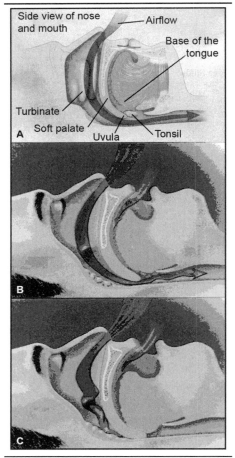

A) Side view of the normal human nasal, oral, and pharyngeal anatomy; B) Snoring results when air flow is partially blocked due to the tongue and soft tissues being sucked down into the throat; C) During sleep apnea, air flow is completely blocked by this soft tissue obstruction.

sive: You can't do both at the same time. Brief episodes of sleep are like swimming underwater, and arousals are like coming up for a few breaths before diving down to sleep without breathing again. Instead of resting, the brain is involved in an unconscious struggle to keep the throat open. In addition to drops in oxygen, these events are characterized by surges in panic hormones such as adrenalin. Trying to breathe against a closed throat can also produce large pressure swings in the chest that can affect the heart.

If you think this is pretty bad for the heart and blood vessels, you're right. We know that sleep apnea can contribute to the development of high blood pressure, stroke, heart arrhythmias, congestive heart failure, and heart attacks. Stress hormones can raise blood glucose, and sleep apnea is known to cause insulin resistance. There is evidence of increased blood coagulation, and it is possible that sleep apnea may also contribute to obesity.

Signs and Symptoms of Sleep Apnea

There are a number of signs and symptoms that can be present with sleep apnea. Some of the more common appear in **Table 22-1**.

Obesity

Obesity is one of the more important risk factors for sleep apnea. It turns out that fat is deposited in the throat as well as everywhere else, narrowing the throat and making collapse more likely. This being said, there are plenty of thin people with sleep apnea. This is most commonly seen in small-boned people (especially women) with fine facial features, overbites, or recessive chins, as shown in the photos (**Figure 22-2**).

In addition, sleep apnea may contribute to obesity, though this is less well established. People with sleep apnea are less active, resulting in decreased energy expenditure.

Snoring

Snoring is very common and is often described as loud or constant. Occasionally the bed partner notices the patient actually stop

Table 22-1

Symptoms of Obstructive Sleep Apnea

- Obesity (17-inch neck in males, 16-inch in females)
- Snoring—often heavy and/or witnessed apneas
- Gasping and choking during sleep
- Excessive daytime sleepiness
- Restless sleep
- Irritability
- Depression
- Memory loss
- Lack of concentration
- Morning headache
- Nocturia (nighttime urinating)
- Sexual dysfunction
- Esophageal reflux (heartburn)

breathing or gasping during sleep. While snoring is considered one of the major features, it is often not reported because the spouse sleeps through it. We frequently see patients who deny snoring and when studied in the sleep laboratory, shake the walls!

Excessive Daytime Sleepiness

Excessive daytime sleepiness and/or fatigue is often what causes you to seek medical attention. Interestingly, men more commonly describe sleepiness and women complain of fatigue. This may be why the diagnosis is missed more often in women. A common complaint is waking up unrefreshed even after a seemingly good night's sleep. These symptoms are often attributed by the person (or even the doctor) to other medical problems (such as diabetes), stress, depression, etc. I commonly hear "It's just because I'm getting older." We occasionally see patients who have had extensive evaluations for uncommon conditions, including brain scans, extensive blood testing, and multiple other evaluations before the common problem of sleep apnea is even considered. While there are a number of causes of sleepiness and fatigue, sleep apnea is often last on the list of possible diagnoses.

To make things even more complicated, people often underestimate their level of sleepiness, because the symptom develops so

Figure 22-2

Upper Airway Anatomy in a Thin Woman With Sleep Apnea

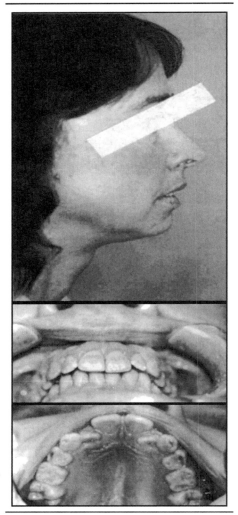

Anatomic abnormalities in a woman with symptoms of sleep-disordered breathing. This woman had a respiratory disturbance index of less than 5 and daytime tiredness. Note her slim neck *(top)*, overbite *(center)*, and high ogival hard palate *(bottom)*.

Annals of Internal Medicine, April, 1995.

slowly that they get used to a certain level of daytime dysfunction. We assume that everybody is as sleepy in the morning as we are. I recently saw a university professor with high blood pressure and snoring who was dragged in by his wife. When he denied sleepiness, his wife pointed out that he falls asleep in a chair whenever he sits down. He had 47 apneas per hour, which is very abnormal.

Restless Sleep

Patients often complain of restless sleep. (What would you do if you were being strangled all night long?) This may be noted only by the bed partner or the bed being torn up in the morning. With treatment, sleep is calmer and quieter. I have occasionally heard of a patient's bed partner panicking because they were afraid the person had died—the snoring and thrashing in bed were gone.

Nocturia

Nocturia (getting up frequently to urinate) is common in sleep apnea and is also often attributed to other things such as prostate problems or diabetes. It turns out that the large pressure swings that occur in the chest can fool the heart into thinking that the body has too much fluid. It then produces a substance that increases urine production (for those who care, it's called atrial natriuretic peptide). Esophageal reflux (heartburn) can occur due to these pressure changes, which can cause stomach acid to be sucked up into the chest.

Other Symptoms of Obstructive Sleep Apnea

Other symptoms that are common are due to the sleep fragmentation induced by the frequent nocturnal arousals. These include irritability, depression, memory loss, lack of concentration, and sexual dysfunction. There is also recent evidence that sleep apnea may contribute to the development of Alzheimer's disease.

Let's not forget auto accidents! People with sleep apnea are three to seven times more likely to be involved in a traffic accident, and the likelihood of a fatality occurring in a "fall asleep" accident is very high. Performance in driving simulators (which measure driving mistakes) is comparable in people with sleep apnea to those who are legally intoxicated.

How Common is Sleep Apnea?

The most conservative estimates for the prevalence of sleep apnea are 2% of middle-aged women and 4% of middle-aged men. The Institute of Medicine (part of the National Academy of Science) reported much higher rates of this disease: 9% of the general population, 34% of the healthy elderly, 27% of patient with high blood pressure, and 55% of patient with coronary artery disease. In fact, in one report, 30% of all patients presenting to a general cardiology clinic at the Mayo Clinic had sleep apnea. With the obesity epidemic, these numbers are probably much higher.

Sleep apnea also occurs in children. This is usually due to enlarged tonsils, however, with the increase in obesity in children, sleep apnea looks much like it does in adults.

How Do I Know if I Have Sleep Apnea?

The most important part of making the diagnosis is thinking of it. Because sleep apnea is so common and is responsible for many health problems, a brief sleep history during a doctor's visit is as important as taking blood pressure. Even though awareness of this condition is increasing among doctors, a routine sleep history is still not very common and 75% to 85% of people with this disorder go undiagnosed and untreated. This is particularly discouraging because treatment is so effective.

Sleep apnea should be suspected in anyone with unexplained sleepiness and fatigue, especially if there is a history of snoring. Because 80% of people with high blood pressure that is difficult to control have sleep apnea, this is an important clue. Most high blood pressure is "essential," which means no underlying treatable cause is identified. Among underlying treatable causes, sleep apnea is the most common. It is also present in a high percentage of individuals with congestive heart failure, and treatment of sleep apnea can dramatically improve heart function. Obesity is a very significant risk factor but is not necessary, and a number of nonobese patients have sleep apnea because of their facial structure (for example, recessive chin).

Because sleep apnea increases the risk of complications of surgery, anesthesiologists developed a very simple screen tool to identify patients who might be at risk for sleep apnea: the STOP questionnaire (**Figure 22-3**).

All this means is that you may have to advocate for yourself (or your bed partner) if you suspect sleep apnea. You need to tell your doctor what your symptoms are and why you think you may have this condition. Don't let anybody dismiss chronic sleepiness and fatigue as getting older or working too hard, especially if there are other signs present.

Figure 22-3
STOP Sleep Apnea: Screening Questionnaire

Obstructive sleep apnea is a common disorder that causes sleepiness and fatigue and can increase your risk for high blood pressure, heart attack, stroke, diabetes, and premature death. The purpose of this questionnaire is to assess your risk for this very common condition.

1. *Snoring*—Do you snore loudly (louder than talking or loud enough to be heard through closed doors)?   ☐ Yes   ☐ No

2. *Tired*—Do you often feel tired, fatigued, or sleepy during the daytime?
                                                                    ☐ Yes   ☐ No

3. *Observed apneas*—Has anyone observed you stop breathing during your sleep?   ☐ Yes   ☐ No

4. *Blood pressure* (high blood pressure = hypertension)—Do you have or are you being treated for high blood pressure?   ☐ Yes   ☐ No

If you have answered "Yes" to two or more questions, there is a high probability you have obstructive sleep apnea.

Name: _____   Date: _____

If the diagnosis is suspected, a sleep study should be performed. The gold standard for the diagnosis is a sleep study performed overnight in a sleep laboratory (known as polysomnography). Many sleep labs have become more like hotel rooms than hospital rooms. A number of physiologic parameters are monitored during sleep, including airflow, oxygen level, and respiratory effort, to determine if apneas are really occurring. Brain waves are measured to assess the quality of sleep and detect arousals induced by apneas. Heart rate and body position, among other things, are also measured.

Because this condition is so common, however, there is a great need for simpler approaches so that more people can be evaluated and effectively treated. Home monitors are becoming more accurate and sophisticated and are being used more commonly. They generally measure almost the same things as the in-lab studies, usually without brain waves. They are most appropriate when the likelihood of moderate to severe sleep apnea is high.

Like any test in medicine, however, the level of expertise and involvement of physicians interpreting the study is most important and may be more relevant than the type of test being performed. A physician knowledgeable in sleep disorders should be involved with the care and the interpretation of your sleep study at some level. The importance of close follow-up in the physician's office cannot be overemphasized.

How Is Sleep Apnea Treated?

Making the diagnosis is just the beginning. Losing weight, avoiding alcohol and sedatives, stopping smoking, and avoiding sleeping on your back are general recommendations for alleviating sleep apnea. Improving nasal congestion may help with people who have mild sleep apnea.

The most widely used treatment is continuous positive airway pressure or CPAP. With CPAP, a mask is worn usually on the nose and is attached to a small air compressor which blows air through the nose and uses pressure to keep the airway from being sucked closed during inspiration (**Figure 22-4**). CPAP is almost 100% effective, has no significant side effects, and is relatively inexpensive (a CPAP machine costs about as much as 3 months of medication for a moderate asthmatic). There are very few treatments in medicine that have all those attributes! In addition, people with symptoms of sleepiness and fatigue often experience dramatic and immediate improvement after CPAP is started. There is evidence that CPAP also is effective at reducing or eliminating most of the cardiovascular risks, may improve control of diabetes, and reduces or eliminates the increased risk of premature death associated with sleep apnea (**Table 22-2**).

The greatest challenge in the treatment of sleep apnea with CPAP is compliance—that is, actually using the device, and there has been a great deal of progress in this area. Improvements in technology have dramatically improved the comfort and convenience of CPAP ma-

Figure 22-4

Examples of CPAP Air Compressors

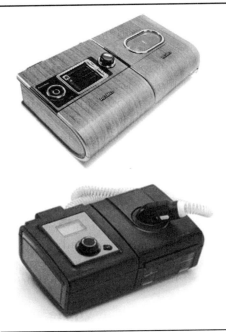

Abbreviation: CPAP, continuous positive airway pressure.

Air pressure applied through the nose by the CPAP prevents the throat from being sucked closed during inspiration.

Table 22-2

Use of CPAP Shown Effective in Improvement of Many Health Issues Associated With Sleep Apnea

Consequences of Sleep Apnea	Effect of CPAP
Daytime sleepiness and fatigue	Improved
High Blood Pressure	Improved
Enlarged Heart	Improved
Congestive heart failure	Improved
Cardiovascular mortality	Improved
Insulin resistance	Improved
Depression	Improved
Increased risk of auto accidents	Improved
Increased health care costs	Improved
Increased risk of stroke	Improved

Abbreviation: CPAP, continuous positive airway pressure.

chines and masks. Because a number of annoyances may occur that can interfere with CPAP comfort, close follow-up by a sleep professional is critical, and most of these issues can be corrected.

The first CPAP machines were vacuum cleaners turned backwards, and earlier commercial models were big, bulky, and noisy. Today, the most commonly used CPAP machines are virtually noiseless, can weigh as little as 3 pounds, and almost fit in the palm of your hand.

There is a large variety of CPAP masks available. Some fit around the nose, some fit in the nostrils, and some can include the nose and mouth for people who are mouth breathers. Selection of the most appropriate mask is purely personal, must be individualized, and greatly increases the likelihood of success (**Figure 22-5**).

The sleep-medicine community is beginning to "wake up" (sorry about the pun) to the realization that sleep apnea should be treated like a chronic disease, similar to high blood pressure, diabetes, or asthma. A number of studies have demonstrated long-term compliance rates are better with close follow-up and individual attention. In our center, we try to review the physiology, clinical implications, cardiovascular risks, epidemiology, and treatment options with every patient. In addition to follow-up visits with the doctor, we involve a nurse practitioner, respiratory therapist, and sleep technologist in an extensive compliance follow-

Figure 22-5

Examples of CPAP Masks

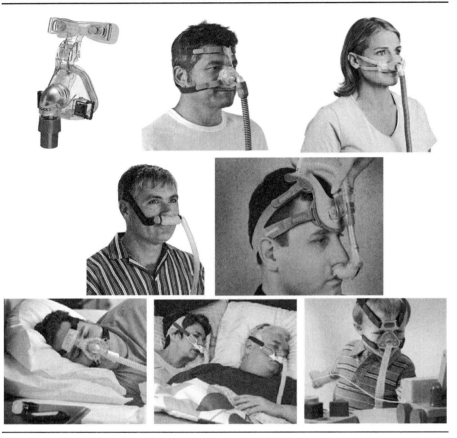

Abbreviation: CPAP, continuous positive airway pressure.

up program. Hopefully, more sleep laboratories that currently focus mostly on testing will evolve into sleep centers that provide comprehensive care for patients with sleep apnea and other sleep disorders.

Because CPAP is so effective, and because close follow-up and some trial and error may be necessary to make CPAP comfortable, no one with sleep apnea should give up on CPAP until this has occurred. That being said, there are a significant number of sleep apnea patients who, even after intensive effort and high motivation, cannot adjust to CPAP. For these individuals a number of alternative approaches exist.

The most commonly accepted nonsurgical approach to treating sleep apnea is a dental mandibular advancement device. This looks somewhat like the mouth guard worn by football players and works by pulling the jaw and tongue forward, providing more room in the back of the throat and decreasing the likelihood of obstruction by the tongue (**Figure 22-6**). It is custom-fitted by a dentist. The device is generally well tolerated with only occasionally minor side effects. The success rate is 30% to 60% and it is most effective for mild to moderate sleep apnea in non-obese patients.

Figure 22-6

Mandibular Advancement Device

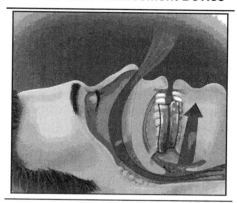

The mandibular advancement device advances the jaw forward, pulling the tongue out of the path of airflow.

Recently, a novel approach to the treatment of sleep apnea has become available which is effective in about half of patient with mild-to-moderate obstructive sleep apnea and somewhat less in those with severe obstructive sleep apnea. These small adhesive pads placed over the nostrils use the patient's own breathing pressure to help keep the airway open (**Figure 22-7**).

A number of surgical approaches exist with varying success rates. One of the more commonly done surgeries, uvulopalatopharyngoplasty (that's a long one!) or UPPP, involves trimming of the uvula, part of the soft palate, tonsils, and other loose tissues in the throat (**Figure 22-8**). The success rate is 40% to 60% and is limited when there is obstruction at the base of the tongue, which is not improved by this procedure. More extensive procedures that involve jaw surgery are sometimes used such as mandibular osteotomy and bimaxillary advancement or some combination of these procedures, which can produce success rates greater than 90%. Before CPAP was available, the only definitive "cure" for sleep apnea was tracheotomy, which may still be appropriate for some patients. Tracheotomy is a permanent hole in the throat that allows air to completely bypass the obstruction. Now, doesn't CPAP sound easier?

There is a great deal of ongoing research to find additional medical and surgical alternatives to CPAP. An implanted pacemaker that activates the tongue muscle to open the airway with each breath is currently in clinical trials.

Figure 22-7
Provent Therapy

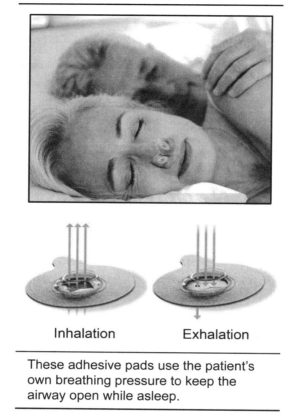

Inhalation   Exhalation

These adhesive pads use the patient's own breathing pressure to keep the airway open while asleep.

Figure 22-8
Uvulopalatopharyngoplasty (Removal of Uvula)

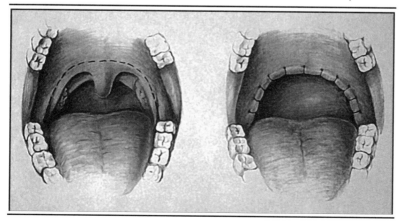

The Bottom Line

There are a number of take-home lessons for you to remember from this chapter:

- Sleep apnea is a common disorder and causes sleepiness, fatigue, and cognitive decline.
- Sleep apnea is a contributing factor in a number of medical and cardiac problems, including high blood pressure, heart attacks, stroke, congestive heart failure, diabetes, and premature death.
- People with sleep apnea have a high incidence of motor vehicle crashes.
- Sleep apnea is associated with high societal and health care costs.
- In the United States, 75% to 85% of sleep apnea cases that could benefit from treatment remain undiagnosed.
- Treatment of sleep apnea reduces or eliminates virtually all clinical consequences.
- CPAP is the treatment of choice and is nearly 100% effective; however, alternatives exist for patients who cannot tolerate CPAP.
- Sleep apnea needs to be treated as a chronic disease with close follow-up after diagnosis.
- A brief sleep history should be as much a part of a doctor's visit as a blood pressure check.

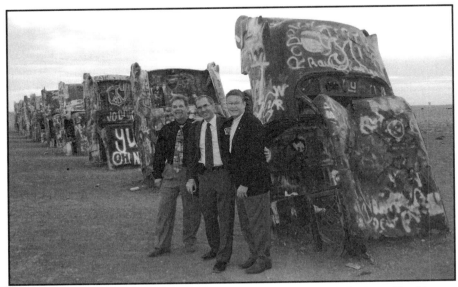

Drs. Ian Blumer, Joe Nelson, and myself at Cadillac Ranch in Amarillo, Texas.

23

Sexual Medicine

Management of the Sexual Health Concerns of Women and Men With Diabetes

By Irwin Goldstein, MD, Rose Hartzell, PhD, EdS, Deborah Cohen, PT, MS, CSCS, COMT, WCS, Catherine Gagnon, CNP, and Sue W. Goldstein, BA, CCRC, IF

Introduction

Women and men with diabetes do not have to accept concomitant sexual health problems. Just as they seek care for their diabetes, they have a right to seek help for their sexual dysfunction if they so choose. All people have a right to sexual health. Too often people with chronic diseases become so identified with the disease that they ignore other parts of their lives. The main purpose of this chapter is to review contemporary knowledge regarding biopsychosocial strategies for women and men with diabetes to improve bothersome or distressing sexual dysfunctions and enhance their quality of life. Often women and men with diabetes are embarrassed and unable to ask for help, and their health care providers do not inquire about sexual problems. It is quite common that the diabetic health care provider is not specifically trained in sexual health management and is uncomfortable providing medical care to such patients. The first principle is to be empowered, to try and get professional biopsychosocial help, even if it requires seeking multiple health care providers until you find the one to help you recover sexual health. The educated patient is the empowered patient.

Persistent and recurrent, distressing and bothersome sexual health changes are common in women, men, and couples afflicted with diabetes mellitus. Studies estimate that up to 50% of diabetic women and men will experience sexual health problems. Diabetes may adversely affect sexual health at all ages, in young and old, and in both genders. In addition, if sexual dysfunction occurs in one member of the couple, this will likely adversely affect the sexual function of the partner even though he or she may not have diabetes.

There are multiple causes of sexual health problems in women and men with diabetes mellitus. Diabetes may adversely influence various psychosocial aspects, including mood, anxiety, depression, panic, stressors, religious, and cultural concerns, and relationship health problems. Biologic aspects include adverse changes in hormones, nerves, and blood vessel function. Other concerns include concomitant health concerns, especially bladder dysfunction, recurrent urinary tract infections, kidney function, heart disease, obesity, and the presence of hypertension, hypercholesterolemia, and/or history of cigarette smoking. Bicycling activities in women and men may contribute to sexual dysfunction. Concomitant prescribed medications (such as antidepressants and antihypertensive agents) and/or concomitant recreational drugs (such as alcohol and mind-altering agents) are usually deleterious to sexual function. In women, conditions such as perimenopause, menopause, pregnancy, polycystic ovary syndrome, endometriosis, recurrent vaginal yeast, treatments for infertility, and hormonal-based contraception can adversely influence sexual function.

There are a gamut of sexual health concerns that diabetes can adversely affect. For women with diabetes, problems may develop in areas of desire, arousal, orgasm, or pain. Sexual desire may decrease, including reduced interest and diminished thoughts and fantasies. Sexual arousal problems include decreased lubrication, reduced engorgement, and absent genital pulsing and throbbing. Orgasms may become reduced in intensity, require increased time and effort to achieve orgasm, or muted with decreased satisfaction by self-simulation or with a partner. Finally, sexual pain may occur, including provoked pain or discomfort with initial penetration, deep thrusting or certain positions, or generalized genital pain occurring in nonsexual situations.

For men with diabetes, complaints of low sexual desire may develop. Reduced sexual arousal may manifest primarily as erectile dysfunction and include issues with decreased erectile spontaneity, diminished erectile rigidity, and poor erectile sustaining capability. Anatomic changes in the penile erection may present in men with diabetes, including shortening and curvatures in various angles and directions that may preclude partner penetration. The erection may also be painful and very distracting. Diabetic men may also have ejaculatory disorders (such as premature ejaculation) that occur without their control or delayed or absent orgasms despite what was once adequate sexual stimulation. Ejaculation may also be retrograde, emptying into the bladder rather than propelling out the urethra. Orgasm dysfunction may manifest as limited intensity, reduced or absent pleasure, or inability to even achieve release of the sexual tension.

For women and men with sexual health problems from any underlying biopsychosocial problem, there are specialized health care providers who focus on the study, diagnosis, and treatment of men and women with sexual health concerns. These health care providers practice in the field of Sexual Medicine. There are dedicated Sexual Medicine journals and Sexual Medicine societies that promote research, education, and patient care in the field. Please check out the following information to identify Sexual Medicine health care providers in your area: International Society for the Study of Women's Sexual Health (*http://www.isswsh.org*) and The Institute of Sexual Medicine (*www.sexualmed.org*). The American Association of Sexuality Educators Counselors and Therapists (AASECT) can be a helpful resource in finding a qualified sex therapist.

Sexual Health Concerns in Women With Diabetes
Low Sexual Interest, Diminished Arousal, and/or Orgasmic Dysfunction

A psychosocial evaluation should be performed with a sex therapist to assess for cultural, religious, and background issues, as well as relationship issues that may be affecting sexual function. A sex therapist can address any of the above psychosocial concerns affecting a couple's sexual function and/or help the woman and her partner adapt to the sexual changes brought on by her diabetes. In addition, a therapist can help the woman to process through how her new diabetes diagnosis has affected her feelings regarding herself and her sexual self-image. Through work with a sex therapist, the couple can learn to communicate regarding what new strategies may need to be implemented in and outside the bedroom in order to adjust to the woman's altered sexual functioning due to the disease or outside factors. For some women, the difficulties with arousal may be helped through the use of a lubricant during sex, and orgasm difficulties can be lessened with the use of a vibrator and/or arousal cream along with any biologic strategies needed.

Hormonal evaluation for diabetic women with low sexual interest, diminished sexual arousal, and/or orgasmic dysfunction should include an assessment of the unbound or free form of testosterone. Testosterone is a forgotten sex steroid hormone in all women but in particular in women with diabetes. Testosterone is as important to overall health, including sexual desire, arousal, and orgasm health, as is estrogen and progesterone. Testosterone is synthesized in the ovary and in the adrenal gland, and aging and chronic medical conditions such as diabetes are associated with reduced testosterone synthesis.

In the blood stream, 98% of testosterone is bound to various proteins, especially sex hormone binding globulin (SHBG). The unbound or free form of testosterone is the biologically active form of testosterone that eventually enters tissues and initiates critical protein synthesis that builds muscles and bones, increases sexual drive, and improves energy and mood. Testosterone that is bound to proteins in the blood (such as SHBG) is not biologically available and instead is in storage form. Conditions associated with increased synthesis of SHBG, such as liver or thyroid disease, and use of medications (such as hormonal-based contraceptives or oral estrogen treatment for menopause) are associated with reduced biologically available testosterone or a condition known as testosterone deficiency syndrome.

Blood tests can be used to measure unbound or free testosterone and determine if the value is below the range associated with healthy sexual function. Women normally have approximately 10% of the testosterone value of men. The condition of testosterone deficiency syndrome includes abnormally low blood tests and the presence of clinical symptoms of fatigue, tiredness, weight gain, depressive mood changes, falling asleep after meals, inability to exercise or perform sports at the same strength level as previously, reduced muscle strength, low sexual interest, diminished sexual arousal, and/or orgasmic dysfunction.

Treatment of testosterone deficiency syndrome involves administration of biologically-identical testosterone hormone thereby raising the testosterone value. A biologically-identical hormone is a hormone that is the exact chemical structure of the testosterone normally synthesized in the body. There are currently no FDA-approved testosterone hormone treatments for women; all current testosterone treatments are "off-label." A common strategy is to use FDA-approved biologically identical testosterone treatments for men at the reduced dose of 10% per day for women. Choices for treatment include daily application of a transdermal gel, weekly intramuscular injections, or administration of a subcutaneous pellet every 4 to 6 months. Frequent blood tests can establish that the selected testosterone hormone strategy has elevated the woman's hormone level into the appropriate range. Improvement of clinical symptoms is typically seen after 6 to 12 weeks of testosterone-hormone treatment. Side effects are usually mild and may include acne, hair loss on the scalp, and facial hair growth. These side effects can be easily treated.

Hormone treatment may also include administration of estradiol and/or progesterone in women in menopause for traditional distressing and bothersome menopausal symptoms of low estrogen, especially night sweats, hot flashes, memory loss, mood swings, insomnia, low sexual interest, poor sexual arousal, vaginal dryness, pain during intercourse, and reduced orgasmic satisfaction.

Concerning estrogen, blood tests can be used to measure estradiol, the major estrogen in the blood stream. Clinically symptomatic low estradiol states in menopause are associated with low estradiol blood values. Treatment of estradiol deficiency syndrome involves administration of biologically-identical estradiol hormone thereby raising the estradiol value. There are numerous FDA-approved estradiol hormone treatments for women. Choices include daily application of a transdermal gel or oral tablet or weekly or bi-weekly administration of a patch. Oral tablets are the least preferred as this treatment is associated with increased risk of blood clots and elevation of the SHBG that acts to lower free or unbound testosterone (*discussed above*). Several intravaginal treatments can successfully treat menopausal symptoms of estradiol deficiency and raise the estradiol blood test. Frequent estradiol blood tests can establish that the selected estradiol hormone strategy has elevated the woman's estradiol hormone level into the appropriate range. Improvement of clinical symptoms is typically seen after several weeks of estradiol hormone treatment. Side effects may include breast tenderness, weight gain, and uterine bleeding. Blood clots are extremely rare with estradiol administered by transdermal delivery.

Breast cancer risk has been overly exaggerated by the now decade-old "Women's Health Initiative" study. The reality is that new research studies have shown that the benefits of hormone-replacement therapy outweigh the risks for women who start hormone therapy at or near the beginning of their menopause, as opposed to starting hormone treatment on average 12 years after starting menopause. Women who start hormone-replacement therapy before age 60 or within 10 years of menopause appear to be different from women who start hormone-replacement therapy on average 12 years after menopause. Starting estradiol-hormone treatment at the beginning of menopause reduces risks of heart disease and bone fractures. Hormone therapy in the early postmenopausal woman is more beneficial than widely used drugs like statins or aspirin. Putting the hormone treatment risk of breast cancer in perspective, it should be noted that being overweight and drinking two alcoholic drinks per day increases the risk of breast cancer as much as using estrogen plus progestin in women who started hormone therapy on average 12 years postmenopause. It should also be noted that women who took estrogen alone had a lower risk of breast cancer.

Concerning progesterone, this hormone has anti-estrogen properties. Women who are taking estradiol and have an intact uterus are usually prescribed progesterone to help prevent thickening of the uterine lining that may lead to unwanted uterine bleeding and/or uterine cancer, known effects of estrogen treatment without concomitant progesterone. Progesterone also has sexual benefits, especially with partner bonding. Treatment of low progesterone involves administration of biologically-identical progesterone hormone thereby raising the progesterone value. There are FDA-approved progesterone-hormone treatments for women. Choices include an oral tablet or intravaginal suppository insert. Side effects may include breast tenderness, weight gain, and uterine bleeding.

Blood tests can also measure progesterone, a hormone that is estrogen in the blood stream, and determine if the value is below the range associated with healthy sexual function.

Sexual Health Concerns in Men With Diabetes
Erectile Dysfunction

Erectile dysfunction is a consistent inability to have an erection firm enough for sexual intercourse. The condition includes the total inability to have an erection and the inability to sustain an erection.

Estimates of the prevalence of erectile dysfunction in men with diabetes vary widely, ranging from 20% to 75%. Men who have diabetes are 2 to 3 times more likely to have erectile dysfunction than men who do not have diabetes. Among men with erectile dysfunction, those with diabetes may experience the problem as much as 10 to 15 years earlier than men without diabetes. Research suggests that erectile dysfunction may be an early marker of diabetes, particularly in men ages 45 and younger.

In addition to diabetes, other major causes of erectile dysfunction include high blood pressure, kidney disease, alcohol abuse, and blood vessel disease. Erectile dysfunction may also occur because of the side effects of medications, psychological factors, smoking, and hormonal deficiencies.

Men who experience erectile dysfunction should consider talking with a health care provider. The health care provider may ask about the patient's medical history, the type and frequency of sexual problems, medications, smoking and drinking habits, and other health conditions. A physical exam and laboratory tests may help pinpoint causes of sexual problems. The health care provider will check blood glucose control and hormone levels and may ask the patient to do a test at home that checks for erections that occur during sleep. The health care provider may also ask whether the patient is depressed or has recently experienced upsetting changes in his life.

Treatments for erectile dysfunction caused by nerve damage, also called neuropathy, vary widely and range from oral pills, a vacuum pump, pellets placed in the urethra, and shots directly into the penis, to surgery. All of these methods have advantages and disadvantages. Surgery to implant a device to aid in erection or to repair arteries is usually used as a treatment after all others fail.

Psychological counseling to reduce performance anxiety or address other issues may be necessary. Since erectile function is often deeply entrenched in most men's feelings of masculinity and sexual virility, the psychological impact of having erectile dysfunction can be difficult on a man and his relationship. It may be beneficial for a couple to consider attending sex therapy when a man is or has been struggling with erectile dysfunction. A sex therapist can help the couple to incorporate any of the biological strategies used to treat the erectile difficulties into the couples sexual script and can help the couple to vocalize and address any of the concerns they may have regarding their new altered sexual relationship with each other (which may now include taking a pill or injection in order to have sex).

Retrograde Ejaculation

Retrograde ejaculation is a condition in which part or all of a man's semen goes into the bladder instead of out the tip of the penis during ejaculation. Retrograde ejaculation occurs when internal muscles, called sphincters, do not function normally. A sphincter automatically opens or closes a passage in the body. With retrograde ejaculation, semen enters the bladder, mixes with urine, and leaves the body during urination without harming the bladder. A man experiencing retrograde ejaculation may notice that little semen is discharged during ejaculation or may become aware of the condition if fertility problems arise. Analysis of a urine sample after ejaculation will reveal the presence of semen.

Poor blood glucose control and the resulting nerve damage can cause retrograde ejaculation. Other causes include prostate surgery and some medications.

Retrograde ejaculation caused by diabetes or surgery may be helped with a medication that strengthens the muscle tone of the sphincter in the bladder. A urologist experienced in infertility treatments may assist with techniques to promote fertility, such as collecting sperm from the urine and then using the sperm for artificial insemination.

Delayed Ejaculation

As mentioned above, in addition to difficulties with ejaculation, men with diabetes may also struggle with delayed ejaculation in which it can become difficult to orgasm. A sex therapist may be able to help the couple overcome this concern. It can be beneficial for a couple to discuss what new strategies may be needed in order to increase the ability to orgasm. It may be necessary for the couple to incorporate stimulating the prostate with the use of a vibrator or finger or increasing sexual communication/novelty into the bedroom, including the use of fantasy. Couples can also learn to have "pleasure" vs "goal-oriented" sex in which they can discover the sensual satisfaction in exploring their bodies/connecting without always having the ultimate goal of orgasm.

Conclusion

Although diabetes can negatively impact both men and women's sexual functioning, it can also provide as the impetus for an individual/couple to further explore/communicate regarding their sexual wants/needs/desires. Through working with a qualified Sexual Medicine physician/ sex therapist, a diabetes sufferer can take control of their sex life and continue to have satisfying sexual encounters.

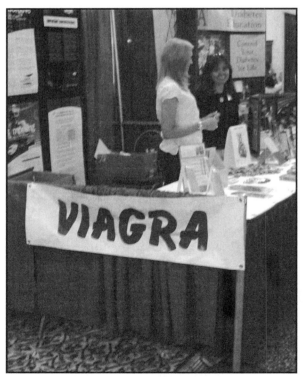

One of the more popular booths in the healthfair.

24

Diabetes in the Bedroom

A Frank Discussion About Diabetes-Related Sexual Complications

by Janis Roszler, MSFT, RD, CDE, LD/N

Introduction

Diabetes, regardless of the type, follows you wherever you go... even into the bedroom! If you think your diabetes has negatively affected your intimate life, you are not alone. About half of all men and women with diabetes develop some form of sexual complications. Men with diabetes may develop a variety of issues including erectile dysfunction (ED), low testosterone, premature ejaculation, and decreased sex drive. Women with diabetes may also experience sexual problems, such as decreased libido, slowed arousal, vaginal dryness, painful intercourse, frequent urinary tract infections, and orgasm difficulties. Both men and women can also have emotional challenges that negatively impact their interest in sexual activity. Let's face it... living with diabetes can be stressful! Unfortunately, few people get an opportunity to chat about sexual issues with their health care providers. So, let's open the discussion now!

Men's Issues
Erectile Dysfunction

If you are unable to achieve or maintain an erection that is firm enough to have sexual intercourse, you have erectile dysfunction (ED). A once-in-a-blue-moon occurrence is nothing to worry about—that is totally normal. But if it becomes an ongoing problem, it is time to seek help. Men with diabetes are three times more likely to develop ED than those who don't have diabetes. If you have trouble in this area, there are many effective treatment options you can try: oral medications, constriction rings, vacuum pumps, penile suppositories, penile injections, penile implants, and counseling. You might even enjoy Tantric Sex, which focuses more on creating sexually-charged moments than on achieving an orgasm. If you have type 2 diabetes, you can also try the Mediterranean Diet, which may reduce your risk of developing ED. Read on, to learn more about all of these great options.

Blood Glucose Control

The better your blood sugar control, the less likely you are to develop ED. If you already have this problem, improved glucose control may really help your performance. Work with your health care team to adjust your diabetes care plan. You may need to increase or change your medication, alter your meal plan, increase your level of physical activity, check your blood sugar more often, and lower your stress level. If you take multiple insulin injections, try an insulin pump. When used properly, it can dramatically improve your control.

Pills

You've probably seen those commercials on television for Viagra, Levitra, and Cialis, which make everything look *so* wonderful. He pops the pill, she swoons, and they walk away, arm-in-arm, into the sunset. The real story is far less idyllic as these pills only work for 50% to 60% of men with diabetes.

I once counseled a patient who tried Viagra several times without any success. Unfortunately, his doctor never asked for an update and he was too shy to complain. That was 10 years ago. During our session, he admitted that he hadn't been intimate with his wife since then. He just accepted the notion that diabetes was going to steal the joy from his life and he was destined to live without sex. The good news is that a different option worked for him and he and his wife resumed their intimate relationship.

If you try one of these pills, follow the timing directions carefully, and take it on an empty stomach, as fat-containing foods make it harder for the medication to enter your system. Most of these pills should not be used if you take any form of nitroglycerin. Side effects include mild flushing, headache, and dizziness. If you notice any change in your vision, contact your doctor. If you already tried them and had no success, don't give up. You have many other options.

Constriction Rings and Vacuum Pumps

A constriction ring is for men who can achieve an erection but have difficulty keeping it. Think of a balloon. When you blow it up, the air will only stay inside if you pinch or tie the end. The constriction ring puts pressure on the base of the penis, so it holds the blood inside. Constriction rings are inexpensive and easy to use. Just don't leave one in place for longer than 30 minutes. While wearing a constriction ring, your penis may be a little wobbly at the base, appear a bit bluish in color, and feel cool to the touch.

Like Austin Powers? If you are a fan, you probably recall that he often carried a penile vacuum pump. The pump is an amazingly effective tool. It creates a vacuum that draws blood into the penis then uses a constriction ring to hold the blood in place. Vacuum pumps range in price, style, and design. Some are manual and others are battery operated. They work extremely well but take some practice to master. Many pumps come with video instructions. Rather than hiding your vacuum pump, introduce it into your foreplay and share the experience with your partner. You can buy a pump without a prescription, but a doctor-ordered pump may be covered by insurance.

Penile Suppositories and Injections

Penile suppositories and injections relax the blood vessels and muscles in the penis so blood can flow into the area more easily. Suppositories are 30% to 50% effective and last between 30 minutes to 1 hour. Penile injections are 70% to 90% effective. They create strong erections that also last between 30 minutes to 1 hour. Be sure to set time aside to learn how to use these options correctly. Do not inject more than three times per week. Suppositories and injected medications both require refrigeration.

Implants

This is another option that is sometimes done when all else fails. Few men, however, find implants to be the best choice for their lifestyle. Men with diabetes also have an increased risk of surgical complications. If you choose this option, be sure to participate in all education and counseling that is available.

There are two main types of implants. One is made up of semi-rigid cylinders that are surgically inserted into the body. They keep the penis in a semi-rigid state that can be difficult to conceal. Most men and their partners find this type of implant highly satisfying. Another implant is made of inflatable cylinders that are attached to a small reservoir/pump that is inserted into the scrotum. When a man wants an erection, he manually squeezes the pump, which sends fluid into the penis and creates the erection.

Penile Sleeves

If you are unable to use any of the options above, yet still wish to engage in sexual intercourse, a penile sleeve is a terrific choice. It is a disposable, rigid sleeve that is worn directly over the penis to hold it in a stiff position. Whether the penis becomes erect or remains flaccid, the sleeve enables a man to actively participate in sexual intercourse. You can purchase penile sleeves without a prescription.

Mediterranean Diet

A group of Italian researchers surveyed more than 600 men with type 2 diabetes who followed the heart-healthy Mediterranean Diet. Those who followed the diet carefully significantly lowered their risk of developing ED. To learn more about this meal planning approach, read the *Mediterranean Diet* section in the discussion of women's sexual complications that follows.

Stop Smoking

If you smoke, cut back or quit altogether. Many men find that their ED improves dramatically after they stop smoking. A great reason to quit!

Low Testosterone

If you have type 2 diabetes, you have twice the risk of having a low testosterone level. A low level can cause the following symptoms:

- Decrease or loss of sex drive
- Difficulty maintaining an erection
- Body changes, specifically increased fat and less muscle mass
- Depressed mood
- Increased irritability
- Lack of energy

If you have any of the symptoms mentioned above, take the quiz in **Figure 24-1**.

Low T Treatments

If your testosterone level is low, don't worry. It's extremely easy to treat with a topical gel, patch, dissolving oral tablets, or even bi-weekly or monthly injections. Once your level returns to normal, you may see a significant improvement in many of the areas listed in **Figure 24-1**.

Premature Ejaculation

Men with diabetes have a higher risk of developing premature ejaculation, which means that they ejaculate before or at the very start of intercourse. For a long time, this issue was thought to be caused by

Figure 24-1
Do You Have Low Testosterone?

1. Do you have a decrease in libido (sex drive)?	☐ Yes	☐ No
2. Do you have a lack of energy?	☐ Yes	☐ No
3. Do you have a decrease in strength and/or endurance?	☐ Yes	☐ No
4. Have you lost height?	☐ Yes	☐ No
5. Have you noticed a decrease in your enjoyment of life?	☐ Yes	☐ No
6. Are you sad and/or grumpy?	☐ Yes	☐ No
7. Are your erections less strong?	☐ Yes	☐ No
8. Have you noticed a recent deterioration in your ability to play sports?	☐ Yes	☐ No
9. Are you falling asleep after dinner?	☐ Yes	☐ No
10. Has there been a recent deterioration in your work performance?	☐ Yes	☐ No

Scoring: _____

If you answered "yes" to questions 1 or 7 or to at least three of the other questions, you may have low testosterone and should see your doctor.

http://www.isitlowT.com.

emotional issues alone. We now know that there may be a physical component as well, especially if nerves in the pelvic area have become damaged.

No medication is currently approved to treat premature ejaculation, but some men find that taking Viagra or another ED pill helps reduce their performance anxiety and enables them to hold their erection longer. Another option is to meet with a qualified sex therapist who can help you run through a series of start and stop erection exercises to help you improve your performance.

Kegel Exercises... for Men

To help improve your ejaculatory control, try the male version of Kegel exercises. Here's how:

1. While you urinate, try to stop or slow down the flow of urine. The muscles you squeeze are the ones you want to tone.

2. Squeeze those muscles for 2 or 3 seconds then release slowly as you count to five. Some men find it easier to contract these muscles when they lay down.
3. Gradually build up to squeezing for a total of 5 seconds.
4. Repeat this exercise 10 times, three times a day.

Herbs

If you are tempted to try an herbal preparation to treat your sexual issues, be careful. Few, if any herbal products have demonstrated real help for ED. If you have a friend who swears by a certain item, it may work for him because of the "placebo effect." That is improvement that happens because a person believes a product really works, when it may have little or no effect at all. There are some herbs on the market that may help, but others may be unsafe for you. Also, many just cost a lot and offer little in return. If you wish to try an herbal product, follow these steps:

• Before you try an herbal product, discuss it with your health care provider to see if it appropriate and safe for you. Always let your doctor know about the herbal preparations you take. Some may affect your health in unexpected ways. Others must be stopped prior to surgery because they may create healing or bleeding problems.
• Only take one herbal preparation at a time and watch for negative side effects.
• Check your blood glucose level often as some herbs may affect your glucose control or alter how your body absorbs your current diabetes medication.
• If you experience any difficulties, stop using the herb immediately.
• Try to purchase herbal preparations that have been evaluated by the United States Pharmacopeia (USP). If a label states that the contents are USP-verified, the ingredients listed on the label can be found in the product. For a list of USP-verified products, visit *www .usp.org.*

Women's Issues

Men joke about how they don't understand women. Unfortunately, when it comes to diabetes-related sexual complications, scientists also struggle to understand how women function. Many women with diabetes complain of having sexual complications, but experts don't fully understand why they occur. Most experts initially believed that poor glucose control and diabetes complications caused sexual problems to develop in women. Not a bad guess as they play a huge role in male sexual dysfunction issues. But women are different. Glucose control plays a big role in the development of urinary tract infections, but other issues are not so obvious. Diabetes complications, such as neuropathy (nerve) and cardiovascular (heart) issues can indirectly cause sexual problems in women, but women with diabetes who don't have these issues can develop sexual complications as well.

Many women with diabetes complain of having a decreased sexual interest, slowed arousal rate, vaginal dryness, painful intercourse, frequent urinary tract infections, and orgasm challenges. Women with diabetes experience the following three things with greater frequency:

- Urinary tract infections
- Vaginal dryness
- Painful intercourse.

Urinary Tract Infections

Women with diabetes have a higher risk of developing urinary tract infections. The symptoms include vaginal itching, pain during urination, pain or burning during intercourse, irritated skin in the vaginal area, and a white, cottage cheese–like vaginal discharge. Symptoms of bladder infections include an increased urge to urinate, unpleasantly-scented urine, pain under the ribcage, and a heavy feeling in the lower abdomen.

To help prevent these issues, try the following:

- Maintain your blood sugar level in your personal target range. If your level is poorly controlled, bacteria can grow quickly.
- Empty your bladder often and urinate right after intercourse.
- Don't wear tight fitting clothes that prevent air circulation.
- Drink plenty of water and artificially sweetened or unsweetened cranberry juice.
- Wear cotton underwear.
- Keep your vaginal area perfume-free. Stay away from perfumed toilet paper, scented tampons, and other scented feminine cleansing products.
- Don't douche. Douching negatively affects your body's natural cleansing process.
- Add healthy bacteria to your diet. Good sources include yogurt with lactobacillus and acidophilus milk.
- Wipe from front to back after using the bathroom facilities to keep harmful bacteria from entering the vaginal area.

Pain and Vaginal Dryness

There are many reasons why you may have vaginal dryness or feel uncomfortable during intercourse. Here are a few:

- You don't produce enough lubrication.
- You need additional time to become aroused.
- You had pain in the past and the memory makes you tense up.
- You feel less attractive because you gained weight from your diabetes medication.
- You are embarrassed about injection bruises or insulin pump infusion set marks on your body.
- You don't feel confident about your choice of birth control and don't want an unplanned pregnancy.
- The relationship you have with your partner is stressed.

Treatment Options

Lubricants

Women with diabetes experience vaginal dryness twice as often as other women. Fortunately, you can purchase many great over-the-counter vaginal lubricants in pharmacies, grocery stores, and online. If the dry area is located inside, in an area that is hard to reach, you may find it helpful to apply the lubricant with a specially-designed, soft foam applicator.

Kegel Exercises

Kegel exercises strengthen the pelvic floor muscles that support your bladder, uterus, urethra, and rectum. When toned, these muscles help improve your sexual response and can reduce any urine leakage you may have as you age. To do Kegel exercises, first identify the muscles you want to tone. Next time you urinate, stop the flow of urine a few times. The squeezing sensation you feel is what you want to duplicate when you do your Kegels. Here are three ways to do them:

- *Option 1*: Squeeze and hold your pelvic floor muscles for 3 seconds. Release for 3 seconds. Repeat this activity six times. As you feel more comfortable, slowly build up to doing this exercise 12 times each day.
- *Option 2*: Squeeze and hold your pelvic floor muscles for 1 second then release for 1 second. Repeat 20 times. Do this version three times each day.
- *Option 3*: Squeeze and hold your pelvic floor muscles for 10 seconds. Repeat this five times. Do this version three times each day.

Since no one can see you do them, feel free to do your Kegels any-time—while standing in line at the grocery store, while seated in a waiting room, etc. They are healthy and easy to do!

Engage Your Imagination

The popularity of the book, *50 Shades of Grey*, was no accident. Many women found that book highly erotic. A woman's sexiest organ is her mind, so use yours to turn up the heat in your bedroom. Invite your partner to watch films with you that contain sensual moments such as *Titanic* or *Body Heat*. Or watch them alone. If you find erotic pictures, stories, or videos sexually exciting, add them to your bedroom fun. Be creative and relax. Intimacy should be focused on communication and fun.

Time

Men are like microwaves and women are like slow-cookers. Each becomes sexually aroused at a different pace. Add diabetes to the mix and you may become aroused even more slowly. Keep that in mind when you plan a romantic evening. Don't rush. Spend time with your partner and take it slow.

For Both Men and Women
Focus on Your Relationship

To enhance your connection, take time to do things with your partner outside of the bedroom. Go for a bike ride, walk after dinner, or see a movie. Build up the part of your relationship that is not physical. I encourage couples to set aside a date night each week. If your evenings don't work for you, do something together at another time of the day. Another great option is to attend a PAIRS seminar together. PAIRS is an interactive program that teaches enhanced communication techniques that can enrich your relationship. For additional information, visit PAIRS.com. If your relationship is stressed and troubled, don't hesitate to meet with a qualified marriage and family therapist who can help you heal and get back on track.

Counseling

We generally think of women as having a strong mind/body relationship when it comes to sexual activity, but men have emotions that can affect their ability to perform sexually as well. Whether you are male or female, if you are nervous about your sexual performance, unhappy with your relationship, or feel stressed out about your diabetes, physical appearance, or other issues, discuss these feelings with a trained mental health professional. As a marriage and family therapist, I have personally seen how effective counseling can be for individuals as well as couples. It is a very worthwhile option.

Tantric Sex

Rumor has it that Sting and Trudie Skyler dabble in it. Jane Fonda says she tried it and wants to learn more. It is an approach to sex that focuses on sensuous connection, not on orgasm. This form of sexual activity offers a lot to an intimate relationship, especially if your ability to achieve an orgasm has changed. Here is an example of a very basic Tantric activity:

1. Wear something that makes you feel sexy (or no clothes at all).
2. Sit, cross-legged and face your partner.
3. Place your hands on your knees. Turn your palms up.
4. Gaze into each other's eyes and breathe softly and deeply. Try to breathe at the same pace.
5. Practice this activity until you can maintain eye contact and breathe in sync for 10 minutes. Once that happens, you are ready to move onto additional activities.

Tantric Sex's enhanced level of intimacy is highly erotic. If you are interested, there are numerous books, CDs, and classes available.

Mediterranean Diet

Recent research showed that men and women with type 2 diabetes may be able to reduce their risk of sexual complications if they follow the guidelines of the Mediterranean Diet. In one study, women with diabetes who followed this style of eating increased their feelings of sexual satisfaction. In addition to the heart-healthy benefits this meal-planning approach offers, research now shows that the Mediterranean Diet helps slow down the development of Alzheimer's, supports bone health, and reduces the risk of some cancers.

The Mediterranean Diet Pyramid (**Figure 24-2**) encourages you to eat certain foods, but doesn't designate portion sizes, so you can use it with your current diabetes meal plan. It encourages the intake of vegetables, legumes, nuts, fish, water, good quality olive oil (extra virgin is best), yogurt, and low-fat cheese, and limits other animal products. If you are accustomed to drinking wine, you can add a moderate amount to your week, with meals, along with daily physical activity and socializing.

Figure 24-2

Mediterranean Diet Pyrdamid: A Lifestyle for Today
Guidelines for Adult Population

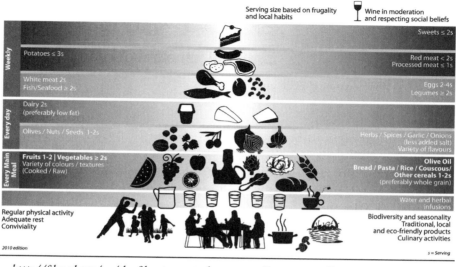

http://fdmed.org/en/the-fdm-presents-the-new-mediterranean-diet-pyramid/.

Conclusion

If your sex life has taken a downturn since diabetes entered your bedroom, don't give up! Take time to ask your health care provider about different treatment options or try some of the options highlighted in this chapter. For additional information, pick up a copy of *Sex and Diabetes: For Him and For Her*, by Roszler and Rice (ADA). It is a fun and helpful book that is filled with expert advice, personal stories, and even contains diabetes friendly recipes that use aphrodisiac ingredients. Another great source of info is the new intimacy section at dlife.com. It contains videos, advice, helpful columns, and links to products you can purchase that can help improve your intimate life. You can even send questions to me via that webpage or contact me at dearjanis.com. I look forward to hearing from you!

25

Dr. Edelman's Corner

Important Issues in Diabetes With a Twist

This chapter consists of the top 10 *Dr. Edelman's Corner* columns that have appeared in our award-winning newsletter (*MyTCOYD*, *www.tcoyd.org*). The different articles are an eclectic collection of important issues in the field of diabetes, as well as some offbeat thoughts that I have had regarding medical education, food, home glucose monitoring, getting activated, prevention, and other topics. One of my favorites is listed first and is titled *Diabetes Is Just Another Raindrop.* Hope you enjoy them and, please, visit our website for more "Taking Control" messages and information.

Diabetes Is Just Another Raindrop
Volume 26, Third Quarter 2008

Since my early years in medical school in 1978 until now, I have observed, spoken with, read about, and treated thousands of people with a wide variety of conditions. Some of these folks had medical diagnoses that were easy to treat, such as hypothyroidism, however, others were very serious and often fatal, such as cancer.

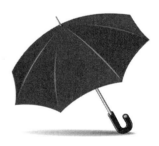

It all seemed so random to me, because I would see hardened criminals who were convicted murderers and rapists escorted to my hospital for routine medical care with absolutely no medical problems and, on the other hand, I have cared for sweet innocent kids who came down with leukemia that, most of the time, eventually took their short lives. After trying to make sense of it all for years, I've come to a realization in my own mind. Getting hit with a disease happens by chance—kind of like a raindrop falling on your head.

In this mindset, being afflicted with a medical condition is like walking in the rain, and each raindrop has a certain disease that you can get if it lands on you. The majority of the raindrops have not-so-serious conditions, however, some of them have illnesses such as diabetes, high blood pressure, abnormal cholesterol levels. Some raindrops carry no problems inside at all, while others hold malignant conditions. The longer you live, the higher the chance you can be tagged by a raindrop containing a serious illness. One would not be exempt from getting multiple problems even if you already have diabetes, which never seems fair to me. Your chances are the same of being affected by any particular raindrop no matter where you live, how much money is in your bank account, what religion you practice, or if you are a good or bad person.

Some conditions can be prevented or the seriousness mitigated by our behavior, like a protective umbrella in a rainstorm. For those of us living with diabetes already, our umbrellas can shield us from other conditions. Our umbrellas consist of achieving and maintaining good blood glucose levels, as well as blood pressure and cholesterol control. A healthy life with regular exercise and good eating habits, is something many of us would not practice if we did not get hit by the diabetes raindrop.

We cannot change the raindrops that have fallen on us, however we can get under the protective umbrella of education, motivation, and self advocacy. Being knowledgeable about your condition is essential for living a long and healthy life, both physically and mentally. Taking Control Of Your Diabetes strives to provide the umbrella of information and inspiration you need to deal with the raindrop that has fallen on your head.

Every Day Should Be World Diabetes Day
Volume 23, Fourth Quarter 2007

November 14th was World Diabetes Day. The theme of the campaign this year was to highlight children and adolescents living with diabetes. There were grand celebrations in major cities around the globe including New York, Sidney, and Tokyo. 246 monuments worldwide, such as the Coit Tower in San Francisco, were lit up to commemorate this day of diabetes epidemic recognition. The United Nations recognized World Diabetes Day for the first time since the International Diabetes Federation established it in 1991. Dignitaries, politicians, and diabetes professionals made speeches to highlight the growing and staggering diabetes epidemic—one of the most important health concerns facing millions of people around the globe. Many diabetes organizations brought attention to this day with email blasts, form letters, media alerts, and requests for donations. Their representatives showed up at events to bring attention to the cause. What a day it was! Yep… 24 hours of incredible festivities.

There are over 245 million people living with diabetes worldwide, and it is estimated that by the year 2027 there will be over 380 million. It is estimated that 200 children a day are diagnosed with type 1 diabetes and over 4000 children and adults are diagnosed with type 2 diabetes each day in the United States. Type 2 diabetes, formerly called "adult onset diabetes" is growing at alarming rates in children and adolescents. In the United States, it is estimated that type 2 diabetes represents between 8% and 45% of new-onset diabetes cases in children, depending on geographic location, and an increasing trend is seen around the world. For example, over a 20-year period, type

> *"There are over 245 million people living with diabetes worldwide and it is estimated that by the year 2027 there will be over 380 million."*

2 diabetes has doubled in children in Japan, so that it is now more common than type 1. In addition, the prevalence in children of native and aboriginal decent in North America and Australia is growing at an alarming rate never before observed.

In addition to the human suffering, the effects of which cannot be estimated, we will spend hundreds of billions of dollars caring for these afflicted people. And don't forget the men, women, and children of developing countries suffering every day from the acute and chronic complications of diabetes. These unfortunate individuals suffer from malnutrition, infections, blindness, amputations, and kidney failure—and cannot even get the basics of care, such as oral medications or insulin. Some advances, such as newer insulins, insulin pumps, and pens, Byetta, home and continuous glucose monitoring are totally out of reach. The difficult lives of these folks are the same every day throughout the year, including November 14th (World Diabetes Day).

The main issue for me is this: What happens on November 15th and thereafter until the next volley of extravaganzas that will occur on World Diabetes Day in 2008? Every health care organization focusing on diabetes, including TCOYD, needs to work together everyday of the year with the common goal of wiping out the devastating effects of diabetes in those afflicted with this increasingly common and deadly chronic condition. We have so many tools to help successfully control type 1 and type 2 diabetes, yet access to these new medications and devices, in addition to knowledgeable caregivers, is severely limited for the vast majority of people living with diabetes on this planet. Increased public and government awareness, ongoing meaningful patient and professional education, access to the basic oral pills, insulin, and glucose testing devices, advocacy and emotional support are all part of a long list of what is needed to make a dent in the amount of human suffering caused by diabetes worldwide. World Diabetes Day is important to re-ignite awareness of diabetes to the public as well as to governmental agencies and the private health care sector. However, it is also important that we do not ever lose sight of the fact that this disease is with every person affected by it every minute of every day, year after year. All of us at TCOYD feel that every day should be World Diabetes Day!

Redefining the Diabetes Doctor Visit
Volume 30, Third Quarter 2009

When it comes to diabetes care in this country, healthcare reform is urgently needed to more effectively and efficiently prevent, diagnose, and successfully treat this increasingly common chronic condition. Careful evaluation of what works and what doesn't work will be needed to properly address the burden of diabetes that currently affects the lives of 23 million Americans, in addition to another 50-60 million individuals with "pre" diabetes.

Of all the different aspects of diabetes care that we need to improve, re-defining the diabetes doctor visit has the potential to allow those precious few minutes in the exam room to make a significant impact on clinical care and overall satisfaction for people with diabetes (PWD) and healthcare providers.

In medical school, we are taught the art and science of performing a history and physical (H&P) exam. The format is fairly rigid, methodically marching through a series of questions and maneuvers in chronological order. It starts off with the history of present illness (HPI), which is a summary of the patient's main problems, going through each one in terms of what has changed since the last visit and the current status. Next is the past medical history (PMH), which requires a listing of all current and past medical and surgical conditions, including medications, allergies, smoking and drinking habits, social situation, and much more. Then there is the review of systems (ROS) in which questions are asked about every organ system in the body from head to toe. You may be asked if you have been having any headaches, chest pain, shortness of breath, skin rashes, stomach problems, etc. All of this is followed by a detailed physical exam (PE) which, if completed in a thorough manner, can take quite some time. The laboratory results are reviewed next and then there is the grand finale, the assessment and plan (A&P) for each individual problem. This last section is a mini-summary of the entire H&P and includes all of the medication adjustments to be made as well as tests and consults that will be needed either immediately or before the next visit. Oh yeah... don't forget that new prescriptions and refills may be needed. I hope you are beginning to see the picture I am painting for you. All of this in a typical doctor visit?

When it comes to dealing with a person living with diabetes, our formal evaluation process is quite ineffective, inefficient and cumbersome, wasting a lot of precious time. Part of the problem is that most health care professionals spend less than 2% of their training learning about diabetes management and do not know what questions to ask or how to ask them. In addition, insurance companies may not pay the provider for services unless there is documentation in the chart that all of the perfunctory items in a typical H&P have been addressed and completed, even if they do not pertain to the most crucial aspects of diabetes care! Lastly, the time allotted for an appointment is too short and should be adjusted upward for a diabetes appointment.

We need to individualize the diabetes visit and prioritize the most important issues in order to address the emotional, physical, and medical barriers limiting successful diabetes management. I believe the patient's questions and concerns should be addressed first and not left to the last few seconds as the doctor hurries off to the next exam room. Listening, instead of asking a series of standard non-diabetes–related questions, is the best way to start an evaluation. The bulk of the available time needs to be spent on what is limiting the PWD from achieving an A1C value below 7%, including reviewing home or continuous glucose monitoring results, addressing dietary struggles and any difficulty maintaining a regular exercise program, as well as achieving appropriate blood pressure and cholesterol levels. I want my patients to walk me through a typical day in their lives in order to get a grasp of what could be the main limiting factors in getting to goal. The sensitive issues of depression, erectile dysfunction, and other psychosocial problems must be discussed openly and as often as needed. If appropriate, the significant other, or "type 3", should be there to listen, learn, and ask questions that relate to their loved one living with diabetes. Diabetes cannot be treated in a vacuum because there are so many other important external influences.

The traditional ways professionals are trained to take care of PWD will not change overnight. As an individual living with diabetes, it is your responsibility to help direct and focus your diabetes doctor visit so that you feel your most pressing problems and concerns have been addressed. On the other hand, you must be careful not to overpower or turn off your caregiver with a barrage of demands and a list of questions that is 10 feet long. There must be a balance between getting what you truly need and still allowing for what your trained professional needs to accomplish during a typical health care encounter. Let's all work patiently and persistently together to redefine the diabetes doctor visit.

Your Own Personal Laboratory in the Palm of Your Hand
Volume 28, First Quarter 2009

Your glucose meter is truly your own personal laboratory in the palm of your hand. Every person living with diabetes should have and use a glucose meter. Finding out your blood sugar level in relation to eating, exercising, sleeping, concurrent medical illnesses, emotional stress, medications, and all of the other many factors that can effect our glucose levels throughout the day and night is truly invaluable.

Home glucose monitoring (HGM) is not just pricking your finger and writing the result in a log book for your health care provider to look at during your next appointment, which may be weeks or even months away. HGM is knowing what your individual blood glucose goals are and then doing something about any abnormal values to get them back into a desirable range. One of the biggest barriers that I see as a diabetes specialist is that people with diabetes are not educated about how to act on their results, leading to frustration, helplessness, inaction, and chronic poor control.

If you are a person with type 1 or type 2 diabetes on insulin, it is impossible to keep your blood glucose values in a desirable range most of the time without testing on a regular and frequent basis. How can you know if you took enough insulin or too much, before your daily meals? How can you correct or know how much extra insulin to take if you were unexpectedly high? How can you avoid hypoglycemia during exercise and other activities like driving a car or caring for a young child? Please, do not tell me that you can "feel" whether you are too high or low, and that you do not need to test!

One of the controversies in the medical arena is whether or not people with type 2 diabetes, treated with oral medications alone, should perform HGM. Besides, those glucose test strips are expensive, and why poke into our limited heath care dollars (and fingers!) if testing does not make a difference? If you have type 2 diabetes treated only with Glucophage (common oral medication for diabetes that does not cause hypoglycemia) and have never had an A1C greater than 6.5%, then you certainly do not need to test on a regular basis. However, if you are a 57-year-old male with type 2 diabetes in poor control and on several oral medications, HGM can help you and your caregiver make the proper medication adjustments and/or additions. The results can also be a powerful behavior modification tool in terms of your food choices and portion sizes as well as seeing the beneficial effects of exercise.

Individualizing your HGM testing schedule is crucial to getting the most out of the results. For example, a person with diabetes taking fast-acting insulin before meals may need to test before and 2 hours after most meals in order to stay off the blood sugar roller coaster. On the other hand, a person on oral medications may only need to test once a day, alternating between first thing in the morning and 2 hours after the largest meal.

Consider this challenge: If you are not content with your A1C, take a look at the average blood glucose feature on your meter. My meter gives me an average for the last 2 weeks, as well as the number of times I've tested in those time periods. If you'd like to use your meter a little more effectively, push yourself to get the 14-day average inside your goal blood glucose value window. As for frequency, if you only have part of the blood glucose picture, challenge yourself to get enough data to get your blood sugars in control.

The key is to test at times that will give you information on how your medications are working and/or how your daily lifestyle is affecting your control. Remember that your glucose meter is your own personal laboratory in the palm of your hand. Know when to test, and know what to do with the number!

Getting Activated
Volume 33, Fall 2010

I have never met a person with diabetes who does not want to live a long and healthy life. However, people with diabetes who do not have perfect glucose control are often labeled as "non-compliant." I see this all too often in the hospital among the medical students, residents, endocrine fellows, dietitians, CDEs, and other faculty and staff.

Once a person with diabetes is labeled as non-compliant in their medical record, healthcare professionals who read the record in preparation for a visit have already developed a preconceived notion that this person does not follow the rules. It is a common situation that is pervasive among healthcare professionals and has been proven difficult to change.

So why is it that many people with diabetes have high A1C values? The reasons are diverse, ranging from emotional and physical barriers to uninformed caregivers. Frequently, there is limited access to the best therapies currently available. Of the many variables that influence glucose control and the eventual development of diabetes complications, the "activation" of the person living with diabetes to take a more dedicated role in his or her care is the most critical. Activation basically means that the PWD has been educated, motivated, and empowered to take control of their diabetes with a positive attitude.

As we spoke about in our previous newsletter, *Extreme Diabetes Makeover (XDM)* will soon be available to millions of people around the globe to view online. TCOYD's *XDM* program successfully addresses how to help people with out-of-control diabetes to become active in their own healthcare. Trust me, it's not rocket science.

For our first *XDM* program, we accepted seven individuals living with diabetes who have extremely poor control of their condition (A1C values mostly between 9% and 11%, indicating an average blood glucose value of more than 250 mg/dL). Over a 5-month period, they greatly improved their control and completely changed their attitudes about living a normal and proactive life with diabetes. TCOYD helped provide them with a dream team of diabetes specialists, including myself; Dietitian Janice Baker, RD, CDE; nurse educator Angela Norton, RN, CDE; exercise physiologist, Larry Verity, PhD, FACSM; and clinical psychologist Bill Polonsky, PhD, CDE. We gave them the attention they needed, gained their trust, and addressed their emotional and physical barriers. This occurred only after we were able to truly connect with the group and develop a meaningful understanding of the issues that were preventing them from living successfully with their diabetes.

There is no question that we helped to activate these individuals who were generally disheartened with the day-to-day frustrations of this chronic condition and all of the demands put forth by our professional community. I have always wondered how well physicians would do when asked to prick their fingers and test their glucose 3 to 4 times per day, follow a consistent and rigid diet, exercise each day with consistent duration and intensity, take medications regularly, including insulin injections, and deal with the requirements to see multiple care professionals throughout the year as part of their diabetes treatment.

What does it take to activate someone living with diabetes? It takes understanding, sincerity, knowledge, and the ability to empathize with individuals in regard to what it is like to live with diabetes on a day-to-day basis. It also takes a conscious shift in attitude from categorizing someone living with diabetes who has poor control as non-compliant, to regarding them as not being active in their own condition.

The answer to improving care in this country is, in part, developing new drugs and devices, but also changing the attitudes of caregivers toward their patients with diabetes by encouraging them to become activated in their own self-management, while addressing their individual physical and emotional fears, needs, and concerns. This takes time and is a multidisciplinary approach. We just allow for these vital requirements within our new healthcare policies to take action. As patients and healthcare providers, let's work together to improve lives and ultimately change the face of diabetes in this country.

How Sweet Is Sweet Enough? What Should Your A1C Be?
Volume 35, Spring 2011

The A1C is the most important test in diabetes management. It tells all of us folks living with diabetes and our caregivers how our blood sugars have been on average over 2 to 3 months. In recent years, a controversy has developed amongst diabetes professional organizations regarding the ideal A1C value.

The American Diabetes Association (ADA) says the ideal goal should be less than 7% (average blood sugar of ~150 mg/dL), while the American Association of Clinical Endocrinologists (AACE) and American Association of Diabetes Educators (AADE) state it should be less than 6.5% (average blood sugar of ~120 mg/dL). There have been many heated debates over these limits with no real consensus to date.

Adding to the differences of opinion came the results of three large clinical trials, all demonstrating that there are no obvious benefits of tightly controlling blood sugar levels in terms of reducing heart disease (medically speaking, macrovascular complications) in people with type 2 diabetes, which happens to be the main cause of death. As mentioned above, there is no argument that proper glucose control will prevent or reduce the incidence of microvascular complications. Adding even more fuel to the fire, one of the three large studies (ACCORD trial) showed a higher death rate in the group of people with type 2 diabetes whose A1C values were the lowest! Researchers are investigating the reasons for this, but they are concluding that severe low blood glucose, or hypoglycemia, may have played a role in these excessive deaths.

"One thing that remains constant is that there is no one perfect value for everyone and individualization is key."

With all these differences of expert opinion and surprising clinical trial results, where should people with diabetes keep their A1C values? One thing that is not debatable is that there is no one perfect value for everyone, and individualization is key.

There are many important variables that may influence what your A1C goal should be, including age, how long you have lived with diabetes, presence of risk factors for heart disease (such as high blood pressure and abnormal cholesterol levels), having heart disease (such as a heart attack), not being able to recognize low blood sugar levels (hypoglycemia unawareness), and what type of diabetes medications you are on.

If you are an older person with diabetes and have heart disease, then it would be prudent to not get your A1C down too low, especially if you are on insulin or other medications that may cause low blood sugar. Concentrating on reducing your cardiovascular risk factors should be one of your highest health priorities.

If you are young and healthy and have a long life ahead of you living with diabetes, getting and keeping your A1C as low as possible is a good idea.

The bottom line is that your A1C should be as low as possible as long as that level can be achieved and maintained safely while avoiding hypoglycemia and not interfering with your lifestyle in an adverse way. This is a statement that all organizations would agree with.

Don't be in the dark when it comes to your A1C. Talk with your caregiver to find out how sweet you should be and how you can improve for the future!

Are We What We Eat or How Much We Eat?
Volume 36, Summer 2011

Millions of people in the United States and other developed countries around the world constantly struggle with weight problems. There are as many weight-loss diets as there are brands of wines or cigars. In addition, the number of unregulated, unproven, and ineffective over-the-counter and Internet-accessible "diet pills and remedies" are too numerous to count.

People with any type of diabetes also struggle with dietary and weight issues every day and with every single meal. For a typical person with type 1 diabetes, even if body weight is not a problem, he or she must calculate the correct insulin dose for the food consumed. This calls for reading food labels, accurate carbohydrate counting, and portion estimates, in addition to knowing blood sugar levels and anticipating exercise after meals.

For a typical person with type 2 diabetes, the main issues include dealing with excess weight and controlling the appetite. Many of my type 2 patients tell me they can smell food and gain weight! For someone living with diabetes, it can be so frustrating and confusing to figure out what to eat.

Let's first tackle the carbohydrate-counting dilemma. I feel it is only a diabetic dietary fad and is seriously flawed in many ways. Since I was diagnosed with diabetes in 1970, there has been the Exchange System, Glycemic Index Scale, and now it has transitioned into just plain "Carbohydrate Counting." I do feel it is important to know the carbohydrate content of the foods we eat, since they get absorbed more quickly compared with proteins and fats, however, it is difficult for the average person to accurately measure carbohydrates. In addition, proteins and fats also have calories in them and will eventually raise the blood sugar levels.

I wish a steak had no calories. A lean, 8-ounce filet mignon has over 450 calories! Underestimation of calories also leads to insufficient insulin dosing and frustrating postmeal hyperglycemia. I feel we need to count calories and not just carbohydrates and also learn how to deal with the different time/course ratio of absorption, depending on the composition of the meal. I realize this may be a big challenge, but relying on carbohydrate counting alone, and ignoring the calories of fat and protein, has contributed to the roller coaster of diabetes management in insulin users.

When it comes to dealing with excess weight, I am a big believer that we are not what we eat, but rather how much we eat. It all comes down to portion control. Most people who develop type 2 diabetes are over the age of 40 and have weight problems. Type 2 diabetes and central obesity go hand-in-hand and are genetically and metabolically linked in a complicated and not fully understood way. It is unreasonable to ask someone who is set in their ways to give up their personal and cultural food preferences just because they now have diabetes. For example, getting your morning source of protein, as directed by a dietitian, in a scoop of cottage cheese or a tablespoon of peanut butter may not be something that you are accustomed to or that agrees with you. Cutting out sugars and fats completely or that occasional big juicy hamburger from the local joint down the street is unreasonable and, if enforced, can lead to a really bad attitude and resentment toward diabetes. This is surely a prescription for failure.

After dealing with my own diabetes and the diabetes of thousands of my patients and TCOYD conference participants, I am more convinced than ever that eating the foods you like (in moderation) is the key to blood sugar and weight control. Eating two to three well-balanced and proportioned meals a day, avoiding simple sugars and saturated fats (most of the time), and sticking to your personal preferences is the diabetes diet for long-term success. There is no question that we are not what we eat, but rather how much we eat.

Bon appétit!

Patient and Professional Inertia: Major Barriers to Taking Control Of Your Diabetes
Volume 37, Fall 2011

Patient and professional inertia refers simply to the delay in appropriate treatment due to a whole host of reasons but mainly ignorance, fear of change, unbreakable old habits. and misinformation.

Let's tackle professional inertia first, as it is a HUGE problem and hampers timely and appropriate care for people with diabetes. When caregivers graduate from medical, nurse practitioner, or physician's assistant school, multiple studies have shown that their practice habits get stuck in the mud. If a new treatment or device comes along, getting providers of care to become knowledgeable about them, and then change their practices enough to prescribe them for their patients, is really tough and takes a long time… sometimes up to 10 years! I spend a lot of my time educating professionals to take better care of all of us with diabetes and it is so frustrating when I speak to doctors who have never prescribed Byetta or Victoza and have never heard of continuous-glucose monitoring. This happens on a very regular basis and I just want to scream OMG, but I don't, unless I am alone in my car!

Patient inertia is different, as the individual living with diabetes is his or her own biggest barrier to achieving control. The best way to define patient inertia is to give you some examples.

First, a young, smart, and dedicated doctor with type 1 diabetes since childhood is still using a syringe and vial to give himself fast-acting insulin throughout the day. The syringe is so old you cannot see the labeling on the side and the needle is extremely dull. The insulin is also being exposed to light, heat, and agitation (all factors that make the insulin less potent). For some reason, he is not using an insulin pen, which delivers very accurate doses, and the insulin is protected from the environment.

Second is a person who has type 2 diabetes and will not take her statin medication to keep her LDL cholesterol at goal, because she read on the internet that her Lipitor causes muscle aches. Give me a break. Heart disease is the number one killer of all Americans, and these very safe statin drugs have done more to reduce heart attacks than any other prescription drug. These medications have been used in 100s of millions of people worldwide and have withstood the test of time.

The third example is a patient of mine who would rather take an herbal remedy from the local vitamin store for his diabetes, even though he does not know what the heck is in it, than an FDA-approved oral medication where we know the pros and cons, as well as the efficacy of the therapy. He tells me that the powder he bought is from

> Knowledge wipes out fear, ignorance, misconceptions and inertia. This is what Taking Control of Your Diabetes is all about.

the East African subterranean, multileaf monkey bush, also known as E.A.S.M.L.M.B. to the crooked company that makes it, and that it is "natural". I tell him that strychnine is natural! Are you getting the picture? Do you have patient inertia?

Reversing patient and professional inertia comes with timely, consistent, and appropriate education as well as eliminating misinformation from family, friends, the internet, and people who work at some of the herbal and vitamin stores. Professionals need to remember to continuously improve upon their original medical education in diabetes and allow more time for mandatory continuing diabetes education. Patients may need the help of a clinical psychologist, but for sure, knowledge is the key. Knowledge wipes out fear, ignorance, misconceptions, and inertia. This is what Taking Control Of Your Diabetes is all about. See you at a conference soon!

Medical Advice Should Always Be Questioned: Knowledge Is Key
Volume 38, Winter 2012

In health care today, it is very important to question the medical advice you are given. NEVER blindly trust what you are told to do by any medical professional. The best thing that you can do for your health is to be your own best advocate, take control, and be informed and involved. This may sound harsh but, as an endocrinologist working at several major medical centers and hearing stories from my colleagues around the country, I have seen first hand the effects of just plain wrong advice given to people with diabetes and, sometimes, that advice is the culprit of severe negative outcomes.

You, the person living with diabetes, will suffer the consequences of poor advice, not the person giving the harmful information. Before I give you some examples, let me say that NONE of these situations was created intentionally, and it just boils down to plain old ignorance on the part of the medical professionals, as well as individuals with diabetes who have not learned to take control!

If you have type 1 diabetes and a surgeon says to you, "Do not take your basal insulin (Lantus or Levemir)" or "Stop your pump" the day before your scheduled operation, would you do it? Believe it or not, this is a very common occurrence. The surgical specialists often do not have a clue about diabetes and especially the difference between type 1 and type 2. A person with type 2 on insulin would probably be okay with this advice, but a person with type 1 will go into the severe metabolic state called diabetic ketoacidosis, or DKA. If it is an elective procedure, the surgery will most likely be cancelled due to high blood sugar levels. Give me a break! One of my colleague's patients had a heart attack while in DKA that was caused by stopping his insulin. My doctor friend, who is a diabetes specialist, even told the patient a week before surgery not to stop his basal insulin even if the surgeon or anesthesiologist tells him to stop. This scenario happens every day multiple times across America. I bet each one of you has a frustrating story about what happened to your diabetes while in the hospital, but this patient should have known better.

This next example is super common but typically not as dangerous. Health care professionals commonly give steroids for many different conditions and, out of ignorance, do not tell their patients with diabetes that their blood sugar levels will go through the roof. What happens is that the person with diabetes, who doesn't have any knowledge about what steroids can do to blood sugar levels, panics and starts calling their diabetes specialist or primary care physician with no idea of what is happening or why! Every person with diabetes should know the basics of which medications can mess with their diabetes control, and steroids are the worst offenders. With a little bit of knowledge, proactive adjustments can be made, especially for those on insulin.

These types of scenarios occur between caregivers and patients in all disease states, some with more serious consequences than others. Diabetes is a condition with a 24/7 presence, and it can be thrown off by many variables throughout the day and night. Medical professionals, including doctors, nurse practitioners, physician assistants, pharmacists, etc, went into medicine to help their patients, but they can not know every single thing about every disease. What it comes down to is that the person with the medical condition needs to be as smart and informed as they can be about their own disease. Knowledge is the key for both the patient and the provider. You owe it to yourself and your family to take control of your diabetes and never blindly trust the medical advice given to you.

It's All About Prevention: Halting the Onset and Delaying the Progression of Diabetes and Its Complications
Volume 39, Spring 2012

Prevention is the key to many chronic conditions. However, it is especially important for people who are at risk for getting diabetes and those who already have diabetes. If you are at risk for getting diabetes, your primary goal should be to hault the onset of the disease, and for those who already have it, the objective is to prevent or delay the progression of complications.

Diabetes complications are typically broken up into two categories: microvascular and macrovascular. Microvascular complications include eye disease or retinopathy, kidney disease or nephropathy, and nerve disease or neuropathy. So, what ultimately causes eye, kidney, and nerve diseases? It is well known from several large clinical trials that microvascular complications are a direct result of the duration and severity of high blood sugar levels, or hyperglycemia. This is why it is so important to try to get your glucose levels, and your A1C value, as close to normal as possible. The challenge is to get your glucose and A1C values down while, at the same time, avoiding hypoglycemia. There is also some research that suggests the ups and downs, or variability of glucose levels, may also contribute to the development of complications.

In addition to glucose control, it turns out that making sure your blood pressure is within in the normal range is of extreme importance when it comes to preventing eye and kidney disease. High blood pressure puts a strain on the blood vessels and other vital structures of the eyes and kidneys. Avoiding drugs that can damage your kidneys and nerves is also part of prevention. Nerves can be affected by numerous factors, including vitamin deficiencies, exposure to toxins, and smoking, which makes the onset and progression of neuropathy less predictable than eye and kidney disease.

Macrovascular complications include heart attacks and strokes, which remain the most common causes of death in all Americans, diabetic or not. People with type 2 diabetes are at the greatest risk for macrovascular complications because of the high rate of cardiovascular risk factors associated with this condition: high blood pressure, abnormal cholesterol levels, propensity to form blood clots, inflammation, and blood vessel abnormalities. The main ways we prevent heart attacks and strokes are to treat each of these risk factors directly: blood pressure medications, cholesterol drugs, anti-inflammatory agents, and blood thinners, such as aspirin. Lifestyle modification is also very important. We need to be constantly aware of not only what we are eating, but, how much we are eating. It is also imperative to incorporate frequent aerobic exercise into our daily routines and to maintain the best body weight that we can possibly achieve.

Diabetes is a treatable condition. One of the most important things to remember is that if you have diabetes, you can prevent complications, and if you are already experiencing complications, you can delay their progression. The key issues to pay attention to and obtain control over are your glucose levels, blood pressure measurements, and cholesterol values. You should also consider a daily regimen of aspirin (only with the advice of your caregiver). It comes down to the ABCs of diabetes management: "A" for A1C and aspirin, "B" for blood pressure, and "C" for cholesterol. Take control of your ABCs and enjoy a long and healthy life with diabetes.

To read all of these newsletters in their entirety, all others that have been published to date, and to keep up with current information published on a quarterly basis, go to *http:// tcoyd.org/landing/my-tcoyd -newsletter.html*.

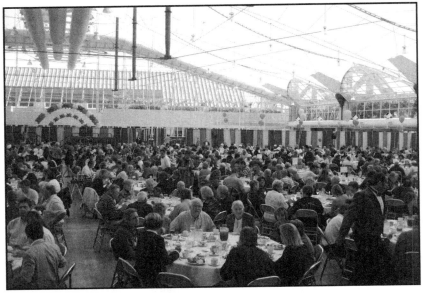

TCOYD lunch crowd in San Diego.

26

Diabetes in the Internet Age

How Getting Networked Can Change Your Life

by Amy Tenderich of
www.diabetesmine.com

If you ask most people what's the hardest thing about living with diabetes, they'll almost always say, "the psychological side." Not in those words, of course. They'll answer with something familiar like: "It's so frustrating—and I never get a break!" Or... "It's so hard to keep motivated when I feel like I'm 'failing' all the time." Or the classic... "None of my family or friends really understands what I'm going through. I feel so isolated!"

For many thousands of PWDs (people with diabetes), having access to a whole new world of connections via the Internet is transforming the experience of being a patient from a horribly isolating one of hopelessness and helplessness to a more positive, social experience that helps them feel understood and empowered!

At this very moment as you read these words, there are scores of PWDs out there chatting via blogs, Facebook, Twitter, and dedicated diabetes communities. They are learning, laughing, and helping each other with practical tips that no doctor who hasn't walked in our shoes could ever know.

We call it the Diabetes Online Community, or DOC, and for many who've discovered it, it is nothing less than a lifeline.

The "Empowered Patient Revolution"

To understand why online connections are such a big deal, it's important to understand the current "e-Patient movement" that's underway.

Don't forget that the traditional notion of a "patient" was someone laid up in a hospital. Their journey either ended there or, if they were lucky, they were cured of their ailment and walked out of the hospital no longer a patient. But today, we have a whole new notion of *survivorship* with chronic illnesses, as popularized by (cancer survivor and cycling champion) Lance Armstrong. Thanks to modern medicine, folks with all kinds of serious health conditions are leading full, active lives.

But the medical establishment hasn't kept up with their needs—certainly not on the emotional side of living your life as a patient or watching someone you love become one. Our needs for coaching and psychological support have *not* been adequately addressed. For the most part, medicine is still seen as a lab science, with professionals trapped in an old-school, patriarchal, and rather patronizing model of health care. If you've ever felt judged or belittled by a doctor, nurse, or other health care provider, you know what I'm talking about.

I personally attend a lot of conferences around the country—focusing on health care reform, health policy, and diabetes events for professional providers—and the term "patient" is volleyed around like it stood for some mysterious block of "other beings" who are often "naughty" because they don't strictly follow doctor's instructions.

But as humans, we all share this experience! We've all been a patient at some point in our lives, whether with a simple case of the flu or even a routine vaccination. We must *all* recognize that life is complicated by work, financial responsibilities, family relationships, etc, etc, etc. This needs to be taken into account when handing out directions for managing our health!

Moreover, when you're stricken with a serious, lifelong health condition (like diabetes), you're expected to suddenly be totally reliant on some magical health care experts... who are going to understand what's happening with your body even when you don't. Nor are you expected to truly understand your condition or be capable of making decisions about it.

e-Patients, or empowered patients, are people who are taking a stand against this approach. They are using social media for what it's best for: connecting, telling their stories, building relationships, helping and mentoring each other, and sharing educational resources. All of this becomes mission-critical when you're dealing with a serious health condition.

So in a way, online communities and the notion of so-called Participatory Medicine (in which the patient is treated like a partner in their own care) are attributes of a Revolution—a fight for rights and respect for people whose health is compromised in some way. And we're talking about a *lot* of people: the Pew Internet Foundation tells us that half of the adults in the United States have at least one chronic condition, and nearly 75% of those people are now going online to do something about it, to "get networked" if you will...

Why Social Media Matters

As new web-based technologies allowing *interactive* publishing started to appear in the early 2000s (blogging software and community platforms), people and organizations quickly began to realize how incredibly powerful this new social media could be. As I'm sure you're aware, nowadays everyone from your kids' daycare center to the supermarket down the street have Twitter feeds and Facebook pages. Why? Because it opens up a whole new world of connections, both between individuals with shared interests who may never otherwise have found each other, and between organizations and their customers or stakeholders.

For people struggling with health conditions, this has been a huge boon! In many respects, because our health care system is so fractured and ill-equipped to deal with our day-to-day needs. Have a look at the circle diagram in **Figure 26-1**. When first diagnosed, we patients are often presented with this idealistic vision of patient-centered care, where *you* are the center of the universe. Supposedly, a whole host of providers (primary physician, certified diabetes educator, nutritionist, etc) will snap into motion working as a coordinated health care team just for you. They'll provide you with a perfect set of instructions to guide you to do just the right thing at all times with your diabetes. And of course, your family and friends will immediately transform into this ideal support network, *right?* NOT!! In reality, it's all pretty messy—starting with the fact that different providers are often at different clinics, and you as a patient have to fight to get them to even communicate with each other. And your poor family and friends are generally at least as clueless as you are...

So using social media, PWDs started creating new online spaces and resources that never existed before— blogs and communities and podcasts and videos—that help fill those gaps, by serving three core purposes. These online spaces provide:

Figure 26-1

Ideal Vision of Diabetes Care vs the Reality

The VISION...

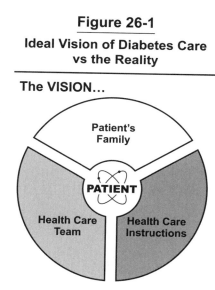

The REALITY...

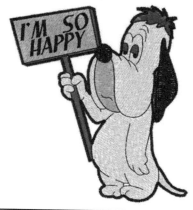

- *Camaraderie/support*—they allow you to socialize with like-minded people and share life experiences.
- *Information/a dynamic education*—you get instant, 24/7 access to all kinds of practical help, and it's completely free.
- *Advocacy!*—by gathering in these online spaces, posting our opinions, and creating petitions and other campaigns online, we patients now have a collective voice we never had before, and the ability to lobby for our own interests.

Evolution of the DOC

I was one of the online pioneers in the diabetes online community (DOC). But my story of being diagnosed with type 1 diabetes as an adult, and feeling lost and overwhelmed, is not unique. It was May of 2003, shortly after I'd given birth to my third child. After losing 20 pounds within 2 weeks and suffering from severe dehydration, I was hospitalized for a week. Because of my age, the doctors thought I was type 2 diabetic, but they put me on insulin anyway—far too much insulin! The glucose lows I experienced were so severe that I felt like I was having a nervous breakdown after every meal! I was afraid to leave the house, afraid to get behind the wheel with my three small children. Eventually I was told I had type 1 diabetes, the "bad kind." And it turned my world upside-down. The whole first year was miserable, and I soon realized: *I can't live like this! There has to be a better way!*

As a San Francisco-based freelance writer and fan of technology, naturally I turned to the Internet, looking for help. But at the time, I found only incomprehensible medical journal articles and bad news headlines… Where were answers to my real-life questions? Where were the other people living with diabetes who could relate to what I was going through?

I was so frustrated and so hungry to learn more about this new illness that I set out to create the website that I myself was looking for, sort of "a diabetes newspaper with a personal twist." I was able to use new blogging software that had just been introduced to create *Diabetes-Mine.com*, a play-on words for "it's mine, I'm stuck with it" and "a gold mine of straight talk and encouragement for people touched by diabetes."

I wrote about my personal struggles. I also put on my journalist hat and treated diabetes like my "beat" at a newspaper, attending industry events and reporting on what I had learned. I wrote product reviews, news analyses, and published testimonials from other patients and their

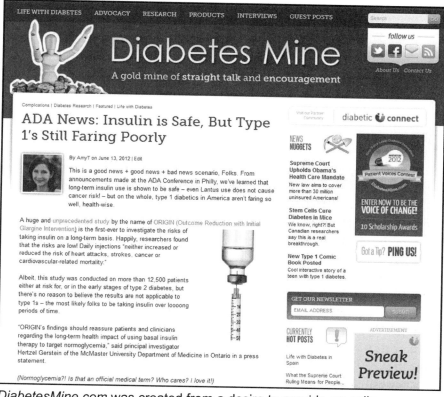

DiabetesMine.com was created from a desire to provide an online venue where people with diabetes could obtain reliable, current information concerning the disease as well as exchange ideas and experiences with others.

---

partners. Reporting on industry news, I tried to act as a "consumer watchdog" for the patient community.

The site quickly turned into an information resource and networking place for patients, caregivers, and folks in the medical and pharma industries. I cannot believe how much I learned myself from interacting with readers, and how incredibly uplifting it was to feel that I was doing something positive about my diabetes!

Soon, all around me dozens (and then hundreds) of new diabetes blogs and online communities started popping up. I found myself in the middle of this movement called Health 2.0 (where Web 2.0 technologies meet new approaches to health care). In 2007, I was approached by a company in Salt Lake City called Alliance Health Networks, which asked me to help them launch a new, Facebook-like community called *DiabeticConnect.com*. The idea would be a dedicated site where PWDs could chat with each other, share videos and recipes and tips and hints and opinions on products, and more. Within a few months, the site had 10,000 registered members, then 20K and 30K, and they are now up to over 700,000 registered members to date! Clearly there is a great need and desire for sites that help connect us!

My blog, *DiabetesMine.com*, was actually acquired by Alliance Health Networks in January 2011, so my job is now to act as Editor in Chief and also head of patient advocacy for this company that's creating powerful social platforms for patients. They've developed over 50 similar sites for other health conditions (*ArthritisConnect.com*, *SleepConnect.com*, *DepressionConnect.com*, etc), but the *DiabeticConnect* community remains the flagship site.

Three other major diabetes online communities you should know about are *TuDiabetes.org* (founded by Manny Hernandez and associated with the nonprofit Diabetes Hands Foundation); *DiabetesDaily.com*, which has an excellent recipe section and hosts a variety of bloggers who publish directly on this community site; and *dLife.com*, which also produces a weekly CNBC cable television show on diabetes by the same name.

A tremendous community of diabetes bloggers has emerged and in recent years, we've banded together to form a grassroots organization

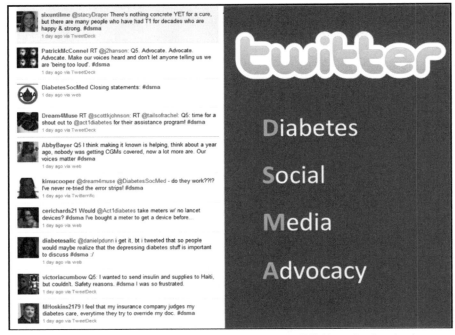

PWDs tweet news and experiences to others using #DSMA and other hashtags.

that can be found at *DiabetesAdvocates.org*, a site where you can browse a roster of various bloggers and learn about advocacy efforts we're working on as a group. Note that a wonderful subset of the blogging community are the D-moms and D-dads, who write about caring for a child with diabetes. In fact, one of the oldest and most robust online communities is *CWD.com*, or Children With Diabetes, an organization that also runs fantastic in-person conferences. *(See their site for details.)*

A newer, very dynamic group is called Diabetes Social Media Advocacy (*Diabetessocmed.com*), which features bloggers, creates awareness videos, and runs a weekly Podcast and Twitter chat under the hashtag #DSMA. Hundreds of PWDs join the chat each week to discuss different aspects of living with diabetes.

One of the recurring themes in the DOC is that of invisible illness, as in, "*Hey, you don't look sick*" But we PWDs are dealing with day-to-day challenges that most healthy people cannot even conceive of. Therefore, sharing images of our rarely seen challenges is powerful! That's why I'd also recommend the Diabetes Made Visible group on *Flickr.com*, a popular photo-sharing site. Social media helps us invisibles find each other. In the immortal words of Mike Hoskins, an early diabetes blogger who now works with me at *DiabetesMine*:

> "*In a way, (the online community) is like Diabetes Camp, but 24/7 and whenever you need it. It's a place where we can be 'normal' and among friends with diabetes.*"

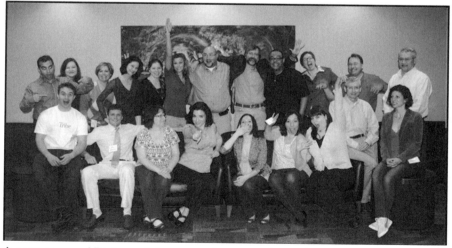

A core group of Diabetes Advocates who met online—they've turned my life around with this illness!

Spotlight on Patient Voices

Online connections can help us with behavior change, too. For example, we all know we're *supposed* to eat healthier and exercise more, but changing habits is hard, isn't it? Networked patients can rally each other, often by creating online support programs like the "Biggest Loser D-Style," one blogger's 16-week group challenge to encourage each other to lose weight and get more physically active. Participants paid $5 or more into a "pool" that paid out the winners (biggest losers) at the end of the program. Check-ins were achieved by submitting photos of your bathroom scale showing your weight loss progress. It was a very fun and popular program.

Product reviews are important too. Think about it: where in the past could you ever get real-life feedback from other patients using various medical treatments?

People want to share the experience of trying new drugs and devices; they want to learn about things like side effects, fine-tuning of dosing, and how one treatment might compare to others—all things you aren't going to get from the pharma company's website, or from your doctor either.

And in the past, if your health insurance denied your claim for a particular treatment, you had no way of knowing what experiences other patients may have had: were they able to appeal a denial? If so, on what basis? An online forum for sharing this kind of information is incredibly powerful.

Now with social media, anyone who wants to raise their voice and become an active advocate can start networking, and even create an online hub or petition to publicize patient protests, and the Powers That Be have taken notice. The pharma industry has been forced to recognize that *we patients* are their customers, not just the clinicians they've typically catered to, and that *we* are talking about them and influencing their relative success. So much so that in 2009, Roche Diabetes actually hosted the first annual in-person Diabetes Social Media Summit, bringing in few dozen outspoken patient advocates for a day of frank dialogue at their headquarters in Indianapolis. It was a risky move in some ways to allow us to confront them on their own turf, but it paid off well

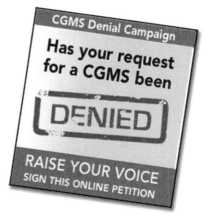

in establishing a much more open relationship between the DOC and the medical companies that we sometimes "love to hate." I give Roche kudos for taking the first step, and they certainly listened to the online community: they changed some of their ad campaigns to look more realistic based on our feedback, and also put more emphasis on Patient Assistance Programs. The Summit was so successful that competitors have followed suit; Medtronic and Eli Lilly have begun similar programs.

The big national advocacy organizations have likewise embraced the online community. JDRF has been in close touch with bloggers and even hosted an "online roundtable," while ADA has more recently begun proactive outreach and even hosting receptions for bloggers at various ADA events.

How to Start Connecting

These days, it seems that everybody is already doing *something* online. Whether you're extremely web-savvy or just getting started, here are the basic options for engagement in various online forums:

- *Blogs*: you can read and comment, or just "lurk" (read without commenting), find contact info and reach out to the author(s), or start your own blog using a platform like Wordpress, Typepad, or Blogger.com from Google.
- *Facebook*: you can follow the pages of individuals or organizations, "like" and comment, post photos, tag people, read news feeds, and more. You can create your own personal profile, or a page to promote your blog or program.
- *Diabetes Community Sites*: you can just "lurk," but will get more out of the experience if you register, make comments, and start your own discussion threads.
- *Twitter*: you can post your own brief 140-character updates, follow people and organizations, "retweet" their updates, and create and use hashtags[a] to find topics that interest you (**Table 26-1**).

Connecting online doesn't have to be tremendously time-consuming. Even if you only have 15 minutes per week to spare, you could get started by...
- Adding some bookmarks to your desktop

---

[a] Hashtags are simply key words that are posted on twitter with the pound sign (#) in front of them. That makes these terms searchable, so you can find discussions that interest you any time of day or night. See the box for a list of some popular hashtags among PWDs.

- Subscribing to a few blogs by email
- Reading for a few minutes each day
- Trying to find a few new resources each week.

If you have a little more time to invest, you could…
- Follow a #DSMA Twitter Chat (Wednesdays at 6pm PST/ 9pm EST)
- Join one or more Diabetes Community sites and create your own online profiles
- Commit to doing something new each week—creating new posting(s), sending outreach emails, or updating your status or photos.

Table 26-1
Diabetes Twitter Hashtags

- #diabetes
- #diabetic
- #PWD (person with diabetes)
- #CWD (child with diabetes)
- #bgnow (blood glucose)
- #bgwed (on Wednesdays)
- #Type2
- #Type1
- #dblog (diabetes blogs)
- #diabetessucks
- #diabetesoutrage
- #ehealth
- #insulin
- #pump
- #epatient
- #insulinpump
- #DSMA (Diabetes Social Media Advocates)

Some Sites You Shouldn't Miss

Hopefully this chapter has convinced you that the Diabetes Online Community is a resource you don't want to miss out on! **Table 26-2** lists some sites that I highly recommend. This is not a comprehensive list, but these are some excellent places to get started.

Table 26-2
Highly Recommended Web Sites

- *DiabetesAdvocates.org*—a collective of individuals and organizations offering expertise, resources, and support to those touched by diabetes. Find links to members and their blogs, and download the DA brochure. Twitter: *@D_Advocates*.
- *DiabetesSocialMed.com*—through varied vehicles this community connects, supports, and educates PWDs. Twitter: *@diabetessocmed*, #dsma (hashtag). Weekly twitter chat: Wed 9-10 PM EST; DSMA live (talk radio): Thurs 9-10 PM EST; monthly blog carnival with featured blogs and more.
- *TheDiabetesResource.com*—a patient-created guide to diabetes sites and resources.
- Diabetes Community Sites—places where PWDs and their loved ones are connecting:
  - *DiabeticConnect.com*
  - *DiabetesDaily.com*
  - *Tudiabetes.org*
  - *dLife.com*
  - *ChildrenWithDiabetes.com* (for kids & families)
  - *DiabetesSisters.org* (for women with any kind of diabetes)
  - *Divabetic.org* (wellness for women)
  - *Juvenation.org* (JDRF's social network for youth)
  - *MyGlu.org* (for type 1 PWDs, sponsored by the Helmsley Trust)
- Diabetes Blogs—these can be personal diaries or more like media sites that publish news and feature stories regularly:
  - *DiabetesMine.com* (the all things diabetes blog)
  - *DiabetesDaily.com/voices/* (composite of many blogs)
  - *DiabetesStopsHere.com* (The ADA's blog)
  - *DiabetesSelfManagement.com/blog/* (magazine blog)
  - *Diabetesaliciousness.blogspot.com*
  - *D-mom.com*
  - *ScottsDiabetes.com*
  - *SixUntilMe.com*
  - *TextingMyPancreas.com*

  …and many, many more!

27

Safe and Effective Uses of Prescription Medications

by Ian Blumer, MD

If you have diabetes, the odds are high that you are taking at least one type of prescription medication. Indeed, you may well be taking a whole bunch of different prescription medicines and quite possibly some non-prescription medications, too.

In this chapter, we look at the most important things you need to know to ensure that you are taking your medications safely and effectively.

Keep Track of The Drugs You're Taking

Living with diabetes, you are likely seeing a primary care provider (be it a family physician, nurse practitioner, or other health care provider) at least several times per year. You may also be meeting with a diabetes specialist from time to time, may be seeing a diabetes nurse educator on occasion, and, depending on your other health issues, may also be meeting with a cardiologist, kidney specialist, or one of a whole host of other health care providers. And, of course, you are likely seeing your pharmacist regularly... quite possibly more than anyone else we've just mentioned. One thing that all of these providers have in common is the need to know *exactly* what medications you are taking in order to ensure that you are taking the right medication in the right dose to best serve your health needs.

In some ideal world, perhaps there is some foolproof system in place where every health care provider assisting a person living with diabetes is always kept abreast of every medication that a person is taking and is always made immediately aware anytime a change is made to a medication or a dose. If such a place exists, I sure haven't seen it. And, truth be told, health care providers are not nearly so good as we should be at sharing information among ourselves about patients whose care we share. So the bottom line is that it is up to you, as the person living with diabetes, to always keep track of exactly what drugs you are taking and in exactly what dose. Keep a list. And keep it current. And take the list with you whenever you see a member of your health care team. On this list, for each drug you are taking record:

- The name of the drug
- The strength of each dose (usually measured in milligrams)
- How often you take a dose

To avoid re-writing the list each time a change is made to your medications, keeping the list on a computer spreadsheet or other electronic document will make it easier for you to keep the list up-to-date. Then, when you need to see a health care provider, you can print off a copy of your list.

Be sure to keep a copy of the list on you at all times so that in case you end up in an emergency room or walk-in-clinic, you will be able to readily tell the doctor what drugs you are taking.

Also, if you travel outside of the country, be sure to write down on your list both the generic name and the trade name of the drugs you are taking since trade names can differ between countries whereas generic names do not. (If you were to ask for your usual drug by its trade name in a different country from where it was originally prescribed, you might wind up with a drug that is different from what you are supposed to be taking.) You will find both the trade name and the generic name for your medications on the pill bottle or box that the drug came in.

Take Your Medicines With You When You See Your Doctor

In the preceding section, I mentioned how important it is to keep a list of your medications. But even the best list in the world does not replace the need for you to take your actual medications with you *in their original containers* when you see certain of your health care providers. Why? Here are some reasons.

First, lists are fallible. Here's an example. I saw a patient who brought in a list of his medications, which he was certain was correct and up-to-date. I looked at the list and it matched with what my chart also had listed. But he didn't appear quite right. He looked tired and he had gained some weight since his last visit to me the year before. I asked him to go home and retrieve his medications, then come back to the office. Lo and behold, he was on a dose of thyroid medication (L-thyroxine) that was only 10% as strong as his list said he was on. I had prescribed (and he had written on his list) that he was taking 0.25 mg daily whereas the bottle stated that the pills were 0.025 mg strength. Ten times weaker than he was supposed to be on! No wonder he wasn't feeling well. The pharmacist had made an error and dispensed to him the wrong dose. He had an excellent pharmacist, but like everyone else on this planet, his pharmacist was not infallible and had made a mistake… a mistake that was detected only because my patient had brought his medications with him to his appointment (even if it did take some arm twisting to get him to do so).

A second reason to bring your medications with you to your appointments with your doctor is so that if your doctor wants to change the dose of one of your medications or have you stop taking a medication, they can note this directly on the bottle so that the directions are crystal clear. It is not a rarity that I will write in big bold letters "STOP" on a patient's pill bottle as I give them a new prescription for a drug to replace the one I am stopping.

Most people I speak with find it a nuisance to bring their medications with them to each appointment with me. Time and time again, I hear the understandable refrain: "But doctor, I brought my medications to my last appointment with you just a few months ago. None of my medicines have changed so why do I have to bring them yet *again*?" This plea makes perfect sense, except that, in truth, *about 50% of the time* (!) some change to a medication in fact has been made between the time of the patient's last visit and their current visit. Often this is unbeknownst to the patient or slipped their memory. Sometimes the patient has been prescribed a new medicine by a doctor in the ER, sometimes a person inadvertently has stopped a medication, sometimes a person forgot to get a medication refilled at the pharmacy, and so on.

This can be terribly dangerous. I've seen patients whose blood pressure became out-of-control because they had inadvertently discontinued a blood pressure medicine. I've seen patients who were having repeated episodes of low blood glucose because they had been prescribed a blood glucose-lowering medicine to *replace* what they were taking but had inadvertently been *taking both*. I've seen patients who had a dangerously slow heart beat because they had seen two different doctors in a short period of time, didn't have their medicines with them, and ended up being prescribed two nearly identical drugs for the same problem, which, when taken together, slowed the heart beat down to a dangerous level. All of these problems could have been avoided if they had their drugs with them and showed them to the physician.

Do you need to take your drugs with you to each and every appointment with your health care provider? Well, if you are meeting with your diabetes specialist, I would recommend it. As for your appointments with other members of your health care team (such as your family physician or your eye specialist or your diabetes nurse educator or…), best to check with them to find out how often they would like you to bring your medications to your appointments.

Know Why You Are Being Treated With A Medication

When your physician or other health care provider gives you a prescription (or, for that matter, a drug sample) make sure you ask why you are being asked to take the medicine. Medicines are serious stuff and you deserve to know exactly why you are being asked to take them.

I would encourage you to discuss this with the person prescribing your medicine *at the time of your visit* with them. This is far better than asking the pharmacist when you go to fill the prescription and is immensely better than looking it up on the Internet when you get home. Why? Because a given medicine can serve many different functions and your pharmacist (and the Internet!) may not know which of these functions is the one that your doctor wants you to benefit from. Here's an example: Let's say you were prescribed an ACE inhibitor (such as ramipril). This drug can be used to prevent a problem (like a heart attack) or to treat a problem (like high blood pressure). Unless your doctor tells you for which reason they are prescribing the medicine, you will be left in the dark.

Know How To Determine If Your Medicine Is Doing Its Job

When you have a headache and take an analgesic ("pain killer") like acetaminophen (Tylenol) or ibuprofen (Advil) and your headache quickly goes away, you know that the medicine did its job. But what about your other medications? How, for example, will you know if your diabetes medicine or your blood pressure medicine or your cholesterol medicine is doing its job? Simply put—you won't… unless, that is, you specifically do a test to find out.

In the case of medications to lower your blood glucose ("blood sugar"), the only way you'll know the drugs are doing their job will be if you test your blood glucose and/or you have your A1C level measured. You cannot and should not rely on the presence or absence of symptoms as a guide to the effectiveness of your diabetes medicines. To know if your blood pressure medicine is working, you will need to have your blood pressure checked. And to know if your cholesterol medicine is working, you will need to have a blood test to measure your cholesterol.

Sometimes, however, it is harder to know if a medicine is working. Let's say, for example, that you are taking aspirin to lower your risk of a heart attack. The only way you'll know the medicine is working would be if something *doesn't* happen; in this case, a heart attack. But maybe you wouldn't have had a heart attack even if you hadn't been taking aspirin. There are very many situations like this; situations where a medicine is prescribed because medical research studies show that there is likely to be a benefit to *most* people taking a medicine, even if it is impossible to prove that the drug is going to help a *specific* individual. Basically, we are playing the odds that you, too, will benefit from a medication, even if we can't know it for certain.

Know What Side Effects To Look Out For

Every medicine has the potential to cause side effects. And if you're like most people, you've likely seen a long, intimidating—or downright frightening—list of possible drug side effects on an information sheet that your pharmacist gave to you when you picked up your prescription medicine. Or maybe you've seen an equally scary list when looking up information on the Internet. Or maybe you saw some article in the newspaper or heard from a friend about the dangers of this or that drug.

So yes, all medicines have the potential to cause side effects and some of these side effects can be very dangerous indeed. However, there's a "but" for you to be aware of… and it's a big but at that. Actually, there are several buts for you to know:

- Although drugs can cause many different side effects, *most people experience no side effects at all.*
- If side effects are experienced, they are usually minor and quickly go away once a drug is discontinued.
- Serious side effects from most drugs occur only *very rarely.*
- For most drugs, if you don't have side effects soon after starting a medicine, they are unlikely to occur later.

The problem with the side-effect information found in drug information sheets or on the Web is that it typically just lists information without putting things in context. Seldom does this information talk about how rare it is for dangerous side effects to occur.

The next time you are prescribed a drug, I would recommend you ask your doctor and your pharmacist the following three questions:

- What are the common side effects of which you should be aware?
- What are serious side effects of which you should be aware?
- What should you do if you think you are having a side effect?

To illustrate this, let's say you have been prescribed metformin and you've asked the preceding three questions. These would be my answers:

- Common side effects: nausea, vomiting, abdominal cramps, diarrhea
- Serious side effects: lactic acid build-up in the body

- What to do if you think you're having a side effect: If you're having only mild nausea, try putting up with it for a few days and see if it goes away. If your nausea is more severe or you're having vomiting or diarrhea, stop the drug and call your doctor. If you're having severe symptoms, such as continuous vomiting, abdominal pain, and muscle aches, go to the emergency department.

What You Need To Tell Your Doctor
When They're Prescribing A Drug For You

In order to help ensure that you get a prescription that will work safely and effectively, anytime your doctor is prescribing a drug for you, make sure you let them know:

- *If you have any drug allergies.* Importantly, if you are allergic to one type of drug within a certain family of drugs, you might also be allergic to other drugs within that family. For example, if you have had an allergic reaction to penicillin, you might also have an allergic reaction to amoxicillin.
- *If you have any drug intolerances.* A drug intolerance differs from a drug allergy in that it is not related to the immune system. An example of a drug intolerance would be injection-site irritation from glargine insulin.
- *If you've taken the same medication before and had difficulties with it.* This may or may not require a different drug be used. For example, if you had a bothersome cough when you took ramipril, there is little point taking perindopril (or other members of the ACE inhibitor family) because that drug will also give you a cough. On the other hand, if you previously had nausea when taking metformin, it may have been that you started on a higher dose than you could tolerate or you took it on an empty stomach. In both these cases, your doctor may be able to prescribe it for you again but have you start taking it in a low dose and with food and, if you tolerate the medicine, the dose can then be gradually increased.
- *If you have other health problems.* Certain other health problems may make it unsafe for you to take a medicine or may require a reduced dose. For example, if you have had problems with heart failure, you should not take pioglitazone (Actos). If you have cirrhosis of the liver, you shouldn't take metformin. If you have reduced kidney function, you will need to take a smaller dose of saxagliptin (Onglyza) than if you had normal kidney function.
- *If you are taking other prescription medications.* Certain prescription medications interact with other prescription medications that can

result in greater or lesser potency of a drug. No one can be aware of all the thousands of potential drug interactions, therefore computer programs are invaluable in helping to keep track of this. Your pharmacist will use such a program when they are filling a prescription for you. You can look this up too; check out *www.drugdigest.org*.

- *If you are taking other nonprescription drugs or "natural" products.* Just because a drug is purchased without a prescription (so-called "over-the-counter" drugs) doesn't guarantee it is necessarily safe to take nor does it mean it cannot cause side effects or interact with other medications. For example, if you are taking iron pills and ingest them at the same time as thyroid medication, the thyroid medication may not be absorbed properly into your body. And if you are taking a "natural" product such as St. John's wort, it can affect how a prescription drug like digoxin is working. Even seemingly innocuous products like Coenzyme Q10 and garlic can cause dangerous interactions with certain types of prescription drugs.

- *If you have a hard time remembering to take your medicines.* If this is the case, get a dosette container that has compartments marked with the day and time of day for a week. You can fill each compartment at the start of each week or, even better, ask your pharmacist to put your drugs in a blister pack.

- *If you are pregnant, are planning on becoming pregnant, or you are breast feeding.* Many drugs are unsafe for pregnant or breast feeding women to take because the drug can get into the fetus or baby's system. For example, ACE inhibitors (such as ramipril or perindopril) are unsafe to take if you are pregnant.

- *If you have a hard time swallowing pills.* If you have difficulty swallowing big pills, your doctor may be able to prescribe a medicine that comes in smaller pills. If that's not possible, ask if the pill can be crushed or chewed, then swallowed. Some medications can, but some cannot, as they lose some of their effectiveness if they are not swallowed whole.

- *For how long you are to take the medicine.* In most cases, if your doctor prescribes a medicine to control a condition that is not going to go away any time soon (such as diabetes or high blood pressure or high cholesterol), you should keep taking the medicine indefinitely, which means that when your prescription runs out, you need to get it refilled. This is in contrast to medicines taken for short-term problems, such as an antibiotic taken for a throat infection or a bladder infection.

- *If you're not actually planning on filling the prescription*. It comes as a shock to most physicians to find out that one out of every five prescriptions they write is likely to go unfilled. There can be a variety of reasons. Perhaps you've never filled a certain prescription because when you went to the drugstore to get the medicine, you found the price to be onerous. Or maybe you remembered that you had previously taken the drug and had side effects from it. Or maybe you simply lost the prescription your doctor wrote for you. In any event, if you aren't planning on filling a prescription or if for some other reason you don't fill a prescription, be sure to let your doctor know. Remember, you and your physician are on the same team and just like for any team, things will go better if everyone works together.

What You Need To Tell Your Pharmacist When They Are Dispensing Your Prescription

Many of the items that I list in the preceding section also fall within the domain of the pharmacist, and you can feel free to discuss those topics with your pharmacist. Other important topics that you should talk to your pharmacist about when you are having a prescription filled are:

- How many times per day should you take your medicine?
- What time of day should you take your medicine? For instance, a drug that is taken once per day may need to be taken in the morning or the evening, depending on the type of drug.
- Should you take your medicine with food or on an empty stomach?
- Are there certain foods—like grapefruit—that you must avoid because they interact with the prescription drug? You can also look this up yourself at *www.drugdigest.org*.
- Are there certain warnings (and warning labels) of which you need to be aware? For example, can the medication make you drowsy, which could make operating a vehicle or heavy equipment dangerous?
- Does the drug have an expiration date? A glucagon emergency kit (used to treat a severe episode of hypoglycemia), for example, needs to be replaced after the expiration date written on the package. (I'd suggest you make a note on your calendar to remind yourself to get your glucagon kit replaced *before* the expiration date.)
- How should you store your medication? Unopened insulin vials or cartridges, for example, should be kept refrigerated until you start using them. Blood glucose test strips should be stored in their original container.

- If a tamper-proof container isn't suitable for you, can the medication be placed in an easy-to-open container? If you have problems with arthritis, for example, you may find that the tamper-proof pill bottle you just picked up is impossible for your sore hands to open. Tell your pharmacist if you think you will need your medications dispensed to you in a container that will be easy to open. (But of course make sure you keep such a container well out of reach of children.)
- What should you do if you miss a dose of your medicine? Or inadvertently took an extra dose? In general, no harm will come to you in either of these events but best to be prepared in advance in case this situation ever presents itself.

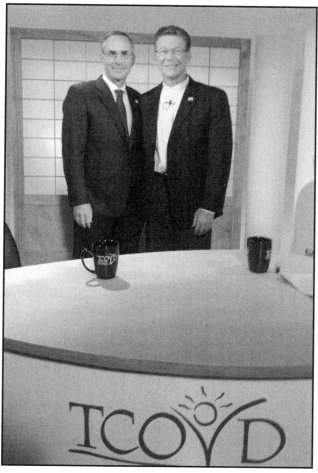

Ian Blumer appearing on a TCOYDtv show.

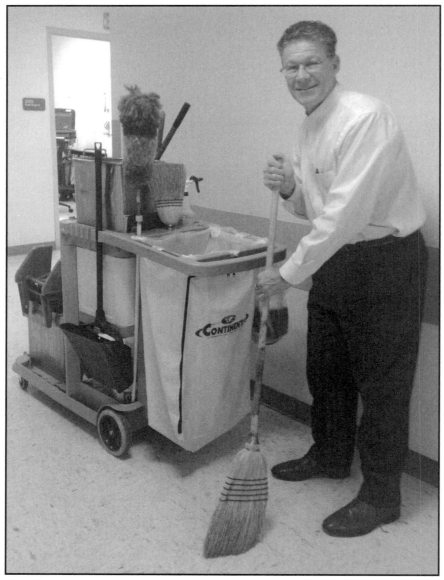

If we find a way to prevent diabetes, I will find a new profession!

28

Diabetes in the Workplace

A Great Excuse to Dodge Buying Cookies

by Urban Miyares

1968 seems like just yesterday. It was then that type 1 diabetes was diagnosed while I was serving in Vietnam with the U.S. Army, 9th Infantry Division, as a platoon sergeant. I had never heard the word diabetes before, and it seemed like I was then the only person in the world who had this disease.

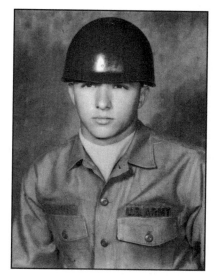

Urban Miyares in 1968 as a 20-year-old sergeant with the 9th Infantry Division in Vietnam.

After almost 6 months of medical care at Valley Forge Hospital, Pennsylvania, I was discharged from the military and returned to my wife and our apartment in New York City, where we began our lives—having been told that, at best, with me being a "brittle" (whatever that word means) diabetic, I had 20 years of productive life remaining. With my life's time-clock now quickly ticking and my wife pregnant, I had to find work right away to support my family. Then, the word "diabetes" was a hush-hush thing, even in family circles, as was the words "Vietnam veteran"—Woodstock was then a year away from happening and the anti-war protests were everywhere. I only wore my military uniform once in the civilian world, and was harassed and called names on the streets of New York City.

In the late 1960s, the workplace, especially in New York City, was lively, with the majority of us "baby boomers" seeking employment from a large corporation to get health care and other fringe benefits. With the help of a friend, I quickly was able to attract employment as a margin clerk trainee with a major stock brokerage firm. It was then, during my apprenticeship, I discovered a 100% mandatory participation health insurance program, and if you were found not qualified (health-wise), you would be dismissed from the company. I deliberately contrived ways to avoid my health exam to protect the identity of my diabetes, a reason for health insurance denial. Secretly, I hid my glass needles and syringes in my desk drawer, along with the blood sugar (urine) testing kit, my emergency stash of favorite sugar-filled candies and snacks. I felt like I was concealing a gun when I went to work at 14 Wall Street each morning, as I needed to take four or more shots of insulin each day. No one, other than my friend who got me the job, knew of my medical and military background. I was still not feeling well, as the urine blood testing method of its day was inaccurate; I intentionally maintained a high blood sugar while at work, to avoid incidents of hypoglycemia and exposure of my medical condition.

This secret life of hiding my diabetes went on for months until, one day, arriving late to work due to a subway delay; someone else sat at my desk to look for a client's file, and uncovered my hidden treasure and told the office manager. When I finally arrived to work that morning, the office manager's secretary met me at the front door and told me her boss wanted to see me right away. I thought I was going to get reprimanded for my lateness that morning or tell me they were going to put me on full-time due to the excellent work I was doing. Going into the manager's office there stood a tall, slim man, finely dressed in one of those executive, pin-striped suits that yelled "authority," I was asked to sit down and the manager, Mr. H, pulled out a box containing my desk's hidden stash and asked "What was this all about?" I responded with my story about being a Vietnam veteran and having diabetes, which required me to take insulin shots during the day, fearful of saying anything else about my other medical conditions. The firm's executive (he never mentioned his name) told me that "This firm is not going to have any needle toting, baby killing, Vietnam veteran working for it," and walked out of the office... telling Mr. H on the way out, "Take care of this." Getting the proverbial "pink slip," I returned home to our apartment, never telling anyone, not even my wife, and the real reason for my dismissal—Welcome home vet!

That was my first employment experience after military service, and what forced me into a career of entrepreneurship. Couldn't wait around to find another job, the time-clock was ticking away, and I needed to create my own employment opportunity immediately.

That was yesterday, and today's workplace is entirely different, thank goodness. As what I experienced in the workplace in 1968-1969 would not only be illegal today, but would be a terrible public relations mark for any business to have on its image or brand.

Today, with both state and federal laws protecting and making accessible and accommodating the workplace, to include those with the (hidden) disease diabetes, as well as many other medical conditions and their unique needs and challenges, along with the historical data of success and productivity of employees with diabetes, there are few trades, professions, or careers a person having diabetes can't enter... and even if there are any vocations a person with diabetes cannot work in, they sure can become its business owner, as I have learned.

Having diabetes is no longer a novelty or an unknown disease in today's workplace. With the growing number of individuals diagnosed and few people not having a family member or knowing someone with the disease, diabetes is no longer that hidden medical condition that was whispered about and had misrepresented causes and remedies. And, with Americans now living so much longer than prior generations, diabetes is already a major health care concern, with the disease having no barriers by age, ethnicity, or gender. With today's high-tech and advancing health care practices and medical devices, individuals with diabetes are able to do so much more in the workplace than 10, 20, and 30 years ago.

People with diabetes, of all ages, are active in most every vocational and professional activity today. And the lists of careers those with diabetes have or are entering are expanding each and every year. Surely technology has had a lot to do with it, but the past performance of those in the workplace having well-controlled and manageable diabetes has opened up the door to so many new employment options and opportunities for the next generation.

Key to Employment Success

The expression of "a healthy business begins with healthy employees and management" is so true. Being sick and having a disability (such as diabetes) is two entirely different things. And being in control of your diabetes is the key to successful employment and/or self-employment and business ownership for, without control, you are sick.

If you are currently employed or now looking to find a job, you need to accept there is a responsibility on your part. Not only does your existing or potential employer have a responsibility to provide the best possible product or service to clients, as well as a responsibility to vendors and you, his/her employees and their families, and then the community and society... but you too have a responsibility to be in control and able to manage your diabetes (and any other medical conditions you may have) so that you can fulfill your work responsibility as efficiently as possible. Being continually sick as an employee is unfair to your fellow workers, your employer, and the goals the company has to fulfill its commitment to others.

As an employer for more than 40 years, also being a business owner with type 1 diabetes and having many of the disease's complications during my entire business career, I have employed dozens of people with diabetes, as well as having employees be diagnosed with diabetes during their employment tenure. In my experience, those who were not in control of their diabetes often made more demands and created more havoc and chaos on the job than those who were in full control and able to manage their medical condition.

Common employment behavior and work issues I've experienced by those with poorly managed diabetes include, but are not limited to:

- The tendency to be late for work, meetings, and breaks more often... and always offering an excuse as to why
- Leaving their desk or work area for breaks (more than the norm) to supposedly test their blood sugars, take medication or insulin, emergency bathroom visits, have a snack, get a drink of water, or take a walk outside, etc
- Seemingly scheduling doctor visits during their work shift, with often emergency doctor visits being more a norm
- Appearring to be tired more often
- Having dramatic changes in mood and personality, especially with co-workers
- Absenteeism—there is a tendency to be absent more and taking longer to recover from an illness than others who have their diabetes under control or than those not having the disease
- More frequent (reported) minor injuries on the job, regardless of job responsibility
- Being less inclined to take on more responsibility in their job with or without the company adding in more benefits or other perks for them personally, eg, making additional personal demands
- Being more likely to request special accommodations and accessibility than others with (controlled) diabetes.

Yes, as an employer these and other issues bring up concern in hiring of those with diabetes, as well as in fulfilling my commitment to existing employees with the disease. But, also, in the businesses I've owned, there have been a number of employees with well-controlled diabetes who have elevated in the company and, in a couple of instances, have actually gone on to become business owners of their own. As a business owner with diabetes who works a minimum of 60 to 80 hours per week, and who seldom is so sick that I am unable to get to the office, you can imagine how I feel and want to react to those employees with uncontrolled diabetes and their excuses, whether directly or indirectly related to diabetes. I am fully sensitive to their issues and concerns and, in my early business career, I learned that letting employees know that I (too) had diabetes, seemed to discourage their excuses... they either took better control of their diabetes and got healthier, or they quit.

Just Diagnosed With Diabetes?

If you've just been diagnose with diabetes. Relax; get your diabetes under control and you'll discover there are few—if any—restrictions in your chosen work or current employment that you are unable to perform. And don't be surprised that with (controlled) diabetes, you may now better perform your work tasks more efficiently.

However, if you find your current or chosen work not compatible, whether or not due to having diabetes, a new or parallel career path might be an option to consider. You can either:

1. Select a new career direction, with your diabetes as a fact, and investigate the requirement (education, vocational training, licenses, etc) that would be needed, or
2. Launch a business in that chosen career or profession—there are many business owners with diabetes who own trucking companies, ambulance services, and even airplane instruction and charter ventures. Again, those with diabetes are involved in almost, if not every profession, business, and vocation.

Personal Note

In one of my previous businesses, I had an employee come to my office to tell me something—he was hiding a secret for months. Sitting down in front of my desk he said, "Mr. Miyares, I have diabetes." Before he could say another word, I enthusiastically jumped up and loudly said, "Congratulations!!! Me too." He worked for me for 3 years before he left to open up his own business.

Tips To Help You in the Workplace

- *Take Control Of Your Diabetes!* There is a saying in business that the key to success of any business is a healthy owner and staff. And with diabetes, maintaining good control and being able to manage your diabetes in all situations is critical. Being sick and having a person with controlled diabetes are two entirely different things.

- *Begin to Take Control Today.* If you have a higher than acceptable A1C blood test reading, having any complications starting or evidence—such as being overweight, retinopathy, neuropathy, kidney disease, etc—and/or have secondary medical issues, getting a firm grip on your diabetes control and management is critical. As I've discovered, it's not too late, regardless of the severity of any medical condition and how long one has had this condition, to get aggressive and make a firm, long-term commitment to better controlling your diabetes. The end result will shock you, and may actually improve or mitigate an existing complication of diabetes or other medical issue. I've discovered this with everything from my kidney disease and neuropathy challenges, to better handling other (non-diabetes related) medical matters.

- *Blood Testing.* It's often not how often you test your blood sugars, but when you test. For me, while at work, I will test my blood sugar before each meal, but also before any decision-making occasion (business meetings, conference calls, appointments, etc.) or when I'm in the creative mood. Getting to know how your body and mind functions best, and at what blood-sugar level, is most important to increasing personal productivity. And even with my blindness, testing my blood sugar takes only a matter of seconds, and can be done comfortably and relatively unnoticed.

- *Food Intake.* I've discovered that I work best with a good breakfast (oatmeal is my favorite); a snack (fruit or food bar) around mid-morning; a light lunch (salad or possibly half a sandwich); an afternoon snack (or appetizers at a "business" Happy Hour); and, then a moderate-sized dinner. If I choose to have dessert, then it's often taken as a before-bedtime snack, depending on what my blood sugar is. Of course, checking my blood sugars beforehand, in most instances. And I drink quite a bit of water, generally a glass (8 oz) before or with each meal, along with a glass of water with each cup of coffee or tea I have.

I readily acknowledge that my work day is quite different than most, with an average work week of 80 hours or more, and traveling 100,000-plus air miles each year. With this, I hope you can see why maintaining control of my diabetes is a more than a full-time concern—it's a life style.

- *Attitude*. Feel good about yourself and having diabetes. If your diabetes is under control, this will be easy. But if control is currently an issue with you, this will be reflected in your workplace attitude, job performance, and how you intermingle with coworkers. Take a serious look at yourself and your attitude. What is your personality like? Do you dress and present yourself as someone who is happy with life and having a job? If not, something has to change, and that's you... and an attitude adjustment may be warranted.

- *Make Sure You're Doing What You Want to Do*. Too often I see individuals with diabetes in a profession or on a career path that might sound good and provide the income they need for personal living expenses and in planning the future, but they really are not happy with their job and its future. If this is your situation and you feel change is in order, a suggestion is to include "diabetes" when thinking of changing career or starting on a new career path. This is where additional education might come into play, or learning a new skill, and talking with someone who is already in that field to learn as much as you can about its requirements and commitment. If it's a consideration of starting your own business, whether full- or part-time, attend a local college or Small Business Administration work-shop, or send me an email: Urban@DisabledBusiness.com.

Personal Note

With a diabetes diagnosis in 1968, I guess, accidentally, I discovered business ownership as my profession of choice. Not necessarily because I had always dreamed of owning businesses, but more associated to me being told I only had a shortened lifespan and the need to support my family. For me, entrepreneurship offered me the opportunity to control my environment, my schedule, my commitments, and my income. I understood early on what my personality traits and what my goals were. And if I lived longer than predicted by the doctors, I would have done so much more than others who took the more traveled path of life.

On A Job Interview, Should You Say You Have Diabetes?

In my opinion, the answer is "No!" If diabetes is not a clearly identified legal or licensing barrier to fulfill a job description in an interview, it should not be an issue for employment consideration. If it is, the job interviewer should state this and all other requirements for that job. Once you've been accepted for employment, then you need to make a decision, based on your job and the work environment, on whether or not you want to tell others you have diabetes. But I do strongly recommend that your supervisor and coworkers know that you have diabetes. This disclosure will help you in the long term and help to eliminate rumors and false statements being spread around the workplace. Besides, I wouldn't be surprised that fellow workers also have diabetes or have a family member with the disease... and remember, as I say in many of my speeches, "Sooner or later, you're going to be one of us."

Legal Issues in the Workplace

Are you experiencing a work-related (legal) issue where you work because of an employer or manager's lack of sensitivity to your needs with diabetes? If so, rest assured that you do have a number of legal rights, both state and federal laws to possibly help you in making your workplace environment more accommodating, safe, and accessible. But first, evaluate yourself and are these personal needs due to you not being in control of your diabetes or because of another workplace barrier or issue that endangers your well-being or workplace performance.

In some instances, your issues with your employer may not be a "disability-related" matter (under the American's with Disabilities Act or other disability-rights laws) or not applicable to the company, due to its size or financial resources. Legal counsel is strongly suggested in any/all employment issues if you firmly believe you need relief.

10 Advantages to Having Diabetes in the Workplace... and Letting Everyone Know

1. You get invited to more parties because they think you're not going to eat or drink as much. (Yeah... Right.)
2. Fellow workers will want you to manage the company softball team, as they think you're too frail to play a competitive sport like softball. (Go and show them who is fragile.)

3. People are hesitant in asking you to buy cookies, even though they now have diet cookies… and you're seldom asked to bake a cake or cookies for a Bake Sale; fearful that no one will buy any diet goodies from you.

4. For Men. Women feel less threatened by you because everyone knows that diabetes causes impotency. (Love those old-aged beliefs.)

5. For Women. When it's one of those moments of anger, frustration, confusion, mood swings, or negativisms, you can always say it was your "low blood sugar." Okay guys, you can use this excuse too.

6. You have a great excuse of cutting a meeting or phone call short— "got to test my blood sugar"—or being later or absent from meetings, appointments, or events.

7. When waiting for a table at a restaurant, you can always say you have a low blood sugar and need to eat right away. If that doesn't get you a table quicker, at least you'll get a glass of juice.

8. If you sport a larger-than-desired belly, having a protruding insulin pump on your waistband/belt will help hide some of the calories (weight) you've been working on getting off your waistline… and you have a good excuse to go out and buy Hawaiian "Aloha Shirts"… wearing them or your others shirts/blouses outside of your belt.

9. When invited to parties, the hostess/host always checks on you to make sure you've had enough to eat and drink, and if there is anything else they can do for you. (Nice.)

10. And, if you have a doctor who also has diabetes, you can always compare your blood tests with his/hers. When your doctor doesn't want to do the comparisons any longer, you know you're doing good and under (better) control with your diabetes than he or she may be.

Closing

With good control of your diabetes, you'll discover that the workplace as well as being involved in any other exciting and challenging activity can be rewarding, regardless of your age or other circumstances. Diabetes is commonplace today, much like asthma, allergies, and other generally-accepted hidden medical conditions. It's when diabetes is uncontrolled and mismanaged that it becomes a complication and issue in the workplace. So put taking control of your diabetes as priority #1, and you too will find the workplace to be a friendly and rewarding activity that will assure you of happiness and good health.

About the Author

Urban Miyares has been an entrepreneur with diabetes, and other medical conditions, since 1968, and has launched or run more than 20 business enterprises. A national-known blinded Vietnam veteran, Miyares, has been recognized for his achievements in business, accomplishments in sports, and service to the community by Presidents of the United States, U.S. Congress and Small Business Administration, state governors, and many others, to include being the recipient of Inc. Magazine's "Entrepreneur Of The Year," "SBA's National Small Business Advocate," "National Disabled Veteran

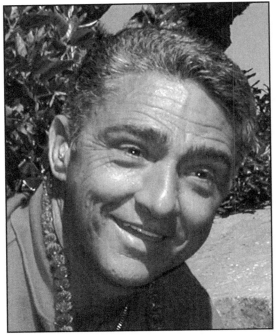

URBAN MIYARES is a nationally recognized blinded Vietnam veteran with type 1 diabetes, an entrepreneur, motivational speaker, writer, media personality, and world-class athlete. Miyares is founder of the charitable Disabled Businesspersons Association, co-founder of Challenged America, and mentor with YEP! (Young Entrepreneur Program).

of the Year," U.S. National (Alpine) Ski Champion, and Transpacific Yacht Race skipper.

Living in San Diego with his wife of 45 years, Urban is founder and president of the charitable Disabled Businesspersons Association (DBA) and its programs: National Disabled Veterans Business Center, Special Kids in Business, and Challenged America

Urban Miyares was the first keynote speaker in the TCOYD program, and continues to attend and participate in many TCOYD Conferences and health fairs around the nation.

Urban can be reached at Urban@DisabledBusiness.com or Port@ ChallengedAmerica.org.

29

Managing Type Zero Diabetes Takes Some Serious Effort

Legal Issues for People With Diabetes

by Kriss S. Halpern, JD

Dealing with Type Zero (Type 0) Diabetes Can Be Tough

Some of us have Type 1 diabetes. Some of us have Type 2. Some of us refer to those in our lives who know what we deal with, who try to help us out, as people with Type 3 diabetes. There is another common type of diabetes that we come across that I'd like to discuss: Type 0.

Type 0 is my term for people who know little or nothing about this illness. They may be our neighbors; our employers, coworkers or employees; people we meet socially, at school, or in stores; folks we deal with professionally, who sell us goods or services; their employees and agents we see in an office or talk with on the phone. I was a Type 0 all my life, until I was diagnosed Type 1 and began having to look at plates of food as numbers and wondering how the heck I was gonna pay for all the stuff the doctors told me I needed so I wouldn't go blind, lose a foot, or have my kidneys check out.

Over the 30 years since my diagnosis, diabetes has been described as an epidemic, especially among those with Type 2 (see **Figure 29-1** for the ever-increasing numbers of US citizens diagnosed with diabetes since 1958). Public awareness about diabetes increased exponentially, along with remarkable improvements in care. The percentage of US citizens diagnosed grew from less than 1% in 1950 to around 7% in 2010. As a result, most Americans know someone with diabetes and most Americans know something about the illness. A little bit of knowledge is not terribly useful if it is not understood. Misinformed and misapplied opinions lead to prejudice and unfair treatment.

Along with needing to learn how to understand and manage this illness for ourselves, we also need to learn how to live and work with the Type 0's among us… the police officer we come across when we have low blood sugar; the boss who doesn't want us taking a shot of insulin at work; the waiter who sees us looking confused but does not know what is going on or how to respond to it.

Figure 29-1

Number and Percentage of US Population With Diagnosed Diabetes, 1958-2010

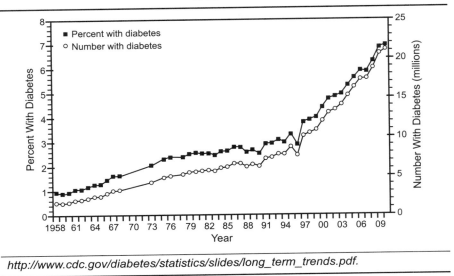

http://www.cdc.gov/diabetes/statistics/slides/long_term_trends.pdf.

Laws exist to help guide and control these interactions so society handles them more fairly. This chapter is a short guide in how to work with some of those laws so you can handle these interactions a little more easily. The best-case scenario is that you learn how to anticipate and avoid problems. If that doesn't work, then it may help to know that solutions may exist to solving problems that cannot be avoided. Having this disease is not only about learning to understand it for ourselves, it is also about having to teach others what we know as an ongoing part of life.

Health Care Reform Helping Overcome Hurdles in Handling Type 0's

Those who have never been diagnosed with a serious chronic illness may have no idea what it means to be refused the right to purchase health insurance. They may have never been forced to face the reality of losing desperately-needed health care, gone months trying to survive a complication setback because they couldn't purchase the most basic management tools for an illness, or forced into bankruptcy when bills became overwhelming and they ran out of luck and resources. People with diabetes are obliged to deal with a kind of societal Type 0 as we struggle to obtain the right to live and work and remain contributing, functioning members of society.

As this book goes to publication, we have learned that the Patient Protection and Affordable Care Act (ACA or "the Affordable Care Act," also known as "Obamacare") has been upheld by the U.S. Supreme Court. There remain extraordinary divisions over those reforms and all we know for sure is that those battles will continue as health care costs remain overwhelming and health care remains out of reach for millions of people. The ACA offers improvements that are real for persons with diabetes and provides us with some meaningful tools to obtain improved care more affordably and remain functioning members of society. Here are some examples:

1. The ACA ends all preexisting condition exclusions for children under age 19. In short, insurers may not discriminate against children of persons enrolled in their plans by excluding or limiting their coverage. Previously, insurance plans could make parents wait 6 months or longer for children to be covered for preexisting conditions when a parent enrolled, or sometimes refused enrollment altogether based on a preexisting condition.

2. The ACA allows all young adults to remain covered on the health insurance plan of a parent until age 26 (**Figure 29-2**).

3. The ACA ends all lifetime limitations in health care coverage plans renewed since it went into effect. Previously, health care plans typically had lifetime limits on insurance coverage so that if you became severely ill and needed extraordinary levels of expensive care, you could reach a plan's limit and receive no further care under the plan. Under the ACA, those limitations are unlawful. The same will be true for annual cost limitations as of January 1, 2014. Annual cost limitations are being decreased until then, with annual limitations no less than $2 million as of September 2012 when this book will be published. Persons on Medicare or Medicaid are already protected since annual health care cost limitations are already banned for them.

4. The ACA places limits on Medical Loss Ratios (MLRs). An MLR is the portion of premiums a policy pays on actual health care for plan participants, as opposed to profits, investments, and costs such as executive salaries, advertisements, insurance company administration and related office expenses. All large group plans must now spend no less than 85% of premiums, and all small or individual group plans no less than 80% of premiums, on actual health care such as office visits to health care professionals, medi-

Figure 29-2

Percentage of Young Adults With Health Insurance, 2009-2011 by Quarter and Age Group

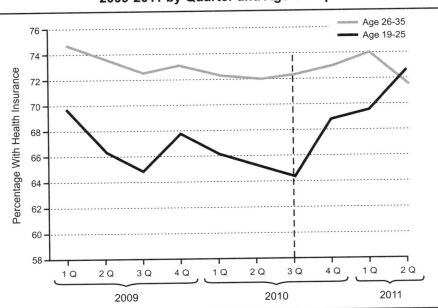

New results from the National Health Interview Survey (NHIS) indicate that 3.1 million additional young adults have insurance coverage as of December 2011, due to the provision in the Affordable Care Act that allows 19 through 25 year olds to remain on their parents' insurance plans.

http://aspe.hhs.gov/health/reports/2011/YoungAdultsACA/ib.shtml.

cations, hospitalizations, and medical equipment and supplies. When annual MLR obligations are not reached, plan members must be reimbursed their premium overpayments.

5. The ACA ends the denial of coverage for persons with preexisting conditions, such as diabetes, as of 2014. See **Figure 29-3** to determine whether the "individual mandate" will apply to your circumstances and require you to purchase health insurance.

For the first time in the history of the United States, no one with diabetes (or any other illness) can be denied the right to purchase health care insurance. The ACA has a wide variety of rules and regulations designed to require that the health care plans offered meet minimum coverage requirements at an affordable cost. We will be allowed to comparison shop among plans on Exchanges set up in each state. Be-

Figure 29-3

The Requirement to Buy Coverage Under the Affordable Care Act
(Created by Kaiser Family Foundation)

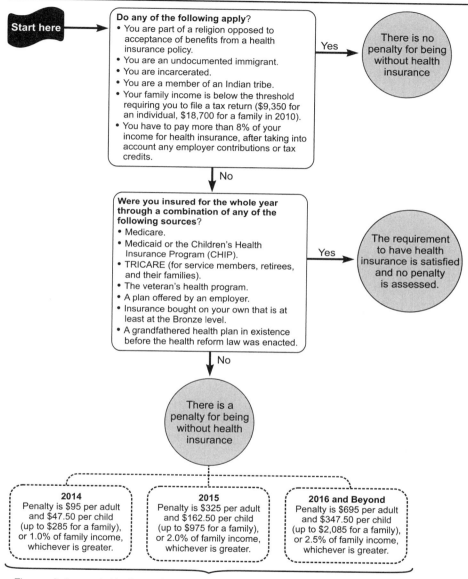

The penalty is pro-rated by the number of months without coverage, though there is no penalty for a single gap in coverage of less than 3 months in a year. The penalty cannot be greater than the national average premium for Bronze level coverage in an Exchange. After 2016, penalty amounts are increased annually by the cost of living.

http://healthreform.kff.org/en/the-basics/requirement-to-buy-coverage-flowchart.aspx.

fore 2014, when the Exchanges begin, certain essential benefits that each plan must provide will be determined by the federal department of Health and Human Services (HHS).

These changes will be of extraordinary benefit to persons with diabetes living in the United States. They will end many of the risks we face from being denied good and affordable health care. But the reforms are very far from perfect and none of us can foresee how well they will protect us in reality. We will need to remain vigilant in remaining aware of our own health care needs. We will need to be able to explain to the Type 0's responsible for managing the plans what our needs are. Understanding diabetes and having the ability to explain what we need to manage our own illness will remain critical tools moving forward. That much is certain.

The Impact of Health Care Reform on Existing Legislation Pertaining to Diabetes Care

Since the 1990s, 46 states passed legislation sponsored by the American Diabetes Association (ADA) mandating coverage for critical diabetes needs such as medical visits, training, medical equipment, and supplies to manage blood sugars. Those laws make it easier for persons with diabetes to receive coverage for visits to doctors, nurses, dietitians, and nutritionists, better training in managing blood glucose, the purchase of newer and better tools such as insulin pumps, sufficient chemstrips, or continuous glucose monitors. Studies show that mandating coverage for improved care improves the long-term health of persons with diabetes and does so at a lower cost.

During the health care reform debate, it was argued by some that state mandates on health insurance coverage were a wasteful expense that increased the cost of health care coverage. In the case of diabetes care and insurance coverage, study after study has shown that this argument is wrong. Insurance coverage that provides care which helps improve blood glucose management dramatically reduces both health complications and health care costs.

This website, www.healthcare.gov, is currently a terrific tool to try and find health care options and compare various plans in your state. Another marvelous site to learn about affordable health care options can be found online at the web site of the Artists Health Insurance Resource Center directory, or www.AHIRC.org.

Once the Exchanges are set up, these Web sites will be even better. By requiring plans to promote and advertise themselves based on health outcomes of plan members, all plans will be encouraged to improve those outcomes at an affordable price compared with other plans. By making health care results easier to assess, the ACA will give us the tools needed to understand what we are buying before we enroll. By giving us the ability to know what coverage we will receive in standard, easy to read formats, the ACA will increase our ability to determine whether the kind of coverage, equipment, and supplies needed to manage our illness will be available to us under a particular plan.

Second, the essential benefits required among insurance plans include, among other things, treatment for management of chronic illnesses such as diabetes. Since the federal government will now be determining what minimum benefits must be provided, there will no longer be the issue of a particular plan deciding to cut costs. Now, the federal government will make these determinations and will have those eventual outcomes and savings as an ongoing concern. It will be in the interest of the federal government to make certain that proper care is provided to persons with a chronic illness in order to avoid expensive complications that would otherwise develop over time.

The list of the types of essential benefits to be included in the ACA includes:

- Ambulatory patient services
- Emergency services
- Hospitalization
- Maternity and newborn care
- Mental health and substance use disorder services, including behavioral health treatment
- Prescription drugs
- Rehabilitative and habilitative services and devices
- Laboratory services
- Preventive and wellness services and chronic disease management
- Pediatric services, including oral and vision care

Third, states may require that insurance plans offered in that state provide certain mandated coverages, such as those sponsored by the ADA and currently approved in 46 states. However, if such mandates cause increased premiums, then states must cover those costs for in-state plan members who qualify for certain types of federal financial assistance.

The benefit to these federal reforms are that persons with diabetes will now receive certain minimal levels of care regardless of where they are living in the United States. It will now be easier for changes to be made in those benefits once evidence demonstrates that they are needed since it will require implementation through rules of a single federal agency rather than passage by each state legislature.

There are, however, risks that go along with these reforms. It has been argued that plans may seek to discourage enrollment of persons with chronic illnesses by not providing coverage that would be beneficial, unless ordered to do so. If, for example, a plan wanted to encourage persons with diabetes to join, it might offer to pay for a Continuous Glucose Monitor when requested. If it wanted to discourage persons with diabetes from joining, it might refuse all such requests. Thus it is argued that persons with a chronic illness that would benefit from such coverage would avoid plans that refused it, allowing that plan to avoid more expensive plan members by discouraging them with lesser benefits. Another argument made is that federal bureaucrats will now be responsible for determining what medical needs are deemed essential. In a time of extraordinary budget deficits, there may be short-term cuts in coverage to pinch pennies, despite the inevitability of higher costs down the road as a result. These risks are real and should not be ignored. However, these same exact risks exist within the Medicare system, and the fact remains that Medicare has been among the most popular and successful government programs of the last 100 years.

It will be critical that persons with diabetes advocate to make certain that our needs are supported under the essential benefits mandated by the ACA. The health care benefits and resulting cost savings from them will continue to be our strongest evidence that the right and healthier decisions will be the same as the more affordable ones.

Federal laws providing additional options to persons with diabetes remain in effect (**Table 29-1**). For example, COBRA laws allowing persons on group plans to continue their health insurance coverage for 18 months after leaving a job will continue. HIPAA laws regarding "guaranteed issue" plans that prohibit an insurance carrier from refusing to sell a policy so long as an application to become a member is made within 63 days of the group plan ending, also remain in force. It may be that there will be better and more affordable coverage available after 2014—especially in comparison to the "guaranteed issue" plans promoted by HIPAA since the cost of those plans are not regulated— but the options provided by these federal laws will remain. In the case of COBRA policies, this will likely continue to be a significant benefit as COBRA coverage allows a plan member to receive what may be high quality care with preferred health care providers at a regulated cost. For many, this may remain a preferred option. The law allowing COBRA coverage for up to 18 months remains in force.

Another federal health care coverage option that will remain includes Health Savings Accounts (HSAs) which allow us to create tax-deductible savings plans that can be used to pay for medical care so long as we purchase a high deductible plan to go with it. A helpful guide to HSAs and how to use them was created by the Mayo Clinic and can be found on its website: *http://www.mayoclinic.com/health/health-savings-accounts/GA00053*. Certain problems with these plans continue to exist. Many people find it much easier to join an existing insurance plan where purchase options and decisions are made for them. There is also frustration in getting actual cost information provided by physicians and hospitals, as well as even being accepted for care by many physicians, if you are not on a plan. The ACA did not seek to address these concerns. To the extent we have found ways to work with these problems and want to use HSAs, we can continue to do so.

For many persons, especially those with fewer health care needs, HSAs remain a tool to consider. All of us can anticipate the approximate cost of a bronze plan under the Exchanges by looking at the cost of high-deductible plans under HSA regulations. Keep in mind that those plan premiums are subject to annual inflation adjustments; and final determinations about premiums for plans that will be available in 2014 have not yet been made as of the publication date of this book.

Explaining Our Illness to Others Remains Critical to Living Well with Diabetes

In virtually every instance of resolving lifestyle problems for folks with diabetes, the key is explaining our needs to people we live and work with on a daily basis.

Identifying ourselves as a person with diabetes can mean the difference between life and death when hypoglycemia becomes overwhelming. Explaining our diabetes management needs is critical to working with a health care plan; maintaining a child's safety in school; keeping safe and secure employment; getting and keeping a driver's license; or receiving proper medical care in an institutional setting.

Receiving Better Care From a Health Plan

Regardless of what type of health plan we are on, understanding and explaining our health care needs will remain critical. Whatever minimal benefits health care reform requires health care plans to provide, we will still need to know and be able to request what we need for our individual care. Doing this continues to require:

- Learning what new tools and treatments are available
- Asking your health care provider about them

Table 29-1

Staying Insured

When a job or other relationship that provided health insurance ends, there are three ways to stay insured other than getting a new job that provides group health coverage:

1. **COBRA**: This 1986 federal law provides continuing health coverage for employees, their spouses, and dependent children when the employee loses a job either voluntarily or involuntarily for reasons other than gross misconduct.

   "COBRA provides certain former employees, retirees, spouses, former spouses, and dependent children the right to temporary continuation of health coverage at group rates. This coverage, however, is only available when coverage is lost due to certain specific events. Group health coverage for COBRA participants is usually more expensive than health coverage for active employees, since usually the employer pays a part of the premium for active employees while COBRA participants generally pay the entire premium themselves. It is ordinarily less expensive, though, than individual health coverage." [Quoted from the US Department of Labor's website at *http://www.dol.gov/ebsa/faqs/faq_consumer_cobra.html*]

   Group health plans for an employer with 20 or more employees on more than 50% of its typical business days in the previous calendar year are subject to COBRA. COBRA lasts for 18 months after the change in employment and that period can be extended in the case of a disability which began within the first 60 days of COBRA coverage if the Social Security Administration approves the application for COBRA extension and this information is timely provided to the health plan.

2. **HIPAA**: This 1996 federal law guarantees the right to purchase new health insurance after coverage under a group plan, such as COBRA, continuation benefits end.

   "HIPAA amended the Employee Retirement Income Security Act (ERISA), to provide new rights and protections for participants and beneficiaries in group health plans. Understanding this amendment is important to your decisions about future health coverage. HIPAA contains protections both for health coverage offered in connection with employment (group health plans) and for individual insurance policies sold by insurance companies (individual policies)." [Quoted from the US Department of Labor's website at *http://www.dol.gov/ebsa/faqs/faq_consumer_hipaa.html*]

If you received health care coverage that ended and you apply for an individual plan within 63 days of the prior coverage ending, you cannot be refused coverage under a new individual plan due to a preexisting condition.

Continued

Table 29-1 *(continued)*

If you received health care coverage that ended and you apply to be included in a new group plan within 63 days of the prior coverage ending, you cannot be refused coverage for a preexisting condition unless you received treatment for that condition in the 6 months before the new coverage began and then coverage for that preexisting condition can only be excluded for the first twelve months of new coverage (unless you enrolled after the time you were first allowed to begin coverage, in which case the preexisting condition exclusion may be extended to 18 months).

Problem with both COBRA and HIPAA: *Cost.* Individuals on COBRA coverage must pay the cost of the insurance themselves; plans selling individuals coverage under HIPAA rules are not limited in how much they can charge for coverage. The cost for COBRA coverage is generally not exorbitant but if you are unemployed and have no savings, that cost can be prohibitive. The cost for HIPAA coverage is often exorbitant and grossly unfair—the law says only that coverage must be offered, it does not prohibit a plan from offering coverage at an unfair and excessive rate.

- If a treatment appears to make sense for you, discussing it with your physician
- Sending a health insurer whatever articles or information you can obtain to show why this new treatment is likely to benefit your care any time a needed request is denied
- Asking your physician to support your request with a letter or note of some kind (if possible, try drafting it yourself and asking your physician to improve it as he or she thinks best and then get it signed and send it to your insurer)
- Contacting the manufacturer of the tool or medication you want and asking what materials they have to support your request
- Sending an explanatory letter to your insurer along with these supporting documents and follow-up with calls to find out what is being done and why; taking notes of who is saying what at your plan about your request (Remember: explain why you need this particular tool or medicine or treatment. Answer these questions: What is it about this item that will likely improve my diabetes care? Why can the same improvement not be achieved with some other already approved item? If you can answer these questions, you have the basis for a good claim.)
- Appealing any denial of needed care to your health plan
- If the denial is not overturned, making sure you understand why and then, if appropriate, appealing to whatever government agency

has oversight over your plan. (This can be a State or Federal agency depending on whether you are on a Medicare plan under Federal authority, or an individual or group plan under State authority.) In 2014 there will be new and simple appeal requirements for all health care plans on the Exchanges.

The idea is to be able to explain what we need and why we need it to someone with little or no understanding of diabetes. These steps more often than not achieve the result requested. Most people give up somewhere along the way in seeking improved health care after an initial denial. It can take real effort to get new treatments approved, but when you refuse to give up on getting something that you need to improve your health care, you are improving health care both for yourself and for others (**Table 29**-1).

Avoiding the Loss of a Driver's License.

The key to ending a suspension is always to make sure the suspended driver truly understands diabetes well enough and handles his or her own diabetes well enough to be able to drive safely. Again, explaining this to someone with little or no understanding of diabetes is key. Realizing that sometimes the person without enough knowledge is ourself is critical.

As an attorney representing persons whose driving license has been suspended, my goal is to make sure my client understands how to drive safely and can explain that ability when questioned about it.

Once I believe my client can drive safely, it is fairly easy for me to prove to the Department of Motor Vehicles (DMV) why I do. I suspect that many of my clients would tell you they had a harder time convincing me they were safe to drive than they did convincing the DMV. By the time I prepare them for a DMV hearing, it should be fairly easy for them to answer questions honestly and accurately in a way that will prove they can drive safely. I may feel sorry for someone who is not allowed to drive, but that is not enough. I need to know they can drive safely before I help them back on the road.

In my fee agreements, I require my clients to sign a Safe Driving Agreement before I will represent them (**Table 29**-2). This part of my fee agreement is not something I could ever enforce. But legal enforcement of this agreement is not the point. I have never represented anyone who did not want to drive safely or who was so irresponsible that they did not care. Usually, it was just a matter of making sure my client was knowledgeable about diabetes and whatever their own personal needs were. Sometimes, it was a matter of getting improved care

Table 29-2

Safe Driving Agreement

You acknowledge your understanding that I am not willing to risk my professional reputation and emotional well-being on behalf of a driver who is not willing to operate a motor vehicle safely to the best of his or her ability. You therefore assure me that you will (*you must initial each numbered statement below or I will not represent you*):

1. Test your blood glucose immediately prior to driving _____

2. Test your blood glucose at least every 2 hours on every occasion in which you drive for more than 2 hours _____

3. Keep your blood test meter with you at all times while driving _____

4. Keep something with you to treat a low blood glucose reaction in sufficient quantities to raise your blood glucose to a safe level at all times while driving _____

5. Never knowingly drive with a low blood glucose level that may impair your ability to drive safely _____

6. Work with a licensed health care provider to assist you to recognize or regain the ability to recognize low blood glucose reactions if at any time it becomes apparent that you are unable to recognize a low blood glucose level _____

for some reason, either because my client was not being treated by a physician with adequate knowledge of the best diabetes care practices or because my client was not adequately trained in knowing how to recognize and avoid hypoglycemia (low blood glucose) incidents. Fortunately, in my experience, DMV officers responsible for suspensions are becoming much more experienced and knowledgeable in understanding and handling diabetes-related suspensions. Regardless of the reason for the suspension or what an attorney needs to be able to do to end one, the truth is that all of us can improve our diabetes care and live more safely by paying more attention day to day. My Safe Driving Agreement is really just a way to encourage my clients to think a little more about what they are doing and to make sure they understand some simple ways to avoid problems.

Preventing Discrimination in the Workplace and Other Public Settings

Sometimes we need to make sure our employer understands our illness and what we need to we manage it. Sometimes we come across businesses or government agencies that do not treat us fairly.

As advances in the treatment of diabetes occur that help us to manage diabetes better and more safely, there are fewer and fewer jobs where having diabetes should ever be a serious issue. Most often, when I have been asked to assist clients with job-discrimination concerns, my role has been to help my client write a letter about diabetes and what the employer can do to provide reasonable accommodations that will allow the employee to handle the job without difficulty. Most honest and worthwhile employers receive these letters without recrimination or difficulty. Some welcome them and are pleased to assist their employee to handle their job well and safely.

Similar issues arise in a wide variety of public settings. I recently represented a child playing volleyball with a club at a recreation center that did not allow the children to take food into the facility. My letter to the facility explained why this was harmful and dangerous for her, as well as why it was unlawful. That was all that was needed. The facility owner listened to my explanation and promptly changed the rules to accommodate children with diabetes who needed better access to food so that they could have an equal ability to take part in athletics.

It is not always obvious or easy to decide when to share your illness with a stranger. There are some occasions when you should not. For example, in the case of telling an employer about your diabetes during a job interview it is sometimes best to leave that information for discussion at a later time. Not only should you not mention it during a job interview (unless, of course, you are applying to work with a pharmaceutical company selling blood glucose meters or something along those lines. In that case, having diabetes might help you get hired so you may as well brag about it and let them know right off), it is usually unlawful for them to ask.

When and how can an employer learn about your diabetes? After they make the job offer, but only if all applicants for this position are treated equally and only if there is some legitimate work-based necessity for the medical information (for example, an applicant to be a police officer may need to demonstrate physical fitness before being hired). Some companies may require that you complete a physical and that they will offer you a job pending satisfactory results. This is lawful if the examination is truly job related. If they then refuse to hire you, there will be clear evidence of why they did so and this can be reviewed to make sure it was lawful and not really a pretext to refuse to hire someone with a chronic illness. Any refusal to hire someone because of diabetes must be based on an actual review of the individual job applicant's health and some legitimate reason why that individual cannot safely and adequately perform the job in question.

Diabetes is sometimes simply misunderstood by a supervisor or employer. Diabetes is sometimes resented out of concern that an employee with a chronic illness may cause an increase in insurance rates for the company or that an employee with diabetes might lead to some unsafe event or a lawsuit of some kind. More often than not, these concerns are completely unjustified and a little effort can explain why.

If explanations and discussions don't help, it may become necessary to file a complaint of disability discrimination with a government agency. The federal agency that enforces workplace discrimination laws is the Equal Employment Opportunity Commission (EEOC). The federal disability law the EEOC enforces is known as the Americans With Disabilities Act of 1990. The Americans with Disability Act outlaws workplace disability discrimination by all private employers with fifteen or more employees. The first thing the EEOC always asks about what happened is what you have done to try and resolve the problem before making a complaint. You will need to show that you have tried to explain your diabetes to your employer and taken fair actions to communicate your needs and request reasonable accommodations to manage them safely while doing your job.

You can contact the EEOC at 1-800-669-4000 and ask them how and where to file a claim. The EEOC will investigate your claim at no charge to you. Remember, you have 180 days from the date the discrimination occurs to file a claim or you lose your right to file a claim under the ADA. (Some states have laws that extend the deadline to 300 days, but filing within 180 days is always a good idea to avoid risking an unintentional loss of rights.)

If the EEOC chooses not to try and prove or resolve your claim of discrimination, it will issue a "right to sue letter" that allows you to file your claim in court. It is often better to have an attorney assist you as you pursue this kind of claim but it is possible for you to pursue your claim directly with the assistance of the EEOC or a state agency. You can read Titles I and V of the Americans With Disabilities Act on the EEOC website: *www.eeoc.gov/facts/qanda.html.*

Some states have laws that go further than federal laws in banning workplace disability discrimination. In California, for example, we have a law that explicitly recognizes diabetes as a disability and bans workplace discrimination against persons with this and many other illnesses. An attorney who practices in the area of disability discrimination can assist you in understanding these laws and, if necessary, making claims of discrimination arising from violations of them. But before you file a lawsuit based on workplace disability discrimination, you will always need to file a disability discrimination claim with a government agency first—either with the EEOC or, if one exists where you live, a state agency that enforces workplace discrimination laws.

One aspect of federal disability law is certain: An individual's specific medical history and needs must be considered in order to determine whether or not that person can be considered disabled under federal law. The fact of having diabetes alone will neither support nor end a claim of workplace disability discrimination. Rather, the medical history of the individual with diabetes must be considered—including, for example, whether that person suffers from impairment of a major life activity resulting from diabetes complications or whether the employer unlawfully treats the individual as if he or she does (**Table 29-3**).

It is not comfortable to consider oneself disabled. Most of us do not want to be looked at or treated differently than anyone else. We just want to be given a fair chance to prove our worth and do our job. Most of us do not think of ourselves as in any way disabled, but I know that when I am sitting at my desk and suddenly am unable to think clearly, read, or speak— when I am nervous and shaky

Table 29-3

Can a Person on Insulin Drive a Truck?

Currently, federal law in place since 1970 prevents persons on insulin from driving trucks in interstate commerce. A diabetes waiver program began in 1993 giving persons the opportunity to demonstrate they can drive a truck safely even though on insulin. But a federal court found a similar law improper and the waiver program was ended in 1996. In 1999, the Department of Transportation (DOT) commissioned a new group of experts to study the issue and make recommendations. The study found that it would be feasible and safe to allow persons with insulin-dependent diabetes to drive trucks if they could demonstrate their ability to control and monitor their diabetes. The report can be found on the Internet at *http://www.fmcsa.dot.gov /facts-research/researchtechnology /publications/medreports.htm*

A division of the DOT known as the Federal Motor Carrier Safety Administration (FMCSA) is currently reviewing and preparing to announce new rules and regulations that would allow persons with insulin-dependent diabetes to drive trucks in interstate commerce. The FMCSA can be contacted at 1-800-832-5660. (At the time of publication, the contact on this issue at FMCSA is Sandy Zyworkarte at 1-202-366-2987.) A few states already allow, or are considering rules that will allow, insulin-dependent drivers to work as truck drivers within their state.

and sweating—there is no doubt that at that moment I am disabled. This kind of temporary disability does not prevent me from performing my work. But it does require that my employer understand my needs and provide me with reasonable accommodations to handle and avoid the problem such as allowing me to test my blood glucose, eat a meal, or even take a break for a while if hypoglycemia actually occurs.

The main issue is not whether or not one is disabled; it is whether or not one is being allowed to overcome it or is being prevented from getting a job and doing one's work despite it. And this is an issue we can and will win. Winning begins with explaining our diabetes and what we need to handle our job safely and properly.

Obtaining Proper Care for Children in Schools

Another situation in which it may be necessary to make sure others understand the need for proper diabetes care and how to provide it is when a child with diabetes is in school. Any school that receives federal funding (including, of course, all public schools but also many private and parochial schools as well) must comply with Section 504 of the Rehabilitation Act of 1973, which provides individuals with disabilities basic civil rights protection against discrimination. The Education for All Handicapped Children Act of 1975, amended and renamed in 1991 the Individuals With Disability Education Act (IDEA), guarantees a free, appropriate public education for all children with disabilities. Children with diabetes are specifically protected under this law.

Parents have the right to meet with school officials to develop a Section 504 Plan or an Individualized Education Program (IEP) under the IDEA to address a child's specific needs to manage his or her diabetes. This may include eating as necessary, participating in school activities without discrimination, assistance with blood glucose monitoring and injections, and other issues that the family and the child's physician raise and explain to the school. The 504 Plan and the IEP plan are used to make sure these issues are discussed, understood, and addressed so that safety is maintained for the child and discriminatory treatment is prevented.

Most public schools are able and willing to assist with these plans and have the experience to do so. The main thing a parent can do to make certain the plan is properly devised is to understand the child's daily needs by speaking with the child and the child's health care provider, then communicating those needs to the school and making sure the school is handling those needs properly after the plan is created. An attorney can be used if there are difficulties in achieving these goals and some attorneys specialize in creating plans for disabled children. If a school is resistant to meeting and creating and implementing a plan, an attorney may be needed to obtain compliance with the law. Sometimes, however, government officials or agencies that specialize in providing advice about children with disabilities may work just as well; information about how to obtain those free services is provided in **Table 29-4**.

Another benefit of the Affordable Care Act is that schools are now being provided with the means of treating chronic illness such as diabetes more readily. The reforms establish school based health centers that will be provided the funding to improve the health care provided to students. These improvements are, again, based on the overwhelming evidence that providing better health care at an earlier age will limit disease complications and allow for the safer and less expensive treatment of illness over time.

Table 29-4
Aiding Children With Diabetes

The National Information Center for Children and Youth with Disabilities provides free information on handling school issues for children with diabetes. Their phone is 1-800-695-0285. Their website is *www.nichcy.org/* and also includes information on how to contact state agencies that may be able to help: *www.nichcy.org/states.htm.*

The US Office for Civil Rights provides free information and assistance on handling school issues for children with diabetes. Their phone is 1-800-421-3481; website is *www.ed.gov /about/offices/list/ocr/index.html.*

Proper Care for Persons Who Are in Nursing Homes or Suffering From a Critical Illness

Persons in nursing homes and person in hospitals suffering from a critical illness frequently are allowed to let their blood glucose level run high. If the person under care is able to make the determination about their blood glucose level preference and allowed to determine their own level of care, this should not be an issue of great significance. But in many instances, the choice is not made by the person being treated; options and consequences are not explained. Simply put, it is far easier for overworked caregivers to allow blood glucose levels to run high in nursing-care and in critical care settings. Often it is assumed that as long as the person receiving care does not fall too low and risk serious hypoglycemia, everything should be all right. Unfortunately, hyperglycemia is both unpleasant and deadly. Those of us who have experienced elevated blood glucose levels know all too well the miserable feeling of urgently and incessantly needing to urinate; the unpleasant and awful taste in one's mouth; the discomfort of simply running too high. To be obliged to lie in bed in such a state day after day is a horrifying thought. Yet that is the reality for many persons with diabetes whose blood glucose levels are under the control of others.

Not only is the experience unpleasant, it can also lead to increased morbidity and ongoing critical health problems. A study published by the New England Journal of Medicine on November 8, 2001, found that after 12 months, well-managed blood glucose levels in critically ill patients reduced mortality from 8% of 1548 patients to 4.6%. That is a nearly 50% decrease in patients dying in the course of 1 year among the group whose blood glucose levels were well managed. Moreover, the improvement in health care success was similarly high across many different areas of care, reducing the need for red-cell transfusions by 50% among well-managed patients, renal failure by 41%, and bloodstream infections by 46%.

Based on this evidence, it is fair to say that allowing blood glucose levels to escalate too frequently, and without a meaningful evaluation and effort to prevent it, may constitute elder abuse or abuse of patients receiving critical care. Of course, such claims need to be reviewed carefully and the evidence of what would constitute proper care under the circumstances seriously considered based on the facts of each case, but this certainly is an area that all of us should be concerned about as all of us are likely to be in this setting at some point in time.

Discussing treatment options with the health care providers who oversee patients in these circumstances is critical. Reviewing blood glucose test results and taking part in how best to manage care is important as well. Persons should not be left to suffer pain or worsened conditions because of laziness and a haphazard approach to managing blood glucose levels—and this is as true for the elderly and the critically ill as it is for those of us still able to care for ourselves.

Living Well Among Those With Type 0 Diabetes

People who are familiar with diabetes may already be sympathetic and understanding. Those who are not so familiar with this disease may be sympathetic and understanding people—but they can't always be so understanding for us until they learn a little about our disease. And, let's be honest, there will be plenty of people who truly do not care about us or our illness, but who we need to deal with whether we, or they, like it or not. Our obligation to manage our diabetes doesn't end with taking care of ourselves. We need to learn to live with, work with, socialize with, and go through life alongside people who may not know a thing about diabetes and may not give a darn about it. Until, that is, we help them learn as best we can, and they allow.

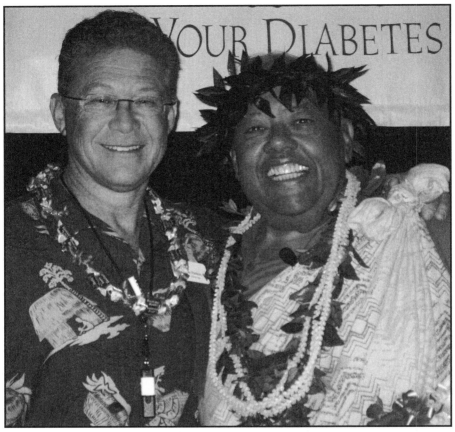

TCOYD serves the people of Hawaii... someone has to do it!

30

Travel Successfully

Don't Leave Your Diabetes at Home

by Adrienne Nassar, MD and
Steven V. Edelman, MD

Travelers should not take a "vacation" from their diabetes management while away from home! Managing your diabetes is a daily part of life, no matter the location. "Travel" may include trips to the gym, grocery store, walks outdoors and, of course, vacationing, whether domestic or abroad. Basically, when someone with diabetes leaves the house, he or she needs to think ahead and take their diabetes supplies (testing strips, glucose meter, insulin syringes and insulin vials, oral medications, glucose tabs, etc). Carrying these supplies in a protective cold case is recommended when in a hot environment. There is no excuse for leaving diabetes testing supplies, equipment, and medications at home! Remember that each and every time that you enter your car, no matter what the destination, you should check your blood sugar since you are responsible for safely operating your vehicle. Diabetes can be managed safely during all types of travel with some universal common sense, pre-trip planning.

Pre-travel Planning

When you plan to travel internationally, it is recommended that you visit with your diabetes health care provider at least 4 to 6 weeks prior to trip departure. At this visit, an updated assessment of glycemic control should occur, along with review of basic diabetes management concepts like sick-day rules and hypoglycemia symptoms, including ways to treat blood sugars. In addition, a physician-generated letter should be written, describing your diabetes regimen and the need to carry diabetes medications and supplies (for example, insulin syringes and sharps) in your carry-on luggage (**Table 30-1**). As such, it would be optimal to have the physician letter translated into the language to be spoken at your destination to allow more easy communication with Transportation Security Agency (TSA) security agents. If you are using insulin pump therapy, a back-up, alternate basal-bolus insulin regimen should be determined by your physician and written out for the diabetes trav-

447

eler, with medications and supplies filled, prior to departure in the event of pump malfunction.

Packing for an upcoming trip can be daunting. Careful planning can help to prevent forgetting your needed diabetes medications and testing supplies. Several recommendations for what to pack are listed (**Table 30-2**). Be sure that these items are packed into carry-on luggage to prevent them from getting lost in the event that the checked baggage never makes it to the final destination. Generally, it is wise to pack about twice as many diabetes supplies and medications as needed, given today's travel delays and in case some get damaged/lost en route.

Dealing With Diabetes Medications and Supplies Overseas

It is important to know that diabetes medications and supplies are not universal and actually differ in various parts of the world. While the insulin concentration is U-100 in the United States, other countries may carry insulin in the U-40 or U-80 concentrations. The diabetes

Table 30-1

Physician Letter Components for the Diabetes Traveler

- Letter should be in English and in the native language of the country to be visited
- Specify whether you have type 1 or type 2 diabetes
- Medications and dosages; if using an insulin pump, include settings and also basal-bolus backup regimen should the pump malfunction
- Emergency glucose supplies (glucose gel, tablets, glucagon pen with label on box)
- Supplies (glucometer, testing strips, lancets, syringes, batteries)
- Need to carry sharps (needles and lancets)
- Physician's name and contact phone number

Table 30-2

What to Pack

- Physician letter
- Identification/medical alert bracelet
- Health insurance card
- Diabetes medications and prescriptions for them
- Rescue diabetes medications (glucose gel, tablets, glucagon pen)
- Supplies (syringes, lancets, test strips, sharps container, and insulin carry case)
- Two glucose meters (in case one fails) with extra batteries
- If on insulin pump, twice as many pump supplies as may be needed
- Small first aid kit
- Comfortable, broken-in shoes to prevent foot ulcers
- Protective clothing, depending on destination climate

traveler should be aware that the units of insulin to draw up will not be the same with differing insulin potencies. This also holds true for different gauge and incremented insulin syringes (but may not necessarily be a concern for those who use insulin pen therapy). Another example of international variation would be the unit of glucose measurement, which is important to know when purchasing a glucose meter in a foreign country. In the United States, the unit is (mg/dL) but in other countries may be (mmol/L), and checking the units of measure on the glucose meter (and changing it accordingly) will allow for consistency when checking point-of-care glucose measurements. Basically, if you multiply the blood sugar value in mmol/L by 18, you will get the approximate blood sugar value in mg/dL.

Likewise, diabetes medications in the United States may not be available in other countries or, if they are, may be named differently altogether. Travelers with diabetes should have a list of their diabetes medications with doses on hand at all times in order to present this information to a physician overseas in case additional diabetes medications are required. It is important to note that even if your US physician provides you with prescription scripts for diabetes medications or supplies, the scripts aren't universally accepted at pharmacies overseas and will likely need to be prescribed by a local physician.

For those individuals with diabetes who are on an insulin pump, calling the pump company to inquire about a loaner insulin pump is a good idea. Some companies will loan an extra insulin pump for international travel (usually for a small price) so that if one's pump malfunctions overseas, a backup pump is readily available. However, if your insulin pump does malfunction oversees, call the company number on the back of the pump to discuss troubleshooting and possible expedited delivery of a new insulin pump while overseas.

Vaccinations

Something perhaps not on one's radar before departure is making sure travelers with diabetes are up to date on recommended vaccinations (influenza, pneumococcal, etc). Diabetes (especially uncontrolled) can place individuals at a higher risk for infection. Furthermore, being ill can pose its own challenges in terms of diet and diabetes medication management (for example, decreasing insulin if needed when oral intake of food is not normal). Vaccination schedules per area of the world are available on the Centers for Disease Control and Prevention at *wwwnc.cdc.gov/travel/* as well as other important health-related information, such as disease outbreaks in certain regions.

Protecting Yourself and Your Diabetes
Medications and Supplies

Prior to departure, travelers can do some homework on the areas to which they will be traveling. For instance, look up the weather conditions ahead of time, knowing that hotter temperatures may require diabetes medications and supplies to be carried in a cold pack to ensure optimal functioning. It may be a good idea to be sure hotel accommodations include a refrigerator in order to properly store insulin if needed. Likewise, diabetes medications and supplies should be protected from cold temperature extremes as well. Remember that cold temperature extremes may exist in airplane luggage compartments below the cabin, so placing insulin vials inside socks (to protect from breaking) and in one's carry-on luggage is recommended instead of in your checked baggage. Furthermore, if ice crystals have formed in an insulin vial, it is recommended to throw this vial away since the insulin potency may have been altered. Injectable diabetes medications typically have optimal storage temperatures between 2°C and 8°C (36°F and 46°F) while oral medications should generally be stored between 20°C and 30°C (60°F and 86°F). Insulin pumps generally have temperature tolerances from 5°C to 40°C (41°F to 104°F) and glucose monitoring devices from 10°C to 40°C (50°F to 104°F), but specific temperature ranges vary by manufacturer. In addition, blood glucose testing strips should be kept in their manufacturer's sealed containers to avoid exposure to moisture (which could decrease their accuracy of reading blood sugar levels). The package inserts for oral and injectable diabetes medications, in addition to optimal temperature ranges for testing strips and glucose meters, are good resources to review and follow.

Don't forget to pack appropriate personal protective clothing depending on the travel climate (sunscreen, gloves, boots, hats), especially if you already have diabetic peripheral neuropathy, since you may not fully be able to feel temperature extremes in your hands and feet. Especially important is comfortable and correctly fitted shoes to prevent foot ulcers. Remember, with diabetes, it is not a good idea to walk around barefoot, so be sure to pack socks, and wear sandals even when at the beach. Last, be sure to stay hydrated (especially in warmer climates), and choose safe water sources to help prevent traveler's diarrhea and possible dehydration that may ensue.

When sitting for long periods of time whether in a car or airplane, it is recommended to take frequent breaks to stand and walk to help prevent blood clots. While sitting, you can point your toes toward the ceiling (similar to walking on your heels), then push your feet toward the ground (similar to pushing on the gas pedal) to help keep the blood circulating in your lower legs during longer periods of sitting.

Diet

Food options may be somewhat limited while traveling through airports, so packing snacks in your carry-on bag allows quick dietary access if needed. In addition, normal eating times may be interrupted or changed according to travel itineraries. Especially important is to remember to pack glucose tabs or other glucose sources in carry-on luggage if needed to correct low blood sugars at any point prior to or during travel. Should one-on-one dietary counseling be desired prior to departure, this could potentially be arranged by your diabetes health care provider if nutritionists and diabetes educators are available for referral.

While on board an airplane, food options are limited, so calling an airline ahead of time to request specific diets (such as low-carbohydrate) is an option. This is likely not as big of an issue if traveling by car since more dietary options are generally available en route to your final destination. Remember protein sources like chicken, eggs, nuts, fish, and cheese are low in carbohydrates and are likely available in most travel destinations.

Travel Insurance and Safety

Do not forget to call and discuss travel health coverage with your health insurance company before departure, in case an additional plan needs to be purchased ahead of time. This will prevent large out-of-pocket costs should medical care be required abroad. Important to note: Medicare doesn't cover medical care outside of the United States, so supplemental travel health insurance is necessary. Furthermore, do not forget to take your health insurance card with you each and every time you leave the house, whether traveling to the grocery store or abroad, since unforeseen emergencies can arise.

With travel overseas, you can obtain a list of health care facilities overseas through either the local American embassy (*http://www.usembassy.gov*), US Department of State, foreign tour offices, and from the International Association for Medical Assistance to Travelers (*http://iamat.org*). In addition, the US Department of State posts up-to-date information regarding safety concerns for Americans traveling abroad at *http://travel.state.gov/travel.*

Insulin Use in Airplanes

Depending on flight durations, insulin may need to be administered in flight. For those using insulin vials, due to cabin pressurization, it may be more difficult to draw up insulin using a syringe. For individuals utilizing insulin pen therapy, cabin pressure differences may cause insulin to leak when inserting the pen needle in preparation or injection.

For individuals utilizing insulin pump therapy during flight, recent preliminary data suggests that unintended insulin delivery can occur during take-off and, likewise, less than intended insulin can be delivered during descent. While this needs further investigation, the take-home message is to check your blood sugars frequently during in-flight time to account for such circumstances.

Airport Security

Take several minutes and review TSA rules and regulations regarding carrying diabetes medications and supplies through security checkpoints and on board airplanes (*www.tsa.gov/travelers/airtravel/specialneeds /editorial_1374.shtm#3*). Basically, travelers with diabetes should alert the TSA officer that they have diabetes and are transporting needed diabetes medications and supplies. This would be the optimal time, if asked, to provide the physician letter clearly stating your diabetes diagnosis and the need to carry the listed medications and supplies with you (including sharps, such as syringes and lancets). Remember, insulin vials and glucagon kits need to have the pharmacy labels attached and visible according to Federal Aviation Administration guidelines.

For those diabetes travelers with insulin pumps and/or continuous glucose monitors (CGMs), it is important to contact the manufacturers for specific instructions regarding radiation exposure (radiation is the technology utilized for metal detectors, carry-on luggage x-ray machines, and whole-body scanners). Several insulin pump and CGM manufacturing companies allow their products to safely pass through the metal detectors but strictly recommend against their products from being run through the luggage x-ray machines or whole-body scanners due to the potential risk of radiation-induced pump or CGM malfunction. The traveler should remind TSA agents that insulin pumps and CGMs should not be removed or disconnected since they are attached via intradermal catheters. However, you must ultimately abide by whatever is asked by TSA security. Showing them your physician letter will help your efforts of getting through security with all of your diabetes medications and supplies.

Adjusting Insulin Therapy During Travel

Diabetes management is based on a 24-hour period, and overseas travel can sometimes change the timing of diabetes medication administration. When traveling from west to east, the day actually "shortens" while when traveling from east to west, the day actually "lengthens." Adjustments to insulin dosing are not usually necessary when crossing fewer than five time zones. Generally, oral diabetes medications are taken once or twice daily and thus time zone differences don't prove too difficult when adjusting administration times for these types of diabetes medications during travel. As a reminder, if meals will be missed, you should not take sulfonylurea medication to avoid low blood sugar levels and potential hypoglycemic events. Generally speaking, oral agents like metformin (Glucophage), DDP4 inhibitors (Januvia, Onglyza, and Trajenta), or thiazolidinediones (Actos) can be safely continued. However, diabetes travelers who are insulin-requiring may take as many as five or more injections of insulin per day, so adjusting timing of doses proves to be more difficult. Specific recommendations regarding insulin-administration times and dosing changes should be made by your diabetes health care provider on a case-specific basis during the pre-trip diabetes appointment.

Following are some general examples of how to dose insulin when traveling in different time zones:

- *Example 1*: East bound flight from Los Angeles, CA to Frankfurt, Germany. Flight departs at 7:00 PM Los Angeles, CA time (which is 4:00 AM Frankfurt time) and arrives at 2:45 PM Frankfurt time (which is 5:45 AM Los Angeles, CA time). Total flight time is 10 hours and 45 minutes.

  - *Basal-Bolus Insulin Regimen*: Diabetes traveler normally takes 20 units NPH and 8 units aspart before breakfast and 14 units NPH and 8 units of aspart before dinner. Since the flight is an evening flight, the traveler can take his 14 units of NPH and 8 units of aspart prior to the dinner served on the flight. Since this is an international flight, breakfast will be served several hours prior to landing, and the diabetes traveler can take half of his morning NPH (10 units) with the full dose of aspart insulin (8 units). After landing, later that evening around dinner time (Frankfurt time), the diabetes traveler can take the other half of his NPH (10 units) and the full dose of aspart insulin (8 units). The following morning (Frankfurt time) he can resume his normal insulin dosing according to local time.

- *Basal Only Regimen*: Diabetes traveler normally takes 24 units of lantus at bedtime, metformin 1000 mg twice daily, and glipizide 10 mg twice daily. This means she takes her full lantus dose (24 units) on board the airplane shortly after departure (10 PM). When she arrives the following day in Frankfurt, she can take half of the normal lantus dose (12 units) at bedtime local time (don't want to stack the doses, since it won't quite be a full 24 hours since the previous lantus dose). The following evening, she can resume the full dose of 24 units of lantus at bedtime local time (keep in mind blood sugar levels may be transiently elevated during the day prior to resuming the full dose of lantus). Oral diabetes medications can still be taken 12 hours apart with meals but if a meal will be skipped, then the sulfonylurea should be skipped as well so as not to cause hypoglycemia. Metformin is unlikely to cause hypoglycemia and can therefore be continued.

- *Example 2*: West bound return flight from Frankfurt, Germany to Los Angeles, CA. Flight departs at 10:00 AM Frankfurt, Germany time (1:00 AM Los Angeles, CA time) and arrives at 12:40 PM Los Angeles, CA time (9:40 PM Frankfurt, Germany time). Total flight time 11 hours and 40 minutes.
  - *Basal-Bolus Insulin Regimen*: Diabetes traveler normally takes 20 units NPH and 8 units aspart before breakfast and 14 units NPH and 8 units of aspart before dinner. He should take his 20 units of NPH and 8 units of aspart with breakfast (either on the plane if breakfast will be served or prior to departure). He will be served lunch prior to landing and should take half of his NPH (7 units) with this meal (since the last NPH dose will likely be wearing off if it was taken almost 10 hours prior during departure). Then later that evening (Los Angeles time), the traveler should give the other 7 units of NPH this time with 6 units of aspart when he eats dinner. The following morning (Los Angeles time), he can resume his normal insulin dosing according to local time.
  - *Basal Only Regimen*: A diabetes traveler normally takes 24 units of lantus at bedtime, metformin 1000 mg twice daily, and glipizide 10 mg twice daily. This means she would have already taken her full lantus dose the night prior to departure (10 PM Frankfurt time would be 1:00 PM Los Angeles, CA time). She will arrive in California the following day and not need her lantus dose until 1:00 PM (Los Angeles time). It would be easiest to take her full lantus dose at dinner (about 28 hours since the last dose, so be advised of transient hyperglycemia). Then the following day, she can go

back to taking her 24 units at bedtime (to be on a nighttime basal insulin schedule). Again, oral diabetes medications can be taken 12 hours apart but if meals will be missed, the sulfonylurea should be skipped (to avoid hypoglycemia), while metformin can be continued (since it is unlikely cause hypoglycemia).

This chapter was adapted from a publication in a medical journal we authored. Nassar AA, Cook CB, Edelman S. Diabetes management during travel. *Diabetes Management*. 2012;2(3):205-212.

Summary

Some say life is about the journey, not just the destination. Likewise, traveling with diabetes should be an enjoyable experience and can be with proper pre-trip planning. Travel can pose particular challenges with unfamiliar environments, new cuisines, time zone changes, altered living conditions, etc. However, diabetes is a self-managed disease and can be done successfully with good communication between you and your diabetes health care providers. No destinations are "off limits" to travelers with diabetes and you should remember that while you may be going on vacation, there is no "vacation" from managing one's diabetes while away from home.

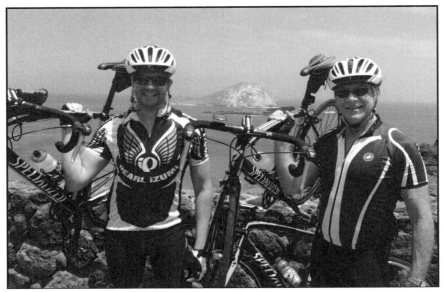

Two famous type 1s, Jeremy Pettus and Steve Edelman, on a long bike ride, while travelng in Hawaii.

31

Adult Onset Diabetes Becomes a Disease of Our Children and Youth

by Francine R. Kaufman, MD

This excerpt from my book, *Diabesity*, remains relevant 7 years later. During that time period, we have become aware that type 2 diabetes accounts for about a third of the diabetes that develops in those older than 10 years who are Hispanic, African American, or Asian/Pacific Islanders; and it is seen in two thirds of Native American youth who develop diabetes. Over 90% of youth who develop type 2 diabetes have two or more cardiovascular disease risk factors. This is a serious condition, and it takes serious measures to prevent it and treat it.

Drinking sweetened beverages, lack of physical activity, and exposure to an excess of advertising that promotes unhealthy food options to youth all contribute to this epidemic of diabesity. Each of us must play a role to make the environment more supportive, to make the healthy choice the easy and affordable choice, and to model appropriate lifestyle habits. We all influence those around us: in our families, in our communities, at work, and at school. Raise your voice, and make a difference now and for the children of the future.

Excerpts from *Diabesity: The Obesity-Diabetes Epidemic That Threatens America—And What We Must Do to Stop It* by Francine R. Kaufman, MD. Copyright 2005 by Francine Ratner Kaufman. Reprinted by permission of Bantam Books, a division of Random House, Inc.)

My greatest joy as a physician is to be with a patient when they have an "Ah-ha" moment. Watching an epiphany develop and emerge is exciting. I remember a 10-year-old boy with diabetes who decided to do his own experiment about the effect of food on his blood glucose level. He took his shot, ate an egg, and monitored his glucose level hourly over 3 hours. It stayed relatively flat. The next day he ate a hamburger on a bun, and he had a late glucose peak. The third day he ate a candy bar and drank a soda. His glucose level skyrocketed. "Ah-ha," he said, "I get it."

As a physician, I have also had a number of "Ah-ha" moments myself. That moment in time when the right diagnosis flashes into my mind, when I say just the right thing to a family as they watch their child slip away from a devastating illness, and when I realize that there has been a paradigm shift in the world. I witnessed a paradigm shift in diabetes in the mid-1990s. In the middle of a spring day in 1995, I received a call from an emergency department doctor, asking if I could see a 13-year-old patient named Tanesha right away. Tanesha's blood glucose level was 427 mg/dL, at least five times higher than normal for a young teen.

I was already in the diabetes clinic. The waiting room and all of the examining rooms were filled with patients and parents, but that didn't matter. I had to see Tanesha immediately because of her dangerously high blood glucose. Hearing the number, I pictured a typical type 1 patient referred from the emergency department: thin, severely weakened by dehydration, nausea, and fatigue, or even comatose. But I soon learned that Tanesha and her family looked nothing like this picture.

"Tanesha has been hyperglycemic for at least 2 weeks," the ER doctor told me. "I can't figure out why she still looks so good. And you won't believe how big this girl is. She's the largest kid with diabetes I've ever seen." Despite her elevated blood glucose, Tanesha was barely symptomatic. She didn't feel weak or exhausted; she hadn't vomited. Instead, she was hungry. While Tanesha waited in the ER, she had eaten a bag of fries and downed a regular soda. "By the way," the ER doctor added, "Tanesha is African American." This too was puzzling. Type 1 diabetes is rarer in nonwhite children.

Even though I'd been told that Tanesha was overweight, and even though she was not sick after a long bout of hyperglycemia, it didn't dawn on me that she might have type 2 diabetes. Not in 1995. Only when I walked into the examining room did it become apparent that my thinking was all wrong. Tanesha was there with her mother and her grandmother. Each of them weighed at least 250 pounds. I realized that I might be walking into a whole new world.

Tanesha was not merely overweight, she was huge. Her height—5-foot, 3-inches—was normal for a girl of 13. But she weighed 267 pounds. She had extensive darkening of the skin around her neck. I'd seen this condition, called acanthosis nigricans, in adults with type 2 diabetes. Could this 13-year-old girl have type 2 diabetes? As I questioned Tanesha about her symptoms, her answers confirmed the possibility.

"Are you thirsty?" I asked.

She told me she had been drinking a lot of juice and soda. "My mama told me to stop drinking so much, but I told her I was just thirsty all the time, day and night," she informed me.

"How about urination?" I asked. "Do you have to pee at night?"

"Only 'cause I get up to drink," she explained. "If I didn't need to drink so much, I mightn't need to pee so much."

She actually had it backward. Her body was trying to rid itself of excess sugar by urinating. And because she lost so much water, she was constantly thirsty.

I asked, "How long have you been waking up at night to urinate?" This would tell me how long her blood glucose had been elevated.

She thought and then answered, "At least for this whole year."

Her response crystallized my thinking: Tanesha had type 2 diabetes. How could that be? And then I looked over at her grandmother, and thought: "Just like her grandma."

I didn't need to see blood test results to guess that Tanesha's grandmother, Thelma, had type 2 diabetes. She was obese and sat in a wheelchair. Her face drooped on one side and her left foot turned in, suggesting that she'd had a stroke. People with diabetes have an elevated risk for stroke and heart attack. Her right foot had been amputated, probably a result of the blood circulation and nerve problems that can develop from diabetes.

I asked Thelma about her medical history, half expecting her daughter Joyce, Tanesha's mother, to reply on her behalf. But Thelma's physical problems had not diminished the force of her personality. Joyce stood silently as her mother answered my questions. Tanesha watched and listened.

"They told me I had the sugar in 1966," she said. "They took my foot in 1987. Gangrene." In 1990 she'd had a mild heart attack, followed by a stroke in 1993. The stroke had left her left leg spastic and her left arm paralyzed. "I've been going to therapy for 2 years pretty regular. Still can't open my hand," she said.

"What medications do you take?" I asked.

"Them doctors tried to get me to take insulin. But insulin makes you sick," she said defiantly.

Joyce rolled her eyes at this. She pulled a sheet of paper from her purse and handed it to me. Thelma was supposed to take three medications to control her blood glucose, two more to lower her blood pressure, aspirin to prevent heart attacks and strokes, and a cholesterol-lowering drug. I wondered how many of those pills she actually took.

"Tanesha will be okay, Doc," Thelma continued. "Everybody has a little bit of the sugar in our family, 'cept Joyce. We don't need to pay it no mind. And we don't need to think 'bout putting her on no insulin shots. Don't you worry, Tanish," she said turning to her granddaughter. "You don't need none of those shots, and we don't need to pay the doctor no mind either."

I was shocked. Thelma needed handsful of medicines and had every possible diabetes complication. If that was only a "little bit of the sugar," I thought, what would be a lot? I had not expected her to attempt to thwart me. Tanesha would require insulin injections, at least at the beginning of her treatment.

I turned my attention to Tanesha's mother, Joyce. I needed to inform her and win her over to my side. I also needed to convince Tanesha.

"The blood tests show that Tanesha has diabetes," I explained to Joyce. I quickly turned to Tanesha and added, "Tanesha, there is no doubt about it. A blood glucose level above 400 mg/dL is diabetes. We now must determine what kind of diabetes you have."

"Although almost all children with diabetes have what we call type 1 diabetes, Tanesha may actually have type 2, just like her grandmother," I explained, swinging back to Joyce.

I didn't want to get too technical and lose their attention. "If Tanesha has type 2 diabetes, we may be able to treat her with pills eventually. But her blood glucose is too high now for the pills to work. The first step is to get her blood glucose level normal, to stop all that drinking and urinating." Then I added, "We must get her well again, so that she doesn't ever have to face what her grandma has faced because of her diabetes."

I looked at Joyce to see if I had made an impression. She remained expressionless for what seemed like a lifetime. Finally, she responded in a quiet but very firm voice: "We will do what you say, Doctor Kaufman. My whole life, I've watched diabetes eat my mother to pieces, because she doesn't take care of herself. No way will I let that happen to Tanesha." Thelma glared at her, but remained silent.

I sighed with relief. The first battle was won; I would be allowed to treat Tanesha with the medications she needed. But that was just one small battle. There was a war yet to win. We would have to get Tanesha to change her eating habits and become more active. She needed to lose weight. I hoped Joyce would do the same for her own sake. It seemed unlikely that Thelma would change, but maybe I could persuade her not to stand in Tanesha's way. Then there would be the constant battle with the rest of the world. Everywhere Tanesha turned, she'd be surrounded by the junk food and soft drinks and candy that threatened her health.

In that clinic room in 1995, I knew that a world of battles would have to be fought for Tanesha. What I didn't know was that this skirmish was the harbinger of a much larger war to come.

The waiting room in my clinic at Children's Hospital is always filled with people—children, parents, nannies, grandparents. When I look at them, I see the changing face of type 2 diabetes. And I see the cause: obesity. Families like Tanesha's are common now: a massively obese child and that youngster's equally heavy relatives, some of whom already show the terrible long-term effects of diabetes. We must do something to try to reverse this trend. But what can we do?

We can all do something—whether we have diabetes or not. Even if we have type 1 diabetes, maintaining a healthy lifestyle and a healthy weight makes a big difference in glucose control and in avoiding diabetes complications; particularly, in avoiding cardiovascular disease.

We can start with our own life and our own home. Commit to a healthy lifestyle. Start to eat healthy portions of healthy foods. Eat fruits and vegetables, whole grains, low-fat, and high-nutrient foods. Stop eating at fast food restaurants and instead eat together as a family. Eating together gives you a chance to touch base and check in with your children and spouse. Eat breakfast, drink water. We weren't meant to drink calories, so get sweetened sodas out of your life. Limit juice; it is nothing but sugar and you are better off eating an orange than drinking a glass of juice. Turn off the TV and the computer games. Get physically active; wear a pedometer and commit to working to get 10,000 steps a day. It might take a long time to get to that many steps, but it is a goal worth achieving. Do this with your whole family. For those with diabetes, those high blood glucose levels may come screaming down. For those without diabetes, but at risk because of family history and other factors, it might be just what is needed since it is the best diabetes preventive.

Make your workplace a healthy environment, too (**Table 31-1**). After all, how much time do you spend there? Each day on your way to work, plan how you can optimize your health. Take a walk at lunch; park far away in the parking lot. Use the stairs; it's a waste of time waiting for the elevator. Be sure water is available, demand healthy food options, stop bringing in junk food and candy, and band together to have a healthy workforce.

We need to be sure our homes, our schools, our communities, and our health care institutions promote health rather than deteriorate it— particularly for people with or at risk for diabetes. To achieve that end, we all have to raise our voice, change our habits, and work toward a healthier future. If not, more and more children like Tanesha will develop diabetes and imperil their life. If we commit now, who knows what the next "Ah-ha" moment might be. If we change our course and opt for health, it might be that we are healthy and vibrant through to old age.

Table 31-1
What to Do at the Workplace

- Wear a pedometer—you need to take 10,000 steps a day and you need to get a lot of them at work
- Park far away—fight for the farthest spot and walk those extra minutes
- Take the stairs—up one and down two
- Take a walk at lunch—you'll have more energy in the afternoon
- Take a walking meeting—your colleagues will be amazed and invigorated
- Don't drink calories—drink only water at work; it will keep you hydrated and alert
- Put resistance bands or 2-lb weights on your wrists and use them when you are on the phone
- Bring your lunch—a salad, healthy leftovers, healthy foods
- Have healthy snacks—don't go to the vending machines
- You need five to nine fruits and veggies a day—get three or more at work
- Make your workplace value health and healthy behaviors

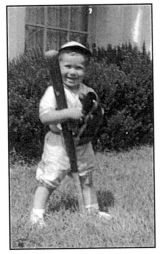

"Play Ball!"... Steve Edelman at 27 months of age.

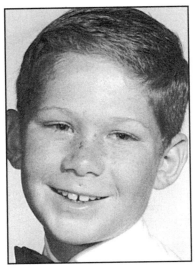

School Days photo of Steve Edelman.

32

Can Diabetes Be Prevented?

A Resounding Yes for Type 2 and Not Quite Yet for Type 1

by Steven V. Edelman, MD and Juan P. Frias, MD

The best way to avoid diabetes complications is to prevent them in the first place. The United States spends our limited health care dollars on treating the complications of diabetes: eye, kidney, nerve, and heart disease. These conditions are common in our diabetic population; complications appear several years after the diagnosis and can lead to tremendous suffering for both the patient and loved ones living with diabetes. Why not demand that the United States repositions itself toward prevention? Over the long term, health care costs are reduced with a strategic emphasis on prevention and quality of life. One of the major obstacles to this strategy is that the people who control the purse strings argue that it will cost more money in the short term. They commonly say, "Since people change insurance companies every few years on average, why spend money today to save the next company from losing money down the road?" This is a strategy for disaster.

One of the more striking facts is that most of the money spent to care for people with diabetes is for inpatient or hospital charges due to end-stage complications: heart attacks, strokes, amputations, and dialysis. About 13% of health care dollars is spent on drugs and devices such as insulin, diabetes pills, glucose meters, continuous glucose monitoring devices, and insulin pumps. I think a uniform policy that included prevention as a shared-cost commitment could reduce overall spending long term.

Can We Prevent Type 2 Diabetes? Absolutely, YES!

Prevention strategies are usually based on the etiology or cause of the disease. In the case of type 2 diabetes, prevention strategies have mainly targeted insulin resistance, which is recognized as one of the main problems. The different types of interventions that have been evaluated or are currently being studied include intensive lifestyle changes (long-term weight-loss and exercise programs) and various medications, such as Glucophage (metformin), the "glitazones" (Avandia [rosiglitazone] and Actos [pioglitazone]), carbohydrate absorption inhibitors (Precose [acarbose] and Glyset [miglitol]), insulin secretagogues (Starlix [nateglinide], and weight loss agents such as Xenical (orlistat). In addition, there are ongoing studies on the prevention of type 2 diabetes with the newest class of agents called the incretins (see *Chapter 7*); however, at the time of writing this edition, they are not yet completed.

Table 32-1 lists several of the more important type 2 diabetes prevention trials conducted worldwide, which will be discussed more. It is also important to note here that since the causes for type 1 and type 2 diabetes are so very different, the prevention strategies are also completely unrelated.

Table 32-1
Primary Prevention Trials of Type 2 Diabetes

Study	Treatment	Relative Risk
ACT NOW	Pioglitazone vs placebo	↓ 72%
DREAM	Rosiglitazone vs placebo	↓ 62%
DPP	Intensive diet and exercise vs placebo	↓ 58%
	Metformin vs placebo	↓ 31%
	Troglitazone vs placebo	↓ 75%[a]
FDPS	Intensive diet and exercise vs control	↓ 58%
STOP-NIDDM	Acarbose vs placebo	↓ 25%
XENDOS	Orlistat vs placebo	↓ 37%

Abbreviations: ACT NOW, Actos Now for the Prevention of Diabetes [study]; DPP, Diabetes Prevention Program; DREAM, Diabetes Reduction Assessment With Ramipril and Rosiglitazone Medication [trial]; FDPS, Finnish Diabetes Prevention Study; STOP-NIDDM, Study to Prevent Non–Insulin-Dependent Diabetes Mellitus; XENDOS, Xenical in the Prevention of Diabetes in Obese Subjects [study].

[a] Average treatment of 10 months.

Definition of Prediabetes

Figure 1-2 shows how we define normal, prediabetes, and diabetes, primarily based on blood glucose levels at two different times. The fasting blood glucose level, measured first thing in the morning after an overnight fast (nothing to eat for approximately 8 hours), should be less than 100 mg/dL. If the fasting value is 126 mg/dL or greater, that is in the diabetic range. Prediabetes is diagnosed if the value is greater than 100 mg/dL and less than 126 mg/dL. This basically means that the individual is at high risk for developing diabetes. The medical phrase for prediabetes based on the morning fasting glucose value is called impaired fasting glucose or IFG.

The other important time to measure the glucose value in order to diagnose prediabetes is 2 hours after swallowing 75 grams of a very sweet substance. This test is called the 2-hour oral glucose tolerance test or OGTT. This test is primarily used for research purposes or in the assessment of women during pregnancy to determine if they have pregnancy-related or gestational diabetes. The medical phrase for prediabetes based on the 2-hour OGTT value is called impaired glucose tolerance or IGT. These criteria were used to screen potential research volunteers for the prevention trials described below.

Most recently, the ADA added a new way to diagnosis prediabetes using the HbA1c or A1C test. An A1C level between 5.7% and 6.5% is another way to define prediabetes.

FDPS

The Finnish Diabetes Prevention Study (FDPS) was one of the first large studies to look at lifestyle modification and how it can prevent someone with prediabetes from progressing to full-blown type 2 diabetes. The study conducted in Finland over a 3- to 4-year period, demonstrated a significant reduction (58%) in conversion rates from prediabetes to diabetes compared with the placebo group which received no lifestyle modification counseling. The active-treatment group was given diet and exercise instructions at the beginning of the study and every year thereafter. The study subjects alternatively were given up to seven individual appointments per year. They were asked to exercise 30 minutes a day, cut their total daily fat intake to less than 30% of their total daily calorie intake, and eat more fiber in their diet. This study set the stage for a larger prevention study conducted in the United States called the Diabetes Prevention Program (DPP).

DPP

The DPP was a powerful, well-conducted, and highly funded government-initiated (National Institutes of Health) study to prevent the development of type 2 diabetes in people who may be at risk for this condition (people with prediabetes). The DPP was conducted at 25 major universities around the country. Subjects who were identified with several risk factors for developing type 2 diabetes were brought in for an OGTT. In order to efficiently screen large populations to be potential

465

research volunteers, it is important to identify those individuals who may be at the highest risk. If they had prediabetes, they were asked to volunteer for the trial. Approximately 4000 subjects who agreed to be in the study were then placed into one of the four following groups:

- Intensive lifestyle changes alone
- Metformin (also called Glucophage) plus minimal lifestyle changes
- Troglitazone (also called Rezulin) plus minimal lifestyle
- Placebo (fake pill) plus minimal lifestyle.

The study subjects placed in the intensive lifestyle changes group were given lots of attention by nurses, dietitians, exercise trainers, and clinical psychologists in order to help them achieve the goals of losing 7% of their body weight and exercising 30 minutes a day for 5 days a week. The other three groups took their oral medications and were simply given some general recommendations on diet and exercise.

The results were so impressive and convincing that the study was stopped early after 2.8 years (originally it was suppose to run for 4 years). The intensive lifestyle changes group had a reduction of 58% in the risk of converting from prediabetes to type 2 diabetes compared with the placebo group. The group that took Glucophage had a 31% risk reduction compared with the placebo group. It is interesting that Glucophage worked primarily in younger (less than 45 years old) and overweight people, whereas intensive lifestyle changes worked to prevent diabetes in all age and weight groups. The other big lesson in this study was that the earlier you can identify people at risk for type 2 diabetes, the better interventions work, whether they be lifestyle interventions or oral medications.

ACT NOW and DREAM Trials

The Actos Now for the Prevention of Diabetes (ACT NOW) was another impressive study that looked at how well a type 2 diabetes medication called Actos (pioglitazone) compared with a fake pill (placebo) in converting from prediabetes to type 2 diabetes in people with prediabetes. Actos is a medication in the same class of drugs as Avandia. It is in a class of medications called insulin sensitizers and is approved by the FDA for the treatment of type 2 diabetes. As explained in *Chapter 7*, insulin sensitizers reduce insulin resistance. In the ACT NOW study, there was not an intensive lifestyle changes group like there was in the DPP.

The results demonstrated that volunteers who took Actos experienced an impressive risk reduction (72%) of converting from prediabetes to type 2 diabetes compared with the placebo group. Of the 602 subjects with prediabetes who were in the study, 50 taking placebo developed type 2 diabetes, while only 15 taking Actos developed diabetes. If they had included a group with intensive lifestyle modifications, like the DPP, just think of the possibilities!

The Diabetes Reduction Assessment with Ramipril and Rosiglitazone Medication (DREAM) trial results were almost as impressive, demonstrating that Avandia could reduce conversion from prediabetes to type 2 diabetes by 62%. Due to the potential side effects of Avandia, the FDA has restricted its use for type 2 patients where other medications are ineffective or intolerable.

STOP-NIDDM, XENDOS, and NAVIGATOR Studies

There have been other prevention trials looking at other diabetes and obesity medications. The Study to Prevent Non–Insulin-Dependent Diabetes Mellitus (STOP-NIDDM) demonstrated that Precose (acarbose), an oral medication that delays the absorption of carbohydrates in the gut and lowers postmeal glucose levels, reduced risk of conversion to type 2 diabetes by 25%. It also reduced the risk factor for heart disease.

In the Xenical in the Prevention of Diabetes in Obese Subjects (XENDOS) study, the obesity drug Xenical (orlistat), which blocks the absorption of fat in the gut, led to an impressive 37% risk reduction (**Table 32-1**).

There was also the Nateglinide and Valsartan in Impaired Glucose Tolerance Outcomes Research (NAVIGATOR) study, which looked at how well a blood pressure drug called Diovan (valsartan) and an insulin secretagogue Starlix (nateglinide) prevented type 2 diabetes.

The number of oral medications currently available that have been proven to prevent people with prediabetes from converting to type 2 diabetes is impressive (Glucophage, Actos, Precose, and Xenical). There is no question that lifestyle modification with or without one of these safe and well-proven medications can prevent type 2 diabetes. It is important to note that the FDA has not given formal approval to any medication to be used for the prevention of type 2 diabetes. The American Diabetes Association (ADA) recommends that individuals with a high risk of developing type 2 diabetes consider starting Glucophage if they are below 60 years of age and obese. Please discuss these issues with your caregiver before starting any of these medications. The pros and cons must be explained to you in detail.

How Do You Know if You Are at Risk for Type 2 Diabetes?

There are a number of factors that may put you at increased risk of type 2 diabetes (**Table 32-2**). These risk factors include being overweight or physically inactive, age (higher risk with increasing age), having high blood pressure or abnormal cholesterol levels, having immediate family members with type 2 diabetes, having had gestational (pregnancy-related) diabetes, being of a certain ethnic group (Latino, African American,

Table 32-2

Risk Factors for Developing Type 2 Diabetes

- *Having someone in your family with diabetes, especially a first-degree relative.* Because type 2 diabetes runs so strongly in families, even if a second- or third-degree relative has diabetes, your risk goes up. There is really no such thing as "old-age diabetes," which a lot of people refer to and do not consider as a familial risk factor.

- *Being overweight, especially with central obesity, commonly referred to as a "beer belly."* People with insulin resistance develop a certain type of fat in the abdominal area giving the person "the apple shape" or upper-body obesity versus "the pear shape" or lower-body obesity.

- *Having some or all of the other associated conditions commonly seen in type 2 diabetes, such as high blood pressure or high cholesterol levels.* These conditions may appear many years before the diagnosis of diabetes and contribute to the high rate of heart attack and stroke.

- *Being a member of an ethnic group that has a high incidence of diabetes.* These include African Americans, Hispanics, Native Americans, Asian Americans, and Pacific Islanders. We do not know the reason for the high incidence of type 2 diabetes in these ethnic groups, but it is probably related to genetic makeup and our westernized lifestyle.

- *Having had diabetes during pregnancy (gestational diabetes).* Most of the time gestational diabetes goes away shortly after delivery of the baby. However, the chance of that woman developing diabetes in the next 5 to 10 years is high (25% to 50%), depending on the ethnic group, degree of obesity, and family history.

- *Having had a baby weighing over 9 pounds.* When a mother's blood glucose level is high during pregnancy, her baby is physically large but internally abnormal. The mother is at risk for developing type 2 diabetes, and recent research suggests a delayed adverse effect of her offspring.

- *If any caregiver ever told you that you had a "touch of diabetes" or "borderline diabetes."* This is a common scenario. So many caregivers do not take diabetes seriously enough. Most of the time, when a person is told they have a touch of diabetes, his or her diabetes is fairly advanced, and therapy is warranted immediately. Having a touch of diabetes is like having a touch of pregnancy.

Native American, Pacific Islander, Asian American), and/or having pre-diabetes (as defined earlier in this chapter). Most people with prediabetes do not even know they have it! For this reason everyone, including the lay public, people with diabetes, medical students, student doctors (interns and residents), and primary caregivers, should be familiar with and knowledgeable about these risk factors for developing type 2 diabetes.

The ADA recommends that your caregiver screen you for type 2 diabetes or prediabetes with a blood glucose or hemoglobin A1C test if you are overweight and have any of the risk factors mentioned above or starting at age 45. If the test shows that you do not have diabetes, it should be repeated every 1 to 3 years, depending on the results of the initial test and your risk factors. If you are at high risk, these tests should be repeated once a year.

A fast and simple Diabetes Risk Test was recently developed by the ADA (*www.stopdiabetes.com*). It helps inform you of your risk of developing type 2 diabetes. These results should be discussed with your health care provider. Based on the initial results, your provider may request a blood test to check for prediabetes or diabetes.

If you are found to have prediabetes, there is a relatively new blood test called the PreDx® Diabetes Risk Score (Tethys Bioscience, Inc.), which can determine your risk of developing type 2 diabetes within the next 5 years. The test results are provided on a scale of 1 to 10—the higher your score, the higher your risk for type 2 diabetes within 5 years. If you have prediabetes, you and your caregiver may find this test useful when planning and following the progression of your diabetes prevention program.

What Do You Do if You Are at Risk for Type 2 Diabetes?

Although there are no proven medications and/or techniques to 100% prevent people from developing type 2 diabetes, there are proven strategies that help reduce your risk.

1. *Improve your eating habits and try to get down to your ideal body weight.* There have been two large studies published (the FDPS and the DPP) that have clearly demonstrated that lifestyle intervention (weight loss and exercise) can reduce the incidence of type 2 diabetes in people who are at risk. Making small changes to your diet over time is the best strategy; cutting out that favorite donut at breakfast, switching from regular soda to diet, and making better choices in the composition of the food you ingest. A well-balanced diet with limited sugar and fat, regardless of your body weight, is a healthy preventative strategy. The results of the DPP demon-

strated a dramatic reduction in the incidence of type 2 diabetes in people at risk just by their participating in mild aerobic exercise 30 minutes a day for 5 days a week and losing just a few pounds. It is important to note that even relatively moderate reductions in body weight (5% to 10% reduction, or 10 to 20 pounds in someone who weighs 200 pounds) can have a big benefit.

2. *Regular exercise is the key.* I recommend doing anything that is enjoyable to you. Don't just join a fancy health club and only go once a year to pay your dues. If you attempt a sport that you must force yourself to do, your chances of following an exercise program over the long term are slim to none. This is why whenever you go to a garage sale, there is always an almost-new, never-used exercise bike, treadmill, set of weights, or golf clubs for sale... cheap. Think of exercise like the American College of Sports Medicine thinks of it, as a medication (see their website called *Exercise is Medicine* at *www.exerciseismedicine.org*). Exercise will reduce your risk of developing type 2 diabetes, help with your weight, blood pressure, cholesterol, and overall well-being. Check with your caregiver before starting an exercise program.

3. *Obtain your own glucose meter.* You should get a glucose meter and test yourself occasionally in the morning before breakfast and 2 hours after a heavy meal. Your morning blood glucose should be less than 100 mg/dL and your postmeal value should be less than 140 mg/dL. If your numbers start to approach or go above these values on a regular basis, you should notify your caregiver. Also don't forget that these meters are not always perfectly accurate, so don't panic if you get a super high or low value. Just test again.

4. *Look for other conditions associated with type 2 diabetes.* Make sure you are checked for the other conditions that are commonly associated with type 2 diabetes, such as high blood pressure and high cholesterol levels. It is important to control these silent risk factors that lead to heart attack and stroke. It is very common to develop these other conditions before the development of diabetes, so why not treat them aggressively when they appear?

5. *Ask your caregiver about taking one aspirin a day.* As discussed in the chapter on heart disease, aspirin is a super-effective, inexpensive, and easy way to prevent heart attack and stroke. Make sure you check with your caregiver first.

6. *Consider drug therapy.* Consider taking a medication that may help to prevent or delay the development of type 2 diabetes. Until recently, there were no proven drugs to prevent diabetes. How-

ever, the results of the DPP have demonstrated that Glucophage is effective at preventing type 2 diabetes in people who are at risk and especially those who are 60 years of age or younger and overweight. Insulin sensitizers such as Actos may be one of the most effective medications to prevent type 2 diabetes. Every drug has its pros and cons, and a serious discussion with your caregiver is definitely a must if one is considering this option. Remember that lifestyle modification is the most powerful tool that we know of to delay or prevent the development of type 2 diabetes. You should never substitute one of these medications for lifestyle modification, but use them in addition to diet and exercise strategies after you and your caregiver consider the benefits and possible risks.

7. *Consider getting involved in a research program.* Consider being a volunteer in a research protocol that is a prevention trial. There may or may not be one going on in your area, but if you live near a university medical center, you can easily find a listing of the various studies being conducted. Also keep your eyes and ears open to the media since many national studies have public-relations firms that work to get the word out. Read the protocols carefully and discuss the details with your caregiver to make sure the study is right for you.

8. *If you have been diagnosed with prediabetes, consider getting the PreDx test (discussed above).* It is a simple blood test that measures seven blood markers associated with diabetes and reports your 5-year likelihood of developing type 2 diabetes *(Dr. Juan Frias, the co-author of this chapter, is currently the Chief Medical Officer of Tethys Bioscience, Inc).*

Can We Prevent Type 1 Diabetes?
So Far the Answer Is No.

(This section was updated by Dr. Jeremy Pettus, who is currently working at one of the top type 1 research centers in the world—The La Jolla Institute for Allergy and Immunology.)

Before we can talk about preventing a disease, we need to know what causes it and you probably cannot find two things more opposite than the etiologies of type 1 and type 2 diabetes. In type 1 diabetes, the immune system essentially gets confused and begins to attack and kill the insulin-producing cells in your pancreas (the beta cells). What causes the immune system to do this is something we still do not know. Your genes certainly have something to do with it, but genes aren't the whole story. For example, if one identical twin gets the disease, there is about a 50% chance that the other twin will get it. In identical twins, every single gene in the body is exactly the same. That means that even if you have the same genes as somebody with type 1 diabetes, it is basically a coin flip whether you will get the disease. Put another way, your genes can explain only half of the reason people get diabetes, but what explains the other half? If it isn't all in our genes, that means there is something in our environment causing the disease. Some researchers believe that a viral infection in childhood could trigger the disease. Others are looking into the effect of formula versus breast milk or the effect of vitamin D deficiency. There are many theories, but the bottom line is, we don't know. One major research effort is The Environmental Determinates of Diabetes in the Young (TEDDY) study. This group is following about 8000 children at risk for the disease and looking at what features in their environment might cause the disease (*http://teddy.epi .usf.edu/*).

So the bad news is that we still don't know what exactly causes the disease. The good news is that we are getting better and better at predicting who will get the disease, which is important. Before the onset of symptoms, individuals with type 1 diabetes produce auto-antibodies in the body that we can find and measure with blood tests. These antibodies can appear years before the disease takes effect. For example, if you have two or more of these antibodies, your risk of developing type 1 diabetes in the next 5 years is between 25% and 50%. By screening family members of patients with type 1 diabetes, researchers can identify people at high risk for developing the disease and attempt interventions to stop the abnormal autoimmune process from destroying the beta cells. Unfortunately, no interventions to date have had any effect on preventing or delaying type 1 diabetes.

Despite the recent failures in being able to prevent the disease, many researchers (including myself) still believe that preventing the disease will be the best way to "cure" type 1 diabetes. Reversing the disease once it has started has proven to be extremely difficult, therefore, our best approach may be to focus on not allowing it to start in the first place. Research trials on prevention are still underway. These trials require large screening efforts and long periods of time to follow the research participants. If you are interested in getting a screening test or for more information, check out the TrialNet website at *www.diabetes trialnet.org*. This is a group of researchers dedicated to preventing this disease and are currently looking to enroll more patients in prevention trials. Alternatively, the Juvenile Diabetes Research Foundation (JDRF) is an excellent resource. You can enter your information and they will tell you about trials in your area. Check them out at *https://trials.jdrf.org/patient/*.

If you or someone close to you test positive for being at risk for type 1 diabetes, there is no real list of things to do, such as there is for people at risk for type 2 diabetes. Lifestyle changes have not been shown to make a difference. Basically, it comes down to being involved in a clinical trial. Screening or being involved in a study may not be for you or your child. If your child is at risk for type 1 diabetes, you may or may not want to have your child tested. If you do not want your child to be involved in a clinical trial after carefully reviewing the protocols, then it comes down to personal preference. If you would worry too much if the test is positive, it may not be worth it. If you are the type of person who likes to know and prepare for the eventuality, testing may be for you.

Case Presentations
Case #1: Prevention of Type 1 Diabetes

I can tell you my family's story. I have two teenage daughters, Talia and Carina. When Talia was 7 and Carina was 3, we decided to have them tested for the antibodies that cause type 1 diabetes. We are the type of people who wanted to know if one or both of our children could eventually develop type 1 diabetes. Talia and Carina still remember getting their arm poked for blood, but I tell my friends that our Christmas present that year (even though we are Jewish) was that they both tested negative. They are supposed to be retested every 3 years but I have not been able to drag them back to the laboratory. Talia is now 23 and Carina is 19 with no diabetes yet in either of them!

Case #2: Prevention of Type 2 Diabetes

Mike is a 51-year-old white male who has been one of my best friends since 1987. He came to me many years ago with blood glucose levels in the prediabetic range (morning level in the 110 mg/dL range and the 2-hour postmeal level around 160 mg/dL to 180 mg/dL). His A1C at that time was in the upper normal range of 5.9%. Type 2 diabetes runs strongly in his family and he also had a weight problem, high blood pressure, and abnormal cholesterol levels just like his dad, who has type 2 diabetes and is also my patient. Other than that, he is a pretty healthy guy; however, he is very sedentary. He came to me because he did not want to get diabetes! Mike once said to me that if he got diabetes, it would be a poor reflection on me... the doctor.

Mike is in the food business, he loves to eat and is always fighting to keep his weight down. He has also tried every diet known to man. He usually loses some weight at first but typically gains it back in the following few months. Fortunately, he does like to play golf and even though he rents a golf cart, there is a lot of walking.

We did have a serious conversation recently about taking a medication, in addition to lifestyle efforts, to prevent diabetes when his blood test showed once again that he had prediabetes. I explained quite clearly to him the pros and cons of taking either metformin or Actos and that the FDA has not officially approved any drug for the prevention of type 2 diabetes. The ADA did have a consensus conference on prediabetes and they clearly stated that medications used to prevent type 2 diabetes are appropriate if they prove to be effective, have a good safety and tolerability profile, and are cost-effective.

Even if Mike develops diabetes, he will be on the right track for early treatment and aggressive therapy before any complications develop and become apparent. Remember that the next best thing to preventing diabetes is being the first to know about it.

Summary

The best way to prevent the terrible complications of diabetes is to prevent diabetes in the first place. Diabetes does not have to be a costly and devastating disease. It is not only the health care professionals who must be informed about who is at risk for diabetes; it is also the responsibility of anyone living with diabetes to notify and encourage their relatives to be tested for either type 1 or type 2 diabetes. There are no symptoms in the early stages of the development of diabetes, which makes screening programs even more important. We now can say without a shadow of a doubt that type 2 diabetes can be prevented with lifestyle modification and medication. Unfortunately, up until now type 1 diabetes prevention strategies have failed, but many more studies are in progress. Even if diabetes is found at the time of screening, or if you develop diabetes while participating in one of the prevention studies, being the first to know you have diabetes is the next best thing to not having it. Early and aggressive treatment of diabetes is the single most important message that I can convey to you.

33

It's Never Too Late to Take Control of Your Diabetes

You Owe It to Yourself and Your Family

The Essentials for Taking Control of Your Diabetes: Keep Yourself Healthy Until a Cure Comes Along

The essentials for taking control of your diabetes can be broken down into these main parts:

1. Blood glucose control
2. Blood pressure control
3. Cholesterol control
4. Following a diabetes warranty program
5. Constantly seeking out new information on how to best control your diabetes.

These basic areas have been covered extensively in this book and should be the backbone of your diabetes care. Controlling your blood glucose level will not only reduce the incidence and severity of the complications of diabetes but will also allow you to feel better on a day-to-day basis. Since the last edition of this book was published, the goals for glycemic control have been lowered. In fact, all of the major diabetes organizations, such as the American Diabetes Association (ADA), have now said that the ultimate goal is to have the A1C in the normal range (4% to 6%) and not just below 7%, if it can be done safely and without excessive hypoglycemia. New research has also shown that we must individualize our A1C goals, because one size does not fit all. Working toward your goal can be difficult and fraught with obstacles, however, remember that this is not a sprint, it's a marathon.

We now have so many impressive and effective tools to control our diabetes, including home glucose and continuous glucose monitors, designer insulin analogues, smart insulin pumps, and an even larger variety of new oral and injectable medications that work well alone and in combination with each other. I strongly believe that continuous glucose monitoring is having a huge impact on the lives of people with type 1 and insulin-requiring type 2 diabetes, however, only a minority of these folks has access to this technology. With more widespread availability of these new medications and devices, along with knowledgeable health care providers, a much higher percentage of people will be able to take control of their diabetes.

Blood pressure control will not only help reduce the microvascular complications of diabetes (eye and kidney disease), it will also greatly reduce your chance of having a heart attack or stroke. People with diabetes should have a home blood pressure cuff for periodic measurements. High blood pressure is commonly found in people with diabetes and there may be no obvious symptoms, however, it can lead to serious complications if left untreated. We have many different types of blood pressure medications that work well alone or in combination and are also well tolerated with few side effects. The goals for blood pressure control have been lowered (less than 130/80 mm Hg) because of excellent clinical research studies demonstrating major health benefits.

Over the past several years, the bar has also been lowered in terms of acceptable cholesterol levels. Getting a yearly fasting lipid panel or cholesterol screening is of utmost importance. Untreated abnormal cholesterol levels (LDL or bad cholesterol, HDL or good cholesterol, and triglycerides) can lead to heart attack and stroke, which are very common in people with diabetes. Once again, there are no symptoms of abnormal cholesterol levels, which make screening very important. Experts in the field now advocate aggressive cholesterol control because extensive and well-conducted clinical studies demonstrate that it results in large reductions in the occurrence of these serious life-threatening and life-altering events. One of the most important guideline changes is to get the LDL (or bad cholesterol) less than 100 mg/dL for all people with diabetes and less than 70 mg/dL if you already have heart problems. Just as is the case with blood glucose and blood pressure control, there are some fantastic, safe, and powerful drugs to bring abnormal cholesterol levels into the normal range.

Following a diabetes warranty program helps you stay on top of your health issues in terms of the tests and examinations that you need regularly in order to stay healthy. It follows the same philosophy of the warranty program for your car. If you take your car in for servicing, according to the recommended maintenance schedule, your car will most likely run better and last longer. It is the same for our bodies. Make a chart, keep good records, and know what the values mean.

And finally, the last and most important step is to take action if the values are not in the ideal or near-normal range. In our current era of restricted care, you must be super proactive in getting the medications and services you need to stay healthy. This is where education, motivation, and self-advocacy play important roles.

Education, Motivation, and Self-Advocacy

Diabetes control in this country and around the world is still inadequate for the majority of people living with this chronic condition. However, there have been numerous advances in the field of diabetes that can potentially wipe out or greatly reduce the amount of human suffering associated with this disease. Why is it that advances in the diabetes medical field have far outpaced care at the community level? I believe one of the greatest missing links is that patient education and motivation have been seriously lacking or nonexistent. We, the people who are living with this condition, need to be the most knowledgeable members of our health care teams and take the main responsibility for our health. We are our own best advocates. We must find out what needs to be done to live a healthy and productive life with diabetes and then go out and do everything we can to achieve it. Be smart and be persistent.

Spreading the Important Messages of TCOYD

In my many years of experience as a diabetes specialist, I have never met a person with diabetes who did not want to live a long and healthy life. I can't tell you how many times I have heard a doctor say, "So many diabetic patients are noncompliant, and they just do not care about their own health." I believe these patients have either never been properly educated and motivated to be their own best advocate and to take control of their diabetes or that their caregivers just do not understand the barriers that these patients face.

TCOYD is a not-for-profit organization whose mission statement is: Guided by the belief that every person with diabetes has the right to live a healthy, happy, and productive life, Taking Control Of Your Diabetes educates and motivates people with diabetes to take a more active role in their condition and provides innovative and integrative continuing diabetes education to medical professionals caring for people with diabetes.

TCOYD promotes its mission through several information portals. These include a national series of conferences, our award winning TCOYD educational television series, our quarterly *MyTCOYD* newsletter, this 4th edition of the *TCOYD* book, our Sweet Member membership program, the Extreme Diabetes Makeover program, The Edelman Report as part of our online presence, and the one-of-a-kind Making the Connection continuing medical education (CME) series of programs that offer the health care providers of our country cutting-edge information about the advances in diabetes care, as well as providing them with an understanding of what it is like to live with diabetes on a day-to-day basis.

TCOYD Conferences and Health Fairs

TCOYD was founded on the core principle that when it comes to education, motivation, and self-advocacy, nothing replaces face-to-face interaction. This is why our on-going national series of conferences remain the foundation of how TCOYD fulfills its mission. The TCOYD conferences and health fairs are held in major convention centers in cities across America and, to date, we have touched the lives of well over 450,000 people. The conferences are normally held on Saturdays from 9 am to 5 pm and consist of general sessions for all attendees in the morning, a banquet lunch with an inspirational speaker, a variety of afternoon workshops, hands-on sessions offering one-on-one time between experts and patients, exercise programs, an extensive health fair, and a closing general session to end the day on a

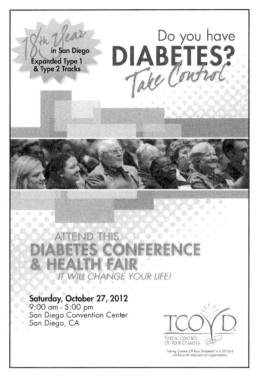

hopeful and motivating note. In addition, we address ethnic groups hit hard by diabetes, including African Americans, Native Americans, and Latinos by producing conferences appropriate to their backgrounds, cultural beliefs, and heritages. Recruiting diabetes professionals and speakers with the same ethnic backgrounds as these groups accounts for a major part of our success in truly reaching and touching these folks.

{ "I laughed, I cried, I was educated, and now I am inspired."

TCOYD Conference Attendee }

TCOYD conferences have changed the lives of countless thousands of people with diabetes and their loved ones, empowering them to be on the diabetes offensive. You can view an 8-minute documentary on the TCOYD conferences and learn more about them on our website (*www.tcoyd.org*). I would encourage you to try to not only attend a conference, but also to bring your loved ones and other friends and relatives living with diabetes. You can help spread the word as well.

TCOYD also offers other live, face-to-face programs, such as the Mini Series programs held in the San Diego area, as well as our Latino initiative led by Antonio Huerta. Please visit our website or call our office for more information on all of our services.

TCOYD Television Show

The first season of the TCOYD TV show aired in 2006/2007 and was the culmination of over 8 years of thinking without having the time to act on those thoughts. The TV show finally became a reality and has enjoyed five successful seasons to date. Although the live conferences are the mainstay of our organization, we are not able to reach the large numbers of people that we can via television. Our current TCOYD TV show reaches a potential of approximately 27 million viewers on the University of California television network that is uploaded to DISH satellite network television. Yours truly is the engaging and handsome host.

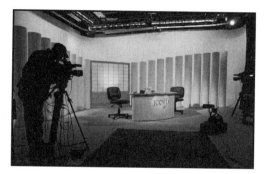

Our topics range from the basics of diabetes care to more advanced and cutting-edge topics, including continuous glucose monitoring, prevention strategies, joining the online community, sexual concerns, and much more. Every episode features the always-interesting and practical cooking and exercise tips. TCOYD pulls together the top professionals in the field of diabetes, as well as real folks who have been successfully living with this condition. Real, substantive content presented in our taking-control format is the main difference between our show and others that have come and gone. Thinking outside the box is our norm at TCOYD. Please visit our website (*www.tcoyd.org*) for 24-hour global viewing of all of our previously aired programs and to find out how you can view TCOYD TV on your television or computer. For those of you without access to the Internet, our shows are available for purchase on DVDs.

The MyTCOYD Newsletter

The *MyTCOYD* newsletter is in its 15th year and continues to fill an important role for our Sweet Membership program. When we visit a city in America to present one of our live conferences, the participants are so motivated at the end of the day that they are happy they have diabetes! We may not return to that city for 1 or 2 years, so the newsletter helps to keep our taking-control messages current throughout the year. Dr. Edelman's Corner is a regular newsletter feature. I use this opportunity to say what is pertinent, provocative, controversial, and critical to our members. Some people say I must be on a hallucinogenic drug when I write Dr. Edelman's Corner, but that is not true. I am always a little off the wall, anyway. Look for Dr. Edelman's Corner on our website (*www.tcoyd.org*) and in *Chapter 25* for my top 10 favorite pieces since the last edition of the book.

Additional regular features include Ask Your Pharmacist, Product Theater, Know Your Numbers, Question of the Month, Taking Control, and Living Well. Ask Your Pharmacist reviews the latest medications that have recently been approved by the FDA for people with diabetes. This information is written in sophisticated lay terms by talented doctors of pharmacy, such as Candis Morello of the UCSD School of Pharmacy and Veterans Affairs Medical Center.

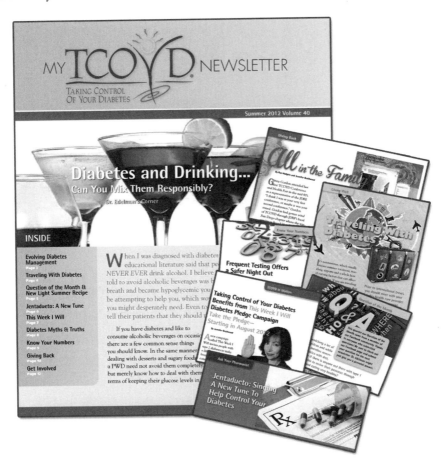

Know Your Numbers shows a real logbook from an actual patient with a detailed explanation of what kinds of trends and patterns are evident. The purpose of this section is to educate our members on how to interpret their own numbers in order to achieve their glycemic goals. We receive many questions throughout the year from our members, and we try to answer all of them within a very short period of time, usually less than 24 hours. I pick one of the more important questions to print in each issue of our newsletter, along with a detailed answer, so that all of our members can learn together (see *Chapter 11*).

Product Theater showcases the latest in products and devices; recently we have spotlighted the new iBGStar blood glucose meter that attaches to the iPhone and also the new patch pumps coming on the market.

Living Well highlights new trends and cutting-edge information in the diabetes sphere, including partner studies, clinical research topics, and new scientific findings as they relate to type 1 and type 2 diabetes.

Taking Control focuses on extraordinary people with diabetes and/or educators who are continuing to make a difference in the fight against this chronic condition.

In order to receive a hard copy of the quarterly *MyTCOYD* newsletter, you need to be a Sweet Member, however, all the issues are posted online, and you can receive an eblast announcing when each issue is available by signing up online.

The Edelman Report
(please do not pronounce the 't' in Report)

I must admit that Stephen Colbert is one of my favorite comedians, and I love his style when presenting the latest news and hot topics in our society. In a similar fashion, I started our new short online video segments on various diabetes-related topics called The Edelman Report.

These videos are meant to give you the real scoop on cutting edge tools and therapies to help you take control. I try to make them interesting, up-to-date, quirky, and with humor. They include topics such as drinking alcohol, steroids, dental care, not letting your doctor kill you while you're in the hospital, the scoop on cold cereals, line pumps versus patch pumps, etc, etc. You can find all of The Edelman Reports at *www.youtube.com/user/TCOYDtv* or just go to our main website at *www.tcoyd.org.*

Social Media

During the last few years, the diabetes online social media community has become an important resource for people with diabetes. Available 24/7 to anyone with access to the Internet, this community seeks to ease the isolation so many with diabetes experience. It offers members connectivity and support through the sharing of videos, photos, and blogging about their lives with diabetes. TCOYD actively engages people with diabetes on Facebook, Twitter, LinkedIn, and YouTube.

The Sweet Membership Program

Every person who attends a TCOYD conference becomes a member of TCOYD for life. If they opt-in, they will receive notices of all TCOYD activities as well as periodic eblasts. The quarterly *MyTCOYD* newsletter is available online for all members. Those who join the TCOYD Sweet Member program for a small annual fee enjoy the advantages of receiving a hard copy of the newsletter each quarter and also this 4th edition of the *TCOYD* book that you are currently reading. When Sweet Members renew each year, they have the choice of another *TCOYD* book or one of several different DVDs of our TCOYD TV show seasons. To become a Sweet Member, go online to our website at *www.tcoyd.org* or simply call our office (800-998-2693). You can also join when you attend any of our conferences.

"Making the Connection" Professional Education Program: Educating the Caregivers of this Country on the Day-to-Day Struggles of Living With Diabetes

TCOYD has taken on a challenge that, to my knowledge, has not been attempted anywhere else. Educating physicians about the most up-to-date treatment strategies in diabetes management is a difficult and slow process, but one of the biggest challenges in improving diabetes care is to improve the attitudes of health care providers toward their patients who are struggling with diabetes and to create an empathetic atmosphere with more open, two-way communication. We have taken on this challenge at TCOYD with Making the Connection (MTC), our innovative continuing medical education program series for health care professionals.

I feel strongly that if the providers in this country really knew what it is like to have diabetes, both emotionally and physically, their level of empathy and genuine understanding would greatly improve. In turn, this would strengthen the communication between doctors and patients, and it would diminish the commonly experienced brow-beating and inappropriate labeling of patients as being "noncompliant."

It is amazing to me when during medical rounds in the hospital, a young resident doctor in training presents a case by starting with some-

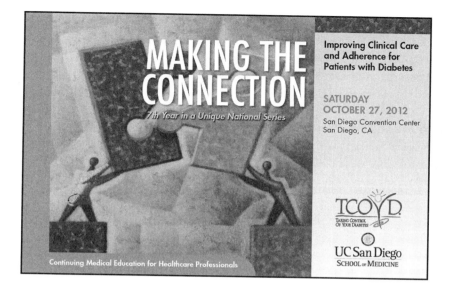

MAKING THE CONNECTION

7th Year in a Unique National Series

Continuing Medical Education for Healthcare Professionals

Improving Clinical Care and Adherence for Patients with Diabetes

SATURDAY
OCTOBER 27, 2012
San Diego Convention Center
San Diego, CA

TCOYD
TAKING CONTROL
OF YOUR DIABETES

UC San Diego
SCHOOL OF MEDICINE

thing like this: "This patient is a 56-year-old, noncompliant male with a 5-year history of type 2 diabetes." After the presentation is completed, I calmly ask the resident, "Why do you say the patient is noncompliant?" The answer is usually, "The last doctor who saw this patient wrote it in the chart, and the blood glucose levels are not under good control." Well, I have never in my life met a person with diabetes who did not want to live a long and healthy life. The residents and interns in the hospital now know very well not to use "that word" when presenting to me... or else!

Our MTC programs are held right alongside our TCOYD conferences and place the medical professionals smack in the middle of the patients as they attend our TCOYD patient conference. Separate from the patient conference during part of the day, they receive several cutting-edge CME approved lectures from experts in the field. Additionally, during other parts of the day, they join the people with diabetes attending the patient conference to hear a discussion about the emotional barriers that are so commonly associated with diabetes. They also have lunch with the patient-conference participants and hear the keynote lunchtime speaker, always a motivational speaker living well with diabetes. During the afternoon, the professionals and a large group of patients attend a workshop that is led by a psychologist, typically my good friend and colleague Dr. Bill Polonsky. This is an interactive and enlightening hour for both the patients and the professionals because they have the opportunity to express both sides of the doctor-patient relationship and come to an understanding of the frustrations faced by both groups. The professionals complete the day in their own classroom and discuss all that they observed and learned during the day from the people who live every day of their lives with diabetes. More information on the TCOYD CME programs can be found online at *www.tcoydcme .org* or by calling our office.

Our Continued Challenge

The vision of Taking Control Of Your Diabetes is for all people with diabetes and their loved ones to have full access to proper education and therapy in order to allow for the prevention, early detection, and aggressive management of diabetes and its complications.

Our vision statement is our future challenge. TCOYD conferences truly touch the lives of the many people who attend. However, the total number of participants nationwide is only a fraction of the people in this country who are living with diabetes. Even though we are now reaching

more people with our television series, electronic newsletter, The Edelman Report, and our other online social media programs, diabetes education and motivation must be seriously recognized by our health care industry as an essential part of an effective treatment program. Successful diabetes education programs must be carefully developed and offered to all people with diabetes and their loved ones. Diabetes education must be informative, humor-

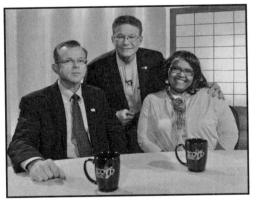

Juan Frias, Steve Edelman, and Renee on the set of TCOYD TV.

ous, practical, adaptable, and compatible with the wide range of ethnic groups and unique individuals that make up our country. It must also focus on methods that enable people to become engaged and activated in their own health and well-being. Just having the information is not enough. Becoming active is key.

In closing, I want to encourage you to take control of your diabetes. It is you and your loved ones who will benefit from you living a healthy life with your diabetes.

I leave you with this:

Take control of your diabetes.
You owe it to yourself and to your loved ones.

34

Appendix

The single best resource I can suggest is a fantastic web site that can really help you find what you want about any topic of your interest. It is called...

GOOGLE

Partnering Organizations

American Diabetes Association
www.diabetes.org

The American Diabetes Association is a voluntary, not-for-profit organization. Their mission is to prevent and cure diabetes and to improve the lives of all people affected by diabetes. Their vision is to make an everyday difference in the lives of all people with diabetes. The ADA's focus is to encourage and educate people with diabetes about the importance of self-management.

JDRF
www.JDRF.org

JDRF is the leading global organization focused on type 1 diabetes (T1D) research. Driven by passionate, grassroots volunteers connected to children, adolescents, and adults with this disease, JDRF is now the largest charitable supporter of T1D research. The goal of JDRF research is to improve the lives of all people affected by T1D by accelerating progress on the most promising opportunities for curing, better treating, and preventing T1D. JDRF collaborates with a wide spectrum of partners who share this goal.

RealAge
www.realage.com

RealAge is a leading health and wellness site centered on the groundbreaking RealAge Test, a highly scientific but simple-to-take test that calculates how old your body thinks you are. The patented test has been taken by more than 27 million people and is backed by powerful new technology that allows it to be constantly updated with the latest medical studies. When you take the test, you will receive a personalized Grow Younger Plan designed to turn back your body clock. The site also offers health tips, dozens of other tests (including the Diabetes Risk Assessment,) and practical, inspiring information to help you become physically younger.

dLife
www.dLife.com

Do you have questions about living with diabetes? dLife has a wealth of information to give you the answers you need to manage your diabetes health! dLife offers an excellent community network and resource for people living with diabetes and their caregivers. dLife also has a great TV show and is part of the online community.

Diabetes Daily
www.diabetesdaily.com

Diabetes Daily is an online community and educational program for people with diabetes. You can ask questions, download free cookbooks, and learn how to live a healthier and happier life with diabetes. Diabetes Daily is also a leading online support community that helps people affected by diabetes live a better life and features one of the largest diabetes forums, as well as meal plans, and educational programs.

Diabetes Hands Foundation
www.diabeteshandsfoundation.org

The Diabetes Hands Foundation is a 501(c)3 nonprofit organization that connects people touched by diabetes (those with diabetes and their loved ones) and raises diabetes awareness. We run two networks for people touched by diabetes: *tudiabetes.org* (in English) and *estudiabetes.org* (in Spanish).

Insulindependence
http://insulindependence.org

Insulindependence is a national leader in the field of diabetes and exercise. Since 2005, this nonprofit organization has empowered thousands of people living with diabetes to take charge of their health through innovative recreation programs. By offering real-world experiences to help individuals with diabetes overcome challenges and fears, program participants gain enhanced self-image, fresh life-perspective, enduring friendships, and deeper self-understanding that lead to improved self-management of their disease. Ultimately, this affords a higher quality of life to individuals and society as a whole.

Behavioral Diabetes Institute

http://behavioraldiabetesinstitute.org

The Behavioral Diabetes Institute is a San Diego–based, nonprofit organization dedicated to addressing the unmet psychological and behavioral needs of people with diabetes. We offer an array of guidance-based clinical programs, all designed to help people overcome the emotional and behavioral obstacles to living well with diabetes.

College Diabetes Network (CDN)

http://collegediabetesnetwork.org

Founded in 2009 by a college student, the College Diabetes Network (CDN) is a 501(c)3 nonprofit organization, which works to empower and improve the lives of students living with T1D through peer support and access to information and resources.

Glu (Bond with others who Match your Mix)

https://myglu.org; info@myglu.org

Glu is an online T1D social network with a purpose to accelerate research and amplify the collective voices of the T1D community. Once registered, you can bond with people who have the same common interests as yourself. It is under the umbrella of The Helmsley Trust and part of the vision of David Panzier.

Riding on Insulin

www.ridingoninsulin.org

Riding on Insulin empowers, activates, and connects the global diabetes community through shared experience and action sports. In addition to establishing a comfortable environment, they strive to help families explore new passions, challenge the illness, and celebrate each other's successes. Specifically, Riding on Insulin hosts a series of ski and snowboard programs for kids and teens living with T1D across the world.

TeamType1

www.teamtype1.org

Founded by my good friend Phil Southerland, TeamType1 is an incredible organization that strives to instill hope and inspiration for people around the world affected by diabetes. With appropriate diet, exercise, treatment, and technology, we believe anyone with diabetes can achieve their dreams. This organization has professional and amateur sports teams (cycling, running, triatheletics) with atheletes with both T1D and type 2 diabetes to lead by example and give hope and inspiration to others.

Bringing Science Home

http://bringingsciencehome.health.usf.edu

This fantastic organization was founded by former Miss America Nicole Johnson. The mission statement is powerful: Empowered by informed research and critical analysis of programs nationwide, this project will co-design solutions to chronic disease education and care with patient audiences. The focus is on learning patient and population needs and desires. Using real life input to drive the creative process, we will then create products to best serve the impacted individuals and groups.

Magazines and Online Resources

Close Concerns

http://closeconcerns.com

Kelly Close has developed one of the most extensive information sites for both professionals and people with diabetes. I rely on Close Concerns almost daily for up-to-date information on hot topics, controversial issues, new drugs and devices, and much more.

Diabetes Forecast

www.diabetes.org

Diabetes Forecast is the magazine of the American Diabetes Association and comes with a membership. Provides an annual "Resources Guide" of products for use by people with diabetes.

Diabetes Health

www.diabeteshealth.com

Diabetes Mine

www.diabetesmine.com

Diabetes Mine was created by founder and editor Amy Tenderich as a "diabetes newspaper with a personal twist."

Diabetes Self-Management

www.diabetesselfmanagement.com

Rick Mendosa's Diabetes Directory

www.mendosa.com/diabetes.htm; mendosa@mendosa.com

This is a directory of articles, columns, and web pages maintained by Rick Mendosa, a freelance journalist specializing in diabetes. The site includes his annotated directory to more than 800 websites about diabetes, which are described and linked in the 15 pages of his online diabetes resources.

Children With Diabetes
www.childrenwithdiabetes.com

An online resource for children, families, and adults living with T1D. This is an excellent site for general diabetes information... it is not just for kids!

National Institute of Diabetes and Digestive and Kidney Diseases (NIDDK)
http://diabetes.niddk.nih.gov

A comprehensive website for an introduction to diabetes, complications of the disease, and treatment. Statistics, clinical trials, guidelines, and research reports are accessible through this site along with additional sources for publications.

The Diabetes Mall
(800) 988-4772; *www.diabetesnet.com*

In addition to information concerning diabetes, this site offers linked information to technology in diabetes, including insulin pumps and infusion sets, meters and monitors, and software to be used in controlling diabetes.

TCOYD's Legal Expert Kriss Halpern: The Diabetic Lawyer
http://www.diabetesattorney.net

Kriss' site is a fantastic place to learn about your rights and the DMV, insurance issues, discrimination, the Americans With Disability act and much more.

Taking Control Of Your Diabetes (TCOYD)
(800) 99-TCOYD (998-2693); *www.tcoyd.org; info@tcoyd.org*

TCOYD promotes education, motivation, and self-advocacy by a multitude of programs and services: our face-to-face, nationwide series of conferences; our award-winning newsletter; *Extreme Diabetes Makeover* online, reality-based documentary; our website, including Facebook and Twitter; the TCOYD Television series; the new *The Edelman Report* (don't pronounce the T!); and much, much more. Check us out online, and see the last chapter of this 4th edition for more details.

General Diabetes Resources

Associations

American Association of Diabetes Educators (AADE)
(800) 338-3633; *www.aadenet.org or www.diabeteseducator.org*

American Dietetic Association
(800) 877-1600; *www.eatright.org*

Centers for Disease Control (CDC)-Diabetes Home Page
(800) CDC-INFO (232-4636); *www.cdc.gov/diabetes*

International Diabetes Center (IDC)
(888) 637-2675; *www.parknicollet.com/diabetes*

International Diabetes Federation (IDF)
+32-2-538 55 11; *www.idf.org; info@idf.org*

National Diabetes Education Initiative (NDEI)
(800) 471-7745; *www.ndei.org; feedback@ndei.org*

National Diabetes Education Program (NDEP)
(800) 438-5383; *http://ndep.nih.gov; ndep@mail.nih.gov*

Diabetes in the Workplace

Disabled Businesspersons Association
(619) 594-8805; *www.disabledbusiness.org*
Disabled Businessperson Association was formed as a charitable not-for-profit organization by Urban Miyares in 1991. As a volunteer-driven organization of and directed by successful business owners, professionals and executives with disabilities, the DBA has the in-house first hand expertise to provide information, counseling, coaching and mentorship from the perspective of someone with a disability in today's, highly competitive business world.

Job Accommodation Network (JAN)
(800) 526-7234; *www.jan.wvu.edu*
An international, toll-free consulting service that provides information about job accommodations and the employability of people with functional limitations. Information concerning the Americans with Disabilities Act can also be found here.

Diet and Nutrition

Calorie King
www.calorieking.com
Setting the food record straight, providing facts that anchor changed thinking about food and result in sustainable behavior improvements and better health.

Nutrition Data
www.nutritiondata.com

Provides complete nutritional information for any food or recipe, and helps you select foods that best match your dietary needs.

Free Diabetes Nutrition Teleconferences
(718) 263-3926; *telediabetes@aol.com*

Pharmaceutical Company Web Sites

Many drug company websites have useful information for doctors as well as patients, including complete descriptions of product features and drug prescribing information.

Abbott Diabetes Care: www.abbottdiabetescare.com

Animas Corporation: www.animas.com

Bayer HealthCare: www.bayerdiabetes.com/us

Becton Dickinson: www.bd.com

Boehringer Ingelheim Corp: www.boehringer-ingelheim.com

Bristol-Myers Squibb: www.bms.com

Dexcom: www.dexcom.com

Eli Lilly and Company: www.lilly.com

GlaxoSmithKline: www.gsk.com

Heal2gether: www.heal2gether.org

Insulet: www.myomnipod.com

Liberty Medical Supply: www.libertymedical.com

LifeScan, Inc: www.lifescan.com

Medtronic, Inc: www.medtronicdiabetes.com

Merck: www.merck.com

Novartis: www.novartis.com

Novo Nordisk: www.novonordisk.com

Pfizer: www.pfizer.com

sanofi US: www.sanofi.us

Schering-Plough: www.sphcp.com

Tandem Diabetes Care: www.tandemdiabetes.com

Travel Resources

Center for Disease Control International Traveler Hotline
(877) 394-8747; *www.cdc.gov/travel*
Provides 24-hour-a-day voice and fax information system of international travel recommendations, information on specific diseases, immunizations, and services.

Highway to Health Travel Insurance
(888) 243-2358; *www.highwaytohealth.com*
Provides travelers' assistance, a worldwide physician list, medical evacuation and repatriation, trip planning, and global assistance services.

International Association for Medical Assistance to Travelers (IAMAT)
(716) 754-4883; *www.iamat.org; info@iamat.org*
Provides a list of foreign doctors who speak English in your destination cities and information on food, climate, and sanitary conditions.

Traveler's Emergency Network, Inc.
(800) ASK-4-TEN (275-4836); *www.tenweb.com*

Travelex Insurance Services, Inc.
(800) 228-9792; *www.travelex-insurance.com*
Provides trip cancellation coverage and medical coverage for physicians and hospitalization during a trip.

Universal Travel Protection Insurance
(800) 694-4311; *www.utravelpro.com*

Worldwide Assistance Services, Inc.
(800) 777-8710; *www.worldwideassistance.com*

Publications
Books Written by Contributing Authors to this 4th Edition

American Diabetes Association. *Diabetes and Pregnancy: What to Expect.* 4th ed. American Diabetes Association; 2001.

American Diabetes Association. *Gestational Diabetes: What to Expect.* 5th ed. American Diabetes Association; 2005.

American Diabetes Association, Lea Ann Holzmeister. *The Diabetes Carbohydrate and Fat Gram Guide.* 3rd ed. American Diabetes Association; 2006.

Ian Blumer, Heather McDonald-Blumer. *Understanding Prescription Drugs for Canadians for Dummies.* Wiley & Sons; 2007.

Ian Blumer, Cynthia Payne. *Diabetes Cookbook for Canadians for Dummies.* Wiley & Sons; 2010.

Ian Blumer. *What Your Doctor Really Thinks.* Dundurn; 1999.

Ian Blumer, Sheila Crowe. *Celiac Disease for Dummies.* Wiley & Sons; 2010.

Ian Blumer, Alan Rubin. *Diabetes for Canadians for Dummies.* 3rd ed. Wiley & Sons; 2013.

Sheri R. Colberg. *Diabetes-Free Kids.* 2nd ed. Muddy Paws Press; 2012.

Sheri R. Colberg. *The 7 Step Diabetes Fitness Plan.* Da Capo Press; 2006.

Sheri R. Colberg. *Diabetic Athlete's Handbook.* Human Kinetics; 2009.

Sheri R. Colberg. *The Diabetic Athlete: Prescriptions for Exercise and Sports.* Human Kinetics Publishers; 2001.

Sheri R. Colberg, Steven V. Edelman. *50 Secrets of the Longest Living People With Diabetes.* Marlowe & Company; 2007.

Lorena Drago. *Beyond Rice and Beans: The Caribbean Latino Guide to Eating Healthy With Diabetes.* American Diabetes Association; 2006.

Sidney Gale (Ian Blumer's pen name). *Unto The Breach.* Lulu Press; 2011.

Cynthia M. Goody, Lorena Drago. *Cultural Food Practices.* Academy of Nutrition and Dietetics; 2009.

Lorena Drago. *The 15-Minute Consultation: How to Enhance Learning and Get Your Message Across Every Time.* Academy of Nutrition and Dietetics; 2012.

Norman O. Harris, Franklin Harris. *Primary Preventive Denistry.* Mayssoun Khoury, trans-ed. Pearson Education, Inc; 2004.

Francine R. Kaufman. *Diabesity: The Obesity-Diabetes Epidemic That Threatens America—And What We Must Do to Stop It.* Bantam; 2005.

William H. Polonsky. *Diabetes Burnout: What to Do When You Can't Take It Anymore.* American Diabetes Association; 1999.

John Walsh, Ruth Roberts. *Pumping Insulin: Everything You Need for Success on a Smart Insulin Pump.* 5th ed. Torrey Pines Press; 2012.

John Walsh, Ruth Roberts, Timothy Bailey, Chandra B. Varma. *Using Insulin: Everything You Need for Success With Insulin*. Torrey Pines Press; 2003.

Diabetes Products
Blood Glucose Meters/Data Management Software

There have been several advancements in the development of home glucose meters since the first edition of this book. Many things should be taken into consideration in deciding which blood glucose meter to purchase. These devices come in many sizes and with a varying range of capabilities. Cost of these devices varies as well. Some companies will provide their meter free of charge, since their money is made on the sale of the device's test strips. Sometimes it is more cost-effective to purchase a meter because the strips for it are more economically priced. Test-result returns can come as quickly as 5 seconds or can take as long as 4 minutes. Many meter companies now offer blood-letting devices that use the forearm and thus avoid the necessity to prick your sore fingertips. Some meters can store results in memory over a period of time and provide test averages. Others have the ability to download their data to a computer for use with software applications that can further your diabetic control by providing graphs that can help you understand your blood glucose readings and determine patterns in your glucose levels over time. Some applications can even provide help concerning diet and exercise based on your meter's stored results. Research the different meters on the market and ask yourself, "How will I be using this meter?" The best meter is the one that is right for you.

Table A-1 provides a partial list of blood glucose meters currently on the market and their features. A comparison of available blood glucose meters can also be found at *http://forecast.diabetes.org/files /images/v65n01_BG_Meters_0.pdf*.

Other Online Medical Resources

These two valuable resources are funded by your tax dollars. They provide a great way to learn about the latest in medical research (Medline Plus) and reliable general information on diabetes (The National Institute of Diabetes and Digestive and Kidney Diseases [NIDDK]) and the National Diabetes Education Program (NDEP):

- Medline Plus: *www.medlineplus.com*
- NIDDK: Diabetes Self-Care on the Internet
- NDEP: *http://ndep.nih.gov*

TrialNet

www.diabetestrialnet.org

A network of 18 clinical centers working in cooperation with international screening sites and dedicated to the study, prevention, and early treatment of T1D.

US Office for Civil Rights

(800) 421-3481; *www.ed.gov/about/offices/list/ocr/index.html*

Provides information and assistance on handling school issues for children with diabetes.

New websites are going up every day for the necessary and inevitable fact that health care information is going to the Internet. This is especially important in our managed-care environment. Only a few of the excellent sites available are listed.

TABLE A-1 — Diabetes Forecast 2012 Consumer Guide: Blood Glucose Meters

Meter Name (Manufacturer)[a]	Blood Sample Size[b]	Battery	User Coding Needed?	A	B	BP	C	K	P
Accu-Chek Aviva (Roche)	0.6	(1) CR2032 lithium coin cell	Yes	—	—	—	✓	—	—
Accu-Chek Aviva Combo[c]	0.6	(3) AAA	Yes	—	✓	—	✓	—	✓
Accu-Chek Aviva Plus (Roche)	0.6	(1) CR2032 lithium coin cell	Yes	—	—	—	✓	—	—
Accu-Chek Compact Plus (Roche)	1.5	(2) AAA	No	—	✓	—	✓	—	—
Accu-Chek Nano (Roche)	0.6	(2) CR2032 lithium coin cell	No	—	✓	—	✓	—	—
Acura (U.S. Diagnostics)	0.5	(2) CR2032 lithium coin cell	No	—	—	—	—	—	—
Advocate Redi-Code Dash (Diabetic Supply of Suncoast)	0.7	(1) CR2032 lithium coin cell	No	✓	—	—	—	—	—
Advocate Redi-Code Duo (Diabetic Supply of Suncoast)	0.7	(2) AAA	No	—	—	✓	✓	—	—
Breeze2 (Bayer)	1.0	(1) CR2032 lithium coin cell	No	—	—	—	—	—	—
Codefree (Gluco Com)	0.7	(1) CR2032 lithium coin cell	No	—	—	—	—	—	—
Contour (Bayer)	0.6	(2) CR2032 lithium coin cell	No	—	—	—	—	—	—
Contour Link (Bayer)	0.6	(2) 3-volt lithium (DL2032 or CR2032)	No	—	—	—	✓	—	✓
Contour Next EZ (Bayer)	0.6	(2) 3-volt lithium (DL2032 or CR2032)	No	—	—	—	✓	—	—
Contour Next Link (Bayer)	0.6	Permanent, rechargeable	No	✓	—	—	✓	—	✓
Contour TS[d] (Bayer)	0.6	(1) CR2032 lithium coin cell	No	—	—	—	✓	—	—
Contour USB (Bayer)	0.6	Rechargeable battery via computer or wall charger	No	—	—	—	✓	—	—
Control (U.S. Diagnostics)	1.0	(1) CR2032 lithium coin cell	Yes	—	—	—	✓	—	—
EasyGluco (U.S. Diagnostics)	1.5	(1) CR2032 lithium coin cell	Yes	—	✓	—	—	—	—
EasyGluco Plus (U.S. Diagnostics)	0.5	(2) CR2032 lithium coin cell	No	—	✓	—	✓	—	—
EasyMax Light (Oak Tree International Holdings)	0.6	(2) CR2032 lithium coin cell	No	—	—	—	—	—	—

Capabilities

Meter		Battery	Coding						
EasyMax No Code (Oak Tree International Holdings)	0.6	(2) AAA	No	—	✓	—	—	—	—
EasyMax Voice (Oak Tree International Holdings)	0.6	(2) AAA	No	—	✓	—	—	—	—
EasyMax Voice 2nd Generation (Oak Tree International Holdings)	0.6	(2) AAA	No	—	✓	—	—	—	—
EasyPlus T2 (Oak Tree International Holdings)	0.6	(1) CR2032 lithium coin cell	No	—	✓	—	—	—	—
Eclipse (Infopia)	1.0	(1) CR2032 lithium coin cell	Yes	✓	✓	—	—	—	—
Element (Infopia)	0.3	(2) CR2032 lithium coin cell	No	✓	✓	—	—	—	—
Element Plus (Infopia)	0.3	(2) AAA	No	—	✓	—	—	—	—
Envision (Infopia)	1.5	(2) CR2032 lithium coin cell	No	—	✓	—	—	—	—
Embrace (Omnis Health)	0.6	(2) AAA	No	—	✓	—	—	—	—
Evolution (Infopia)	0.3	(2) CR2032 lithium coin cell	No	✓	✓	—	—	—	—
Fifty50 Blood Glucose Monitoring System 2.0 (Fifty50 Medical)	0.5	(2) CR2032 lithium coin cell	No	✓	✓	—	—	—	—
Fora D10 (Fora Care)	0.7	(2) AAA	Yes	✓	✓	✓	—	✓	—
Fora D15 (Fora Care)	0.7	(4) AA	Yes	—	✓	✓	—	—	—
Fora D20 (Fora Care)	0.7	(4) AA	Yes	✓	✓	✓	—	—	—
Fora G20 (Fora Care)	0.5	(1) CR2032 lithium coin cell	No	—	✓	—	—	—	—
Fora G71a (Fora Care)	0.5	(1) CR2032 lithium coin cell	No	—	✓	—	—	—	—
Fora G90 (Fora Care)	0.7	(1) rechargeable lithium coin cell	No	—	✓	—	✓	✓	—
Fora Premium V10 (Fora Care)	0.7	(2) AAA	No	✓	✓	—	✓	—	—
Fora V20 (Fora Care)	0.7	(2) AAA	No	✓	✓	—	✓	—	—
FreeStyle Freedom Lite (Abbott Diabetes Care)	0.3	(1) CR2032 lithium coin cell	No	—	✓	—	—	—	—
FreeStyle InsuLinx (Abbott Diabetes Care)	0.3	(2) CR2032 lithium coin cell	No	—	✓	—	✓	—	—
FreeStyle Lite (Abbott Diabetes Care)	0.3	(1) CR2032 lithium coin cell	No	—	✓	—	✓	—	—
Glucocard 01 (Arkray)	0.3	(1) CR2032 lithium coin cell	No	—	✓	—	—	—	—
Glucocard 01-mini (Arkray)	0.3	(1) CR2032 lithium coin cell	No	—	—	—	—	—	—

Continued

TABLE A-1 — *Continued*

Meter Name (Manufacturer)[a]	Blood Sample Size[b]	Battery	User Coding Needed?	Capabilities					
				A	B	BP	C	K	P
Glucocard Vital (Arkray)	0.5	(1) CR2032 lithium coin cell	No	—	—	—	✓	—	—
GlucoLab (Infopia)	1.0	(1) CR2032 lithium coin cell	Yes	—	—	—	✓	—	—
iBGStar[e] (Sanofi-US)	0.5	Lithium rechargeable polymer	No	—	✓	—	✓	—	—
Infinity (U.S. Diagnostics)	0.5	(2) CR2032 lithium coin cell	No	—	—	—	✓	—	—
Maxima (U.S. Diagnostics)	0.5	(1) CR2032 lithium coin cell	Yes	—	—	—	✓	—	—
MyGlucoHealth Wireless (Entra Health Systems)	0.3	(2) AAA	No	✓	—	—	✓	—	—
Nova Max Link (Nova Biomedical)	0.3	(1) CR2450 lithium coin cell	No	—	—	—	✓	—	✓
Nova Max Plus (Nova Biomedical)	0.3 for blood glucose; 0.8 for ketones	(1) CR2450 lithium coin cell	No	—	—	—	✓	✓	—
OneTouch Ping[f] (LifeScan)	1.0	(2) 1.5V AAA alkaline	Yes	—	✓	—	✓	—	✓
OneTouch Select[d] (LifeScan)	1.4	(1) 3.0V CR2032 lithium	Yes	—	✓	—	✓	—	—
OneTouch Ultra2 (LifeScan)	1.0	(2) 3.0V CR2032 lithium	Yes	—	—	—	✓	—	—
OneTouch UltraMini (LifeScan)	1.0	(1) 3.0V CR2032 lithium	Yes	—	✓	—	✓	—	—
OneTouch UltraSmart (LifeScan)	1.0	(2) AAA alkaline	Yes	—	✓	—	✓	—	—
OneTouch VerioIQ (LifeScan)	0.4	Rechargeable	No	—	✓	—	✓	—	—
Precision Xtra (Abbott Diabetes Care)	0.6	(1) CR2032 lithium coin cell	Yes	✓	—	—	✓	✓	—
Prodigy Autocode (Diagnostic Devices)	0.7	(2) AAA	No	✓	—	—	✓	—	—
Prodigy Pocket (Diagnostic Devices)	0.7	(1) CR2032 lithium coin cell	No	—	—	—	✓	—	—
Prodigy Voice (Diagnostic Devices)	0.7	(2) AAA	No	—	—	—	✓	—	—
ReliOn Confirm (Walmart)	0.3	(1) CR2032 lithium coin cell	No	—	—	—	✓	—	—
ReliOn Micro (Walmart)	0.3	(1) CR2032 lithium coin cell	No	—	—	—	—	—	—
ReliOn Ultima (Walmart)	0.6	(1) CR2032 lithium coin cell	Yes	—	—	—	✓	—	—
Rightest GM100 (Bionime)	1.4	(1) CR2032 lithium coin cell	No	—	—	—	—	—	—
Rightest GM300[d] (Bionime)	1.4	(2) AAA	Yes	—	✓	—	✓	—	—
Rightest GM550 (Bionime)	1.0	(2) CR2032 lithium coin cell	No	—	✓	—	✓	—	—

Meter						
Sidekick (Nipro Diagnostics)	1.0	N/A (disposable)	No	—	—	—
Solo V2 (BioSense Medical Devices)	0.7	(2) AAA	No	—	—	✔
True2Go (Nipro Diagnostics)	0.5	(1) CR2032 lithium coin cell	No	—	—	—
Truebalance[d] (Nipro Diagnostics)	1.0	(1) CR2032 lithium coin cell	No	—	—	✔
Trueresult (Nipro Diagnostics)	0.5	(1) CR2032 lithium coin cell	No	✔	—	✔
Truetrack (Nipro Diagnostics)	1.0	(1) CR2032 lithium coin cell	Yes	✔	—	✔
WaveSense Jazz (AgaMatrix)	0.5	(2) CR2032 lithium coin cell	No	✔	—	✔
WaveSense KeyNote (AgaMatrix)	0.5	(2) CR2032 lithium coin cell	Yes	✔	—	✔
WaveSense KeyNote Pro (AgaMatrix)	0.5	(2) CR2032 lithium coin cell	Yes	✔	—	✔
WaveSense Presto (AgaMatrix)	0.5	(2) CR2032 lithium coin cell	No	✔	—	✔
Xpres (Infopia)	0.3	(2) CR2032 lithium coin cell	No	—	—	—
New Technology Pending FDA Clearance (August 2012) (Check *www.presspogo.com* for information on availability)						
POGO BGMS[g] (Intuity Medical)	0.25	(2) AAA	No	✔	✔	✔

Key: A, audio capability; B, backlight on display; BGMS, blood glucose monitoring system; BP, dual meter that measures both blood glucose and blood pressure; C, computer download capability; K, also tests blood ketones; P, communicates with insulin pump.

[a] See **Table A-2** for complete manufacturers' contact information.

[b] Microliters.

[c] Sold and used only with the Accu-Chek Combo insulin delivery system.

[d] Available by mail order only.

[e] Automatically syncs data to the iBStar Diabetes Manager app (DMA) when connected to the iPhone or iPad.

[f] Sold and used only with OneTouch Ping insulin pump.

[g] CAUTION: Investigational device. Limited by Federal law to investigational use. The POGO Blood Glucose Meter requires 510(k) clearance and is presently not for sale.

Adapted from American Diabetes Association. *Diabetes Forecast 2012 Consumer Guide: Blood Glucose Meters.* Diabetes Forecast Web site. http://forecast.diabetes.org/files/images/v65n01_BG_Meters_0.pdf. Accessed July 4, 2012.

TABLE A-2 — Contact Information for Manufacturers of Blood Glucose Meters

Company	Web Site	Toll-Free Phone
Abbott	www.abbottdiabetescare.com	1-888-522-5226
AgaMatrix	www.wavesense.info	1-866-906-4197
Arkray	www.glucocardusa.com	1-800-566-8558
Bayer	www.simplewins.com	1-800-348-8100
Bionime	www.bionimeusa.com	1-858-481-8485
BioSense Medical Devices	www.solometers.com	1-877-592-3922
Diabetic Supply of Suncoast	www.dsosi.com	1-866-373-2824
Diagnostic Devices	www.prodigymeter.com	1-800-243-2636
Entra Health Systems	www.myglucohealth.net	1-877-458-2646
Fifty50 Medical	www.fifty50.com	1-800-746-7505
Fora Care	www.foracare.com/usa	1-888-307-8188
		1-866-563-3764 *(Fora V12 only)*
Genesis Health Technologies	www.genesishealthtechnologies.com	1-888-263-0003
Gluco Com	www.glucocom.com	1-800-678-1446
Infopia	www.infopiausa.com	1-888-446-3246
Intuity Medical	www.presspogo.com	1-408-530-1700
LifeScan	www.onetouchdiabetes.com	1-800-227-8862
	www.animas.com	1-877-937-7867 (One Touch Ping only)
Nipro Diagnostics	www.niprodiagnostics.com	1-800-803-6025
Nova Biomedical	www.novacares.com	1-800-681-7390
Oak Tree International Holdings	www.oaktreeint.com	1-866-994-3345
Roche	www.accu-chek.com/us	1-800-858-8072
Sanofi-US	www.sanofi.us	1-800-981-2491
U.S. Diagnostics	www.usdiagnostics.net	1-866-216-5308
Walmart	www.relion.com	1-800-631-0076
		1-800-992-3612 (ReliOn Ultima only)

Adapted from American Diabetes Association. *Diabetes Forecast 2012 Consumer Guide. Diabetes Forecast* Web site. http://forecast.diabetes.org/files/images/v64n1_Meters_21-23-2.pdf. Accessed September 14, 2012.

INDEX

Note: Page numbers followed by "f" and "t"
indicate figures and tables, respectively.

508

518

538